I0210148

TEACHING ABOUT SEX AND SEXUALITIES IN HIGHER EDUCATION

Edited by Susan Hillock

Teaching about Sex and Sexualities in Higher Education argues that much more can be done in teaching about sex and sexuality in higher education. This edited collection provides key information on professional training and support, and acts as a crucial resource on sex, sexuality, and related issues. With a focus on diversity, this book features expert contributors who discuss key concepts, debates, and current issues across disciplines to help educators improve curriculum content.

This collection aims to provide adequate and appropriate sex education training and opportunities to educators so that they may explore complex personal and emotional issues, build skills, and develop the confidence necessary to help others in their respective fields.

SUSAN HILLOCK is an associate professor of social work and a faculty member in the Department of Social Work and the Department of Graduate Studies in Education at Trent University.

Teaching about Sex and Sexualities in Higher Education

EDITED BY SUSAN HILLOCK

UNIVERSITY OF TORONTO PRESS
Toronto Buffalo London

© University of Toronto Press 2021
Toronto Buffalo London
utorontopress.com

ISBN 978-1-4875-0701-5 (cloth)   ISBN 978-1-4875-3541-4 (EPUB)
ISBN 978-1-4875-2472-2 (paper)   ISBN 978-1-4875-3540-7 (PDF)

Library and Archives Canada Cataloguing in Publication

Title: Teaching about sex and sexualities in higher education /
    edited by Susan Hillock.
Names: Hillock, Susan, 1963–, editor.
Description: Includes bibliographical references.
Identifiers: Canadiana (print) 20210200553 | Canadiana (ebook) 20210200626 |
    ISBN 9781487524722 (softcover) | ISBN 9781487507015 (hardcover) |
    ISBN 9781487535414 (EPUB) | ISBN 9781487535407 (PDF)
Subjects: LCSH: Sexology. | LCSH: Sex (Psychology) – Study and teaching
    (Higher) | LCSH: Sexual orientation – Study and teaching (Higher) |
    LCSH: Sexual ethics – Study and teaching (Higher) | LCSH: Sex instruction.
Classification: LCC HQ60 .T43 2021 | DDC 306.7071/1 – dc23

This book has been published with the help of a grant from the Federation
for the Humanities and Social Sciences, through the Awards to Scholarly
Publications Program, using funds provided by the Social Sciences and
Humanities Research Council of Canada.

University of Toronto Press acknowledges the financial assistance to its
publishing program of the Canada Council for the Arts and the Ontario Arts
Council, an agency of the Government of Ontario.

Canada Council   Conseil des Arts
for the Arts   du Canada

ONTARIO ARTS COUNCIL
CONSEIL DES ARTS DE L'ONTARIO
an Ontario government agency
un organisme du gouvernement de l'Ontario

Funded by the   Financé par le
Government   gouvernement
of Canada   du Canada

Canada

Contents

Preface   ix
SUSAN HILLOCK

Introduction: Let's Teach about Sex   3
SUSAN HILLOCK

Part 1: Current Debates and Hot Topics   15
SUSAN HILLOCK

1 Don't Ask/Don't Tell: Sexuality(ies), Instructor Disclosure,
  and Trigger Warnings in the Classroom   21
  SUSAN HILLOCK

2 Restoring Indigenous Sexuality   36
  CARRIE BOURASSA, BETTY MCKENNA,
  MIRANDA KEEWATIN, SADIE ANDERSON,
  MARLIN LEGARE, MIKAYLA HAGEL,
  DANETTE STARBLANKET, JENNIFER LANGAN,
  AND CARI MCILDUFF

3 Teaching Sexual Consent   52
  TERRY HUMPHREYS

4 What about the Boys? University Students Learning
  about Sexual Consent Talk from Youth in
  Northeastern Ontario   67
  JENNIFER L. JOHNSON

5 The Down Low on Getting Down: Reframing Problem-
Focused Narratives by Focusing on Sex-Positivity and
Desire-Based Education   82
AMIE KROES

6 Transgender Experiences in Healthcare: Addressing
Challenges while Teaching Compassion in Higher
Education   99
COLLEEN MCMILLAN, MIKE LEE-POY,
AND CARYS MASSARELLA

Part 2: At the Margins: Diverse Voices and Perspectives   115
SUSAN HILLOCK

7 Porn and Pedagogies: Reflections on Queer and
Feminist Porn Studies in Academia   121
LAINE ZISMAN NEWMAN, SARAH LIMA,
STUART MACLEOD, OREOLUWA ADARA,
AND IMOGEN TAM

8 Past Practices: How to Think about Sex Historically   133
EL CHENIER

9 Queering Masculinity in Early Childhood and Higher
Education Classrooms: Gendered Regulation and
the Double Bind of Queer Masculinities   148
ADAM W.J. DAVIES

10 Working with Muslim LGBTQ Service Users:
Assessing and Locating Supportive Care and
Teaching Practices   164
MARYAM KHAN

11 Sexuality and Aging   182
HAI LUO AND LORNA GUSE

12 Uncertain Subjects: (Un)Teaching Pain(ful)
Sexualities, Power, and Pedagogy   198
RENEE DUMARESQUE

Part 3: Practical Applications and Recommendations   219

SUSAN HILLOCK

13 Sex and Gender in the Classroom: Lessons from
    (and for) the Front Lines   225
    HEATHER PETERS

14 The Pitch: Teaching Sexuality at Multiple Levels   237
    NICK J. MULÉ

15 Sexual Health Education for Individuals with
    Intellectual and Developmental Disabilities   251
    SHANIFF ESMAIL, MEG TRONSON,
    AND SHEENA CHURLA

16 Teachable Moments: The Intersections of
    Disabilities and Sexualities   271
    MICHELLE OWEN AND BADEN GAEKE-FRANZ

17 Developing a Sexual Education Workshop: Addressing
    a Gap in Social Work Education   285
    CHRISTOPHER STERLING-MURPHY AND
    RICK CSIERNIK

18 Can We Just Stop Faking It? Real Talk about
    Sex and Sexualities in the Classroom   301
    SUSAN HILLOCK

Appendix A: Course Outline for Social Work Elective   319
HEATHER PETERS

Appendix B: An Evaluation of Social Work Students'
Competency Working with Sexuality   329
CHRISTOPHER STERLING-MURPHY AND
RICK CSIERNIK

Appendix C: Taking a Sex History and Related
Sex Education Resources   333
SUSAN HILLOCK

Contributors   337

Preface

SUSAN HILLOCK

Informed by a social justice lens and featuring Canadian content and context, this edited multidisciplinary book focuses on the teaching of sexuality(ies) in higher education. Top Canadian scholars in the sexuality field from various disciplines and fields, including psychology, history, early childhood education, medicine, education, anthropology, occupational therapy, social work, nursing, and community health, as well as Indigenous, queer, gender/women's, porn, equity, and disability studies, bring their experience and expertise to this book. This volume is the first of its kind in North America and its multidisciplinary approach is a rich and untapped area of scholarship, particularly within the helping professions.

Why does this topic warrant an edited collection? As described in more detail in Chapter 1, in the late 1990s, when I was a medical social worker, and patients asked me for advice on sex, sexuality, and related issues, there was little available to me in terms of professional training and support, practical information, patient literature, or resources. More than twenty years later, given the proliferation of sexual content and information across social media and the internet, one might assume that these sex education gaps have been filled by modern research and scholarship. Indeed, it is true that over the last few years, some academic disciplines – for example, psychology, as well as sexuality, public/community health, gender, porn, disability, women's, and queer studies – have made leaps and bounds in sexuality research. However, this has not been the case across all disciplines. I have found that, at least in terms of social work, and what I would describe as professional programs and the helping professions, many educational gaps remain in higher education, especially in teaching about sex and preparing students for future practice in this area.

To fill these gaps, this book provides discussion of current debates and hot topics, celebrates multidisciplinarity and diversity, and offers practical application and recommendations, particularly for those academics responsible for training students to eventually work with vulnerable populations as well as the general public. Thus, this collection is primarily geared toward assisting instructors to provide adequate and appropriate sex education training, knowledge, and opportunities so that their students can explore complex personal and emotional issues; reflect on their attitudes about sex; build skills; and develop confidence so they feel more comfortable with helping others when they are eventually working in their respective fields.

In addition, the book is also aimed at professors and students who are interested in taking on a leadership role in this area, more effectively supporting others, and improving curriculum and the quality of the teaching of sexuality(ies) in their specific discipline. Although not intended specifically as a course textbook, this book, and/or chapters from it, may be of interest to educators in higher education from a variety of fields and can certainly be used as required/recommended reading in a variety of college and university programs and across many generalist courses or in stand-alone sexuality/sexual health courses.

Due to the length constraints of the book, there is limited coverage of sexuality, sexual health, and sex education in field education and placements. This research is necessary and represents a large gap in training and scholarship across multiple disciplines. For future research, some related questions that should be considered are how do we ensure sexuality content is covered in field education; how should field instructors teach/cover this content; how should students be supervised and evaluated for this content and learning; and what activities are best for students to try to learn this content.

Finally, I want to take this opportunity to thank my two daughters, Ashley and Cassie, for their unconditional love and support. I also want to thank the University of Toronto Press and its publishing editor, Meg Patterson, and all the contributors, who worked tirelessly to finish their chapters.

TEACHING ABOUT SEX AND SEXUALITIES
IN HIGHER EDUCATION

Introduction: Let's Teach about Sex

SUSAN HILLOCK

Why did I decide to edit a book collection about teaching sex in higher education? Years ago, as a medical social worker, I worked with many patients who had serious illnesses and operations such as prostate surgeries, mastectomies, colostomies, amputations, spinal cord injuries, and traumatic brain injuries. Although I had not received any sex education training in my bachelor of social work or bachelor of arts, I was comfortable with the topic so regularly included sexuality as part of my bio-psycho-social assessments. As a result, I often ended up fielding patient requests for research, information, and practical suggestions about everything from managing new body tastes and smells to better positioning for orgasm. Indeed, patients would often ask me questions that they were too uncomfortable to ask their nurses or physicians, particularly about issues related to body functions, sexual preferences, desire, and pleasure. Typical examples were: "I now have a colostomy, so how am I going to have sex with my partner without stinking?"; "I have a spinal cord injury – how do I deal with not being able to have orgasm?"; or "This amputation has changed my body image. I feel ugly when I am naked. How do I tell my partner?" Obviously, body changes impact how people feel about themselves, their abilities, and their sense of themselves as sexual beings. These changes also encourage people to adapt and create innovative ways to achieve wellness and experience happiness (Ballan, 2008; Taylor, 2011). In my clinical work, I always tried to reframe what sexuality meant to these folks by assessing how their sexual behaviours, sensory preferences, tastes, and desires had evolved. This included helping them communicate their desires and make requests of partners (if they had any) about what gave them pleasure, expanding their sexual repertoire, and supporting enjoyment of other aspects of sex such as different sensations, touches, smells, and tastes so that they still felt like sexual beings (if that is what they wanted).

In recognition of the intrinsic multidisciplinary nature of sexuality education, when I would receive these inquiries, I would usually ask physiotherapists and occupational therapists for assistance, as at the time, they seemed to be the only other healthcare folks also interested in sexual health and wellness. However, when I asked them if they had any sex research, books, information, examples, suggestions, or advice, they usually had no sources or recommendations. Of course, this was in the late 1990s, in rural northern New Brunswick, before the advent of the internet and information highway. Thus, when I searched high and low for research, books, practical information, and patient literature that I could give service users about various medical conditions, body challenges, and sex functioning, there was nothing available.

More than twenty years later, given the proliferation of sexual content and information across social media and the internet, one might assume that these sex education gaps have been filled by modern research and scholarship. Indeed, there has certainly been increased coverage and development of advanced sex education theory and content, as well as many courses and programs, specifically addressing sexuality in Canadian postsecondary institutions, particularly at the master's and doctoral levels, and within certain academic disciplines such as psychology, public and community health, as well as sexuality, porn, disability, queer, and gender studies. However, across other disciplines, relatively speaking, Werley (2016) still argues that "there has been little discussion around sexuality education at the collegiate level and beyond" (p. 1). Furthermore, what is clear from the current research, at least within professional programs and the helping professions, is that we still have a long way to go in sex education in higher education. Because of this noticeable gap, as a social work professor, I regularly engage with students in discussions about sexuality, not only in terms of assessing sexual health and functioning in service users; providing sexuality-related services, supports, and knowledge; encouraging sex positivity; exploring queer and trans/nonbinary sexuality(ies) and experiences of discrimination; investigating and reporting sexual violence/abuse, but also in terms of exploring their own and others' identities; deconstructing "normative" understandings about sex and sexuality; as well as examining the personal, social, and cultural aspects of how sexuality is performed and understood.

Over time, I have learned that not all students (or colleagues and administrators, for that matter) welcome this openness. Ironically, in an age when students historically have more access and exposure to sexual images, nudity, porn, sexualized images, and sexual information/education than ever before, some students have what I would describe as intense puritanical attitudes and discomfort with any discussion/content remotely related to real talk about sex, bodies, desire, or pleasure. Additionally, when I try to find articles, research, teaching materials, or collegial support on how to best teach this subject or examples of experiential exercises that I can use in the university classroom that would be helpful, there is still very little available within the social work literature. Prior, Williams, Zavala, and Milford (2016) concur, finding that "there has been relatively little attention given to this topic across social work curricula" (p. 55). In addition, the scant content and information that is available tend to be from sex-negative approaches, focusing on problems, differences, and dysfunction, and treating heterosexuality and monogamy as the "norm" (ibid.). In addition, colleagues seem reticent to discuss sex or teach about it (Berry, 2017). Myers and Milner (2007), as cited in McCave, Shepard, and Ramseyer Winter, 2014 (p. 409) agree, stating that "ignoring and pathologizing sexuality has happened all too often within social work education, scholarship, and practice."

Although I am referencing social work sources here, the literature indicates that this generally holds true as well, across other helping professions, including medicine, nursing, child and youth care, and social service programs (Sangra, 2016; Wineberg, 2015; Wylie & Weerakoon, 2010). For example, in medicine, Steinauer, La Rochelle, Rowh, Backus, Sandahl, and Foster (2009) have concluded that in North America "comprehensive reproductive health education is deficient in health professions training and education" (p. 75). They also blame neoconservative and religious influences on higher education for gaps in medical sex education, including a general "lack of contraception and elective abortion education in medical schools" (p. 75). In general, there is a significant lack of theoretical and/or applied literature, research, exemplars, and scholarship available on how to best teach sexuality(ies) within healthcare professions. Indeed, Monteiro-Cesnik and Zerbini (2017) "found that higher education courses in health care do not provide adequate training, and therefore, students are insufficiently prepared to deal with sexuality issues" (p. 7).

Sex and Sexuality(ies)

Historically, the word "sexuality" originated from botanical studies in the early 1800s and referred to "the aspect of reproduction and not … sexual desire and emotionality" (Schultheiss & Glina, 2010, p. 2031). This conceptual link did not occur until at least the early twentieth century. In 1867, the term "sexology" first appeared in print (p. 2031), and originators of this new field of study included Paolo Mantegazza, Conrad Eckhard, Richard Freiherr von Krafft-Ebing, Sigmund Freud, Magnus Hirschfeld, Henry

Havelock Ellis, Harry Benjamin, and Ernst Grafenberg (pp. 2033–2035). They were the founding fathers of what has been called "sexual medicine" (p. 2032) and provided the philosophical foundations of modern day sexual health movements and institutions including the "Kinsey Institute, the International Academy of Sex Research, the Society for the Scientific Study of Sex, and the World Association for Sexual Health" (Fletcher, Dowsett, Duncan, Slavin, & Corboz, 2013, p. 323). These founders in turn, have been critiqued by feminists for their predominant "heavily biomedical and behavioural approaches to sex" (p. 323). Other famous sexuality pioneers soon followed: Kinsey (1894–1956); Masters (1915–2001); and Johnson (1925–2013) (Schultheiss & Glina, 2010). By 1968, Indiana University was the first medical school in North America to introduce a human sexuality course (Westberg & Jason, 1985).

Obviously, times, they were a-changing. Human sexuality was finally being viewed as an important and an integral part of our emotional, physical, social, and psychological well-being. Expressed more strongly, as Brashear (as cited in McCave, Shepard, and Ramseyer Winter, 2014, p. 409) posits, "to ignore our sexuality is to deny our humanity." Correspondingly, given the evolution of various human rights and self-advocacy movements, as well as the advent of the sexual revolution in the 1960s and 1970s, at that time and into the early 1980s, there was a burgeoning of interest in sex research, education, and programming (Berry, 2017; Oswalt, Wagner, Eastman-Mueller, & Nevers, 2014; Satterly & Dyson, 1998; Suarez & Balaji, 2007; Wineberg, 2015), particularly in the area of homosexuality, identity politics, and queer theory (Berry, 2017; Hillock & Mulé, 2016; Knegt, 2011). Across multiple disciplines, scholars were beginning to develop sex education/human sexuality courses, build sex research and theory, and strongly advocate for the inclusion of sexuality content.

Then, due perhaps to the rise of global neoconservatism, right-wing fundamentalism (e.g., just say no/abstinence), and government cuts to spending (including university funding), the late 1980s and 1990s saw a sharp decrease, particularly in the United States, in curriculum content, as well as scholarship and publication in this area, including the 1994 closure of the only North American social work sex journal, Taylor and Francis's *Journal of Social Work and Human Sexuality* (Gray, House, & Eicken, 1996; Wineberg, 2015). In the United States, conservative forces and right-wing fundamentalism also resulted in the long-standing absence of sex education/sexual health/sexuality programming and content, both in Kindergarten-to-grade-twelve (K–12) systems and in most undergraduate and graduate programs, as well as a lack of sexual education knowledge, skills development, and training in various professional programs, including medicine, nursing, social work, counselling, and so on (Dunk, 2007; Sangra, 2016; Wineberg, 2015; Wylie & Weerakoon, 2010).

In contrast, the Canadian K–12 context has been quite different (although there are variations), as provincially most students are taught a compulsory sex education curriculum that tends to be more progressive than the American experience. Even so, Canada's sex education curriculum has periodically also been under attack for being too progressive, particularly by those from the religious right who either object to sex being discussed at school or who do not agree with the topics being covered (e.g., birth control, oral sex, and homosexuality). For example, right-wing parent groups have pushed school boards for years to ban queer-positive books. Fortunately, in 2002, "the Supreme Court of Canada finally ruled these acts as unconstitutional and approved 3 specific children's books" (Hillock, 2016, p. 78). As another example, in 2009, the province of Alberta passed *Bill 44*, the *Human Rights, Citizenship and Multiculturalism Amendment Act*. This bill legally mandated that parents be notified about any upcoming religion, sex, or sexual orientation content and be allowed to withdraw their children from classes when this content was being taught (Hillock, 2016). The ongoing struggle has also been demonstrated by recent events in Ontario, under Premier Doug Ford's administration, that have seen changes to the sex education curriculum that definitely reflect a regressive approach, including a similar exemption protocol for parents to remove their children from classrooms (CBC News, 2019).

Furthermore, even Canada's more progressive lens and mandated K–12 sex education did not mean an automatic carry-over to ensure that this topic continued to be covered or examined in more detail in higher education. I can personally attest to the fact that during this same time frame and across four university degrees, the topic of sex rarely came up in any of my university classes. Moreover, within the helping professions and their professional training programs, there still existed limited information and research on the topic of sex, and what was available focused almost exclusively on the HIV and AIDS crisis, as well as sexual risk, especially the prevention of teenage pregnancy and sexually transmitted infections (STIs) (Wineberg, 2015). Indeed, this sex-negative or risk-based approach, emphasizing vulnerability, violence, and abuse, dominated fields such as social work, nursing, child and youth care, and medicine for several years.

Fortunately, the late 1990s and early 2000s saw an awakening of awareness about the intersections of sexual and gender identity(ies), expression, globalization, anticolonialism, marginalization, and human rights (Hillock & Mulé, 2016). This has led to an increased interest in multidisciplinary approaches to sex research and education (Bancroft, 2000) which can beneficially expand the scope of research by introducing new perspectives and theories while attracting students from many disciplines (Werley, 2016).

There has also been a corresponding growth of women's, gender, queer, disabilities, and sexual-diversity studies departments in academia and the "emergence of a new form of sexuality scholarship ... Critical Sexuality Studies (CSS)" (Fletcher, Dowsett, Duncan, Slavin, & Corboz, 2013, p. 320). Indeed, the last few years have seen what seems to be a renewed interest in sex research and education in higher education (Trotter, Brogatzki, Duggan, Foster, & Levie, 2006). Today, feminism, postmodernism, global human-rights activism; queer, Indigenous, and antiracism theories; and the disability-rights movement have led to a revisiting of the conceptualizations of sexual liberation, desire, and pleasure, opening up new terrain in disability, BDSM, and transperspectives, and deconstructing/reimagining of sexuality discourses, including topics such as global sexual human rights, sex trafficking, pornography, medical research, online technology, intersectionality, consent, vibrator feminism, crip porn, sexual citizenship, and empowerment, to name a few. Indeed, one could argue that Canada has become a hotbed of sex research, no pun intended, as many of the world's top sex researchers are Canadian, including some of our own contributors (The Globe and Mail, 2017).

Additionally, key textbooks have been published that include resources on teaching sexuality, including Hyde, DeLamater, and Byers's (2015) *Understanding Human Sexuality,* Pukall's (2017) *Human Sexuality: A Contemporary Introduction,* and Rathus, Nevid, Fichner-Rathus, and McKay's (2015) *Human Sexuality in a World of Diversity.* In addition, there are now many sex journals. Significant to this book's themes, important journals include the *Journal of Sex Research* (JSR); *Archives of Sexual Behaviour* (ASB); *Canadian Journal of Sexuality* (CJHS); and *American Journal of Sexuality Education* (Berry, 2017). So there is renewed optimism and hope that now is a very good time for educators to assess and evaluate the quality and quantity of the sexuality(ies) discourses and curriculum in their programs (or to add sexuality content, if there is none).

Social Work Education and Sexuality(ies)

Specifically, in terms of social work education, although our Code of Ethics (CASW, 2005) rejects discrimination based on gender or sexual orientation, the CASWE-ACFTS Standards for Accreditation (2014) adds that "Schools of Social Work must encourage and support diversity and social justice related to gender and sexual identities" (pp. 3–4), and International Federation of Social Workers and International Association of Schools of Social Workers Codes of Ethics emphasize an "international requirement to promote social justice for lesbian, gay, and bisexual people" (Fish, 2012, p. 15), the reality is that there is little content, emphasis, guidelines, standards, or teaching related to sexuality(ies) in most North American social work programs (Jeyas-ingham, 2008; Wineberg, 2015). And although we do speak somewhat about violence, sexual assault, and trauma (Wilkin & Hillock, 2015), as well as the social determinants of health and well-being, we rarely discuss basic sex and reproductive facts; referral of service users for services such as abortion, contraception, STI/HIV testing, family plan-ning, and fertility; the link between sexuality and health outcomes; or how to include sexuality in our assessments, let alone teach about our right to have good sex. According to the World Health Organization, sexual health is

> a state of physical, emotional, mental and social well-being in rela-tion to sexuality; it is not merely the absence of disease, dysfunction or infirmity. Sexual health requires a positive and respectful approach to sexuality and sexual relationships, as well as the possibility of having pleasurable and safe sexual experiences, free of coercion, discrimina-tion and violence. For sexual health to be attained and maintained, the sexual rights of all persons must be respected, protected and fulfilled. (WHO, 2006, p. 5)

If we truly support this definition, then we need to view sexual health/wellness as a global human right (Graham & Padilla, 2014). Therefore, teaching about sex, including sexuality(ies) in our assess-ments, and developing sexual citizenship (Weeks, 1998) become our ethical responsibility. Indeed, social workers (and other care provid-ers) have an opportunity to do a great service if they are taught accu-rate knowledge about sex and are willing to ask service users about their sexuality(ies). It is also imperative for educators to continue their efforts to transform their sexuality content/discourses from a risk (and just say no and abstention) perspective to a sex-positive pleasure and desire-oriented discourse (Dodd & Tolman, 2017; Williams, Chris-tensen, & Capous-Desyllas, 2016). Furthermore, we can help service users and students, as well as colleagues and administrators, decon-struct traditional definitions and reimagine conceptions about what sex, bodies, desire, and pleasure can mean, and at the same time help others develop resilience and self-esteem (Glass, 2016).

Teaching Sex and Sexuality(ies) in Higher Education

Consequently, this book elaborates on the argument above: that much more can be done in teaching about sex and sexuality(ies) in higher education. In agreement with Wylie, Hallam-Jones, and Daines (2003), this book focuses on higher education because "undergraduate education in human sexuality is an important developmental link between the sex education that everyone receives at secondary school and the specialist training that is available at the postgraduate level" (p. 294). Furthermore, sex education in higher education can fill gaps in knowledge and change attitudes, particularly if students have had little or inadequate sex education, as well as, if the information they have received has been based solely upon a sex-negative/risk approach. Additionally, as previously discussed, although progress has been made, Fletcher, Dowsett, Duncan, Slavin, and Corboz (2013) still make the point that professional "sexuality training has not kept pace" (p. 321) and that both in North American and globally there still remains a "major gap in the field of advanced sexuality research training" (p. 322).

For this book, although there is no agreed-on definition of sexuality, I draw upon feminist, social work, education, psychological, disability, and queer-theory knowledge bases, definitions, and conceptualizations of sexuality (Braidotti, 2003; Butler, 1990; Bywater & Jones, 2008; Dunk, 2007; Hicks, 2008; Jeyasingham, D., 2008) to emphasize the importance and relevance of teaching sexuality(ies) in higher education, as well as how and why a multidisciplinary approach is best suited for a book of this nature. This book also provides a unique and modern take on more current trends, including developing and promoting sexual well-being, positivity, diversity, mutual consent, and self-efficacy. It also challenges social constructions of what is considered to be "normal" sex; the privileging of penis-in-vagina intercourse; presumptions of heterosexuality, cisgenderism, and monogamy; as well as "the regime of sexuality itself, that is, the knowledges and social practices that construct the self as sexual" (Seidman, 1997, p. 93).

Accordingly, the book consists of multiple contributors who are experts in their individual fields, filling the aforementioned gaps in the literature; discussing key concepts, debates, and current issues; exploring intersectionality and celebrating diversity; presenting exemplars, methods, resources, course outlines, and experiential exercises across disciplines to help educators teach in this subject area and improve curriculum content; and making recommendations about best practices, research, teaching, and supports.

In terms of design, the book has been divided into three thematic sections: "Current Debates and Hot Topics," "At the Margins: Diverse Voices and Perspectives," and "Practical Applications and Recommendations." Although there is some overlap, and some themes, theories, and points clearly intersect, these sections broadly correspond with what the current research recommends related to ideal sex education outcomes: knowledge gains (i.e., cognition); attitude shifts (i.e., affect); and skills development (i.e., behaviour), sometimes referred to as KAS (Monteiro-Cesnik & Zerbini, 2017; Stayton, 1998; Werley, 2016).

REFERENCES

Ballan, M. S. (2008). Disability and sexuality within social work education in the USA and Canada: The social model of disability as a lens for practice. *Social Work Education, 27*(2), 194–202. https://doi.org/10.1080/02615470701709675

Bancroft, J. (2000). *The role of theory in sex research.* Ed. John Bancroft. Indiana University Press: Bloomington, Indianapolis.

Berry, J. (2017). Social workers' perspectives on sexuality in social work practice, Masters' Thesis, University of Calgary, Alberta.

Braidotti, R. (2003). Becoming woman: Or sexual difference revisited. *Theory, Culture & Society, 20*(3), 43–64. https://doi.org/10.1177/02632764030203004

Butler, J. (1990). *Gender trouble: Feminism and the subversion of identity.* New York: Routledge.

Bywater, J., & Jones, R. (2008). Sexuality and social work. *The British Journal of Social Work, 38*(6), September 2008, 1259–1261. https://doi.org/10.1093/bjsw/bcn112

CASW. (2005). Code of Ethics. https://www.casw-acts.ca/en/Code-of-Ethics%20and%20Scope%20of%20Practice.

CASWE-ACFTS. (2014). *Standards for accreditation.* Ottawa, Ontario. https://caswe-acfts.ca/wp-content/uploads/2013/03/CASWE-ACFTS.Standards-11-2014-1.pdf.

CBC News. (August 21, 2019). Parents will be able to exempt children from some of Ontario's new sex-ed curriculum. https://www.cbc.ca/news/canada/toronto/ontario-new-sex-ed-curriculum-1.5254327

Dodd, S. J. & Tolman, D. (2017). Receiving a positive discourse on sexuality within social work. *National Association of Social Workers.* 227–234. https://doi.org/10.1093/sw/swx016

Dunk, P. (2007). Everyday sexuality and social work: Locating sexuality in professional practice and education. *Social Work and the Society: International Online Journal, 5*(2), https://researchnow.flinders.edu.au/en/publications/everyday-sexuality-and-social-work-locating-sexuality-in-professi

Fish, J. (2012). *Social work and lesbian, gay, bisexual, and transpeople: Making a difference*. Bristol: Policy Press.

Fletcher, G., Dowsett, G., Duncan, D., & Slavin, S. & Corboz, J. (2013). Advancing sexuality studies: a short course on sexuality theory and research methodologies. *Sex Education, 13*(3), 319–335. https://doi.org/10.1080/14681811.2012.742847

Glass, S. R. (2016). It's time to talk about sex and social work: Why human sexuality education matters for social work practice. *Theses, Dissertations, and Projects*. 1695. 1–42. https//scholarworks.smith.edu/theses/1695.

The Globe and Mail. (2017, November 22). *Sexuality: The big brains behind Canada's good sex*. https://www.theglobeandmail.com/life/relationships/the-big-brains-behind-canadas-goodsex/article37056097/

Graham, L. F., & Padilla, M. (2014). Sexual rights for marginalized populations. In D. L. Tolman & L. M. Diamond (Eds. in Chief), *APA handbook of sexuality, Vol 2, Conceptual approaches* (pp. 251–266). American Psychology Association. https://doi.org/10.1037/14194-008

Gray, L. A., House, R. S., & Eicken, S. (1996). Human sexuality instruction: Implications for couple and family counselor educators. *The Family Journal: Counselling and Therapy, 4*(3), 206–216. https://doi.org/10.1177/1066480796043004

Hicks, S. (2008). What does social work desire? *Social Work Education, 27*(2), 131–137. https://doi.org/10.1080/02615470701709451

Hillock, S. (2016). Social work, the academy, and queer communities: Heteronormativity and exclusion. In S. Hillock & N. J. Mulé (Eds.), *Queering social work education* (pp. 73–92). Vancouver: UBC Press.

Hillock, S., & Mulé, N. J. (Eds.) (2016). *Queering social work education*. Vancouver: UBC Press.

Hyde, J. S., DeLamater, J. D., & Byers, E. S. (2015). *Understanding human sexuality: Sixth Canadian edition*. Toronto: McGraw-Hill Ryerson.

Jeyasingham, D. (2008). Knowledge/ignorance and the construction of sexuality in social work education. *Social Work Education, 27*(2), 138–151. https://doi.org/10.1080/02615470701709469

Knegt, P. (2011). *Queer rights*. Halifax, Nova Scotia: Fernwood Publishing.

McCave, E., Shepard, B., & Ramseyer Winter, V. (2014). Human sexuality as a critical subfield in social work. *Advances in Social Work, 15*. 409–427. https://doi.org/10.18060/16672

Monteiro-Cesnik, V., & Zerbini, T. (2017). Sexuality education for health professionals: A literature review. *Estudos de Psicologia (Campinas, 34*(1). https://doi.org/10.1590/1982-02752017000100016

Oswalt, S. B., Wagner, L. M., Eastmann-Mueller, H.P., & Nevers, M. (2014). Pedagogy and content in sexuality education courses in US colleges and universities. *Sex Education, 15*(2), 172–187. https://doi.org/10.1080/14681811.2014.991958

Prior, E. E., Williams, D. J., Zavala, T., & Milford, J. (2016). What do(n't) American undergraduate social work students learn about sex? A content analysis of sex positivity and diversity in five popular HBSE textbooks. *Critical Social Work*, *17*(1). https://doi.org/10.22329/csw.v17i1.5895

Pukall, C. (2017). *Human sexuality: A contemporary introduction*. New York: Oxford University Press.

Rathus, S. A., Nevid, J. S., Fichner-Rathus, L., & McKay, A. (2015). *Human sexuality in a world of diversity*. 5th ed. Toronto: Pearson Canada.

Sangra, N. (2016). Let's talk about sex: Counsellors' experiences of actively integrating sexuality into counselling practice, Masters Thesis, Athabasca University, Alberta, 1–154.

Satterly, B. A., & Dyson, D. A. (1998). The use of self-disclosure as an educational intervention in the graduate social work human sexuality classroom. *Journal of Sex Education and Therapy*, *23*(1), 55–61). https://doi.org/10.1080/01614576.1998.11074207

Schultheiss, D., & Glina, S. (2010). Highlights from the history of sexual medicine. *International Society for Sexual Medicine*, *7*, 2031–2043. https://doi.org/10.1111/j.1743-6109.2010.01866.x

Seidman, S. (1997). *Difference troubles: Queering social theory and sexual politics*. Cambridge University Press, Cambridge.

Stayton, W. (1998). A curriculum for training professional in human sexuality using the sexual attitude restructuring (SAR) model. *Journal of Sex Education and Therapy*, *23*(1), 26–32. https://doi.org/10.1080/01614576.1998.11074203

Steinauer, J., La Rochelle, F., Rowh, M., Backus, L., Sandahl, Y., & Foster, A. (2009). First impressions: What are preclinical medical students in the US and Canada learning about sexual and reproductive health? *Contraception*, *80*(1), 74–80. https://doi.org/10.1016/j.contraception.2008.12.015

Suarez, A. E., & Balaji, A. (2007). Coverage and representation in introductory sociology textbooks. *Teaching Sociology*, *35*(3), 239–254. https://doi.org/10.1177/0092055x0703500303

Taylor, B. (2011). The impact on assistive equipment on intimacy and sexual expression. *British Journal of Occupational Therapy*, *74*(9), 435–442. https://doi.org/10.4276/030802211x13153015305637

Trotter, J., Brogatzki, L., Duggan, L., Foster, E., & Levie, J. (2006). Revealing disagreement and discomfort through auto-ethnography and personal narrative. *Qualitative Social Work*, *5*(3), 369–388. https://doi.org/10.1177/1473325006067366

Weeks, J. (1998). The sexual citizen. *Theory, Culture, & Society*, *15*(3–4), 35–52. https://doi.org/10.1177/0263276498015003003

Werley, J. (2016). Sex ed all grown up: The benefits of teaching human sexuality at the collegiate level. *IUSB Graduate Journal*, *3*, 99–102.

Westberg, J., & Jason, H. (1985). Teaching human sexuality. *Medical Teacher*, *7*(1), 53–61. https://doi.org/10.3109/01421598509036791

Wilkin, L., & Hillock, S. (2015). Enhancing MSW students' efficacy in working with trauma, violence, and oppression: An integrated feminist-trauma framework for social work education. *Feminist Teacher, 24*(3). 184–206. https://doi.org/10.5406/femteacher.24.3.0184

Williams, D., Christensen, M. C., & Capous-Desyllas, M. (2016). Social work practice and sexuality: Applying a positive sexuality model to enhance diversity and resolve problems. *Families in Society, 97*(4), 287–294. https://doi.org/10.1606/1044-3894.2016.97.35

Wineberg, H. R. (2015). Social work and human sexuality: An examination of the country's top 25-CWSE ranked MSW curricula. *Theses, Dissertations, and Projects.* 663, 1–41.

World Health Organization. (2006). *Defining sexual health: Report of a technical consultation on sexual health, January 28–21.* Geneva, Switzerland. Retrieved from http://www.who.int/reproductivehealth/publications/sexual_health /defining_sexual_health.pdf.

Wylie, K., Hallam-Jones, R., & Daines, B. (2003). Review of an undergraduate medical school training programme in human sexuality. *Medical Teacher, 25*(3), 291–295. https://doi.org/10.1080/0142159031000100382

Wylie, K., & Weerakoon, P. (2010). International perspectives on teaching human sexuality. *Academic Psychiatry, 34*(5), 397–402. https://doi.org /10.1176/appi.ap.34.5.397

PART ONE

Current Debates and Hot Topics

SUSAN HILLOCK

To start, Part 1, "Current Debates and Hot Topics," presents current research and knowledge about key concepts, debates, and issues related to teaching sexuality(ies) in higher education. In Chapter 1, "Don't Ask/ Don't Tell: Sexuality(ies), Instructor Disclosure, and Trigger Warnings in the Classroom," I describe, as social work professor, my experiences of teaching about sex in social work classrooms. I highlight the benefits of incorporating sex education into higher education, discuss sex as a controversial subject for teaching, and reflect on two examples of student backlash in terms of negative responses to sex education. I further explore instructor disclosure, consider how much, if any, instructors should disclose about their sexuality, sex and gender identity, or sexual orientation, desires, or practices, and also discuss instructor safety in the classroom. Additionally, from a social work lens, I explain the importance of being transparent in terms of instructors' sexuality(ies) and sexual identity(ies).

As well, I examine the emerging trigger-warning trend, analyse the risks that sex education instructors may choose to take, knowing that we tread where no one else may be willing to go, and offer suggestions on how to mitigate risk. As a partial solution, I propose that sex education work requires maintaining a delicate balance between encouraging students to expand their understanding and knowledge, while avoiding ratcheting up the anxiety too high for them to learn. I also recommend steps to prepare students for sex education content and suggest building alliances as a way to build support and mitigate associated risks. Finally, I argue that silence on these topics is not serving our students or society and does not promote effective and ethical social work practice.

In Chapter 2, "Restoring Indigenous Sexuality," authors Carrie Bourassa, Betty McKenna, Miranda Keewatin, Sadie Anderson, Marlin Legare, Mikayla Hagel, Danette Starblanket, Jennifer Langan, and

Cari McIlduff present key teachings, explain progressive Indigenous understandings of gender status and sexual identity, examine contemporary issues of which all educators should be aware when teaching sexuality(ies), and recommend culturally relevant approaches. To accomplish this, they examine current and historical colonial traumas experienced by Indigenous Peoples and how they disrupted traditional methods of passing down health information intergenerationally. This continued disruption changed how Indigenous Peoples view and share traditional sexual-health knowledge and practices. Indeed, Indigenous Knowledges encompass a holistic, multifaceted, nonbinary understanding of health, in which sexual health is an important aspect of holistic health as it includes traditional teachings of gender identity and expression, reproductive roles and responsibilities, and reproductive health. Despite disruptions, the authors maintain that healing practices and traditions have remained resilient through the implementation of traditional rights of passage and ceremony in Indigenous programming and services within Indigenous communities.

They then share traditional teachings from Knowledge Keepers that play an integral role in the maintenance of culture(s) and community health. Furthermore, they describe the role of Knowledge Keepers, who pass on valuable teachings related to sexual health and reproduction. Specifically, regarding sexual health, Knowledge Keepers focus on gender responsibilities, as they play an important role in sharing Traditional Knowledges. They also summarize contemporary issues that Indigenous Peoples face when attempting to access health services, including environmental barriers, lack of awareness about sexual-health services, lack of knowledge or education about sexual health, personal barriers, and a lack of culturally appropriate sexual-health services. Additionally, in response to the increasing rates of HIV among Indigenous Peoples in Saskatchewan, they suggest solutions to restore health that can be found through Indigenous Peoples' cultures and resilience.

Next, top Canadian sex researcher and psychology professor, Terry Humphreys, explores the complexities of teaching sexual consent from numerous perspectives in Chapter 3, "Teaching Sexual Consent," including what is known from the research literature, educational/prevention campaigns, primary/secondary school curricula, and international endeavours. Humphreys argues that sexual consent is conceptually and practically quite complex and outlines how interrelated contextual challenges arise from any attempt to teach sexual consent self-efficacy, including a sex-negative culture, sexual ambivalence and uncertainty, gendered socialization, hetero-centrism, and the lack of a comprehensive sexuality knowledge base. Humphreys brings conceptual considerations and empirical research together to inform the teaching of sexual consent. He also makes the point that sexual communication skills are the foundation of consent education. He suggests that at the postsecondary level, connections between teaching and research are abundant. Most notably, he reports, teachers routinely review the research literature to ensure the content they present reflects the most accurate and up-to-date knowledge on a given subject. Students also have opportunities to interact with research through writing papers and participating in research studies. Humphreys states that this is particularly relevant in the sexuality field where much of our knowledge about consent attitudes and behaviours, as well as sexual assault prevalence rates, is developed through survey-based research conducted with undergraduate students.

Further, research tools and findings can be utilized in the classroom to enhance engagement and make the material come to life. Thus, he recommends that teaching sexual consent to college and university students takes a comprehensive approach that recognizes the social context in which one's teaching exists. He provides specific examples of how to design activities, exercises, and discussions that include aspects of cultural and gender norms, sexual-script theory, legal issues, and sexual orientation that can make lesson plans more inclusive and realistic. He also posits that any approach that does not recognize the cultural backdrop of entrenched sex negativity, as well as sexual and gendered norms, is bound to be ineffective because it will not resonate with the lived experience of those we are trying to educate. Finally, Humphreys emphasizes that it is essential to teach students about the challenges inherent in verbalizing sexual wants and desires to their partners and also to work to break down the discomfort, shame, traditional norms, and media messages that impede a sex-positive approach to teaching sexual consent.

In the following chapter, Chapter 4, "What about the Boys: University Students Learning about Sexual Consent Talk from Youth in Northeastern Ontario," women's and gender studies faculty member, Jennifer L. Johnson queries how sexual violence and consent are discussed in feminist postsecondary classrooms, how these discussions can benefit from the perspectives of men and boys, and why the creative potential of men and boys in challenging toxic masculinity needs to be acknowledged. Johnson argues that new and productive discussions about gender-based sexual violence are enhanced within postsecondary education by acknowledging the vulnerabilities of men and boys and the uncertainties or awkwardness they face while developing their own healthy relationships. Further, she suggests that teaching about sexual violence and consent in feminist postsecondary classrooms requires helping boys become emotionally literate, and that by including sexuality education about consent and violence, instructors can potentially draw on the voices of those who may like to challenge gender-based violence but are not usually seen as knowledgeable about it. In addition, Johnson states that direct interventions in discourses of toxic masculinity for boys at the age of 12 to 13 is not only promising for adolescents but is also an important connection to what should be done in university classrooms. She wonders what would happen to the statistics on sexual assault in Ontario universities if more 12- and 13-year-olds had access to knowledgeable peer mentors and trained facilitators talking about sexual assault. She elaborates by asking educators to consider how postsecondary education can collaborate on and support this type of learning in elementary and high school systems.

In Chapter 5, "The Down Low on Getting Down: Reframing Problem-Focused Narratives by Focusing on Sex Positivity and Desire-Based Education," manager of the Youth Justice Programs at Peterborough Youth Services and former college student rights and responsibilities' coordinator, social worker Amie Kroes offers a feminist review of effective techniques and recommendations to address the issue of sexual violence in postsecondary institutions, promote sex positivity, mutual consent, gender equity, and healthy relationships in higher education, while also analysing continuing barriers and gaps to preventing sexual violence. Part of the problem, as Kroes sees it, is that we live in a society that overtly sexualizes bodies in the name of capitalist marketing, yet openly shames people for participating in, talking about, or learning about acts of sexuality. She hypothesizes that this discrepancy is partly responsible for uninformed sexual exploration that often leads to miscommunication, unrealistic expectations, male entitlement, and sexual violence. As a college students' rights and responsibilities coordinator, she has found that it is often the case that 18- to 24-year-olds receive comprehensive information related to sexuality and sexual violence for the first time in postsecondary workshops. Typically, this is *after* they have had at least one sexual experience in their lives. She proposes that as a time of independence and experimentation, this is an ideal time to be focusing on both the risks and the pleasures related to sex and sexuality(ies). Based upon her understanding of the field, Kroes recommends the implementation of an integrated and comprehensive approach that utilizes a sex-positive approach, encourages conversations related to healthy sexuality, keeps information socioculturally relevant, and provides information that students want. This means providing socioculturally relevant programs, content, and methods for a variety of populations. She also argues that it is important to ensure that all students see themselves represented in awareness-raising campaigns, as well as in the action phase of interventions. Thus, sexual content needs to be not only "open" for anyone but also truly accessible and useful for all.

Finally, in their collaborative interdisciplinary Chapter 6, "Transgender Experiences in Healthcare: Addressing Challenges while Teaching Compassion in Higher Education," social work professor Colleen McMillan and medical physicians Mike Lee-Poy and Carys Massarella attempt to dismantle intersectional barriers that make healthcare unsafe for transgender individuals. Starting with higher education and expanding into legal, political, and healthcare landscapes, informed by the voices of transgender patients, they identify spaces and practices, as well as patient-informed guidelines in which teaching sexuality(ies), guided by the principles of social justice and advocacy, could exist. The authors describe a multitude of systemic factors that converge to make experiences for transgender individuals problematic when attempting to access the basic healthcare rights. Exploring the various terms used to define trans individuals, the authors argue that what transverses all definitions are the multiple and intersecting micro and macro discourses that result in healthcare being experienced as unsafe for some, regardless of definition and practice context. They believe that healthcare and medical education systems hold vast potential to lead the delivery of compassionate, informed, and truly person-centred care for transgender individuals. They propose a specific teaching sexuality(ies) care model, which they call RIANE, that offers practice wisdom about how to work with transgender patients and teach healthcare providers. They recommend that this model be adopted within the classrooms of higher education for both educators and future healthcare providers alike, to normalize the importance of continuing education and professional humility. Further, McMillan, Lee-Poy, and Massarella propose that teaching sexualities is neither static nor definitive but rather an ongoing process of critical reflection, education, humility, and a stance of placing oneself in a position of active learning that is intentional rather than accidental.

1 Don't Ask/Don't Tell: Sexuality(ies), Instructor Disclosure, and Trigger Warnings in the Classroom

SUSAN HILLOCK

Over the last forty years, feminist scholars have contributed much to social work education by critiquing masculine violence, capitalism, the institutions of marriage, monogamy, and patriarchy, as well as by introducing key concepts such as the personal is political, breaking the silence, and sexual liberation (Hanisch, 2009; Levine, 1982). Indigenous, racialized, queer, and Black feminists have in turn critiqued classic feminism for heteronormativity, cisgenderism, and "whitewashing" (Collins, 2000; Hillock, 2011). They have also introduced antiracist, anticolonial, and queer approaches (Hillock & Mulé, 2016; Keating, 2000). By emphasizing "intersectionality" – how various forms of oppression intersect (e.g., race, gender, and class) (Collins, 1991, p. 18) – they have encouraged social work educators to critically reflect upon where they stand, in terms of the implications of their social locations and identities, in what Collins (1991, 2000) views as a matrix of domination.

If we hold that to be true, how much then, if any, should instructors disclose about their social locations and identities (e.g., sexuality, sex and/or gender expression and identity, and sexual orientation, desires, or practices)? What topics should be or can be addressed in the classroom? How do academics negotiate the risky business of teaching subjects that many students, and perhaps colleagues and administrators, find controversial, upsetting, or triggering? Moreover, are there limits to what a professor can say or do related to these topics, particularly in this current neoconservative climate? Accordingly, this chapter will highlight the benefits of incorporating sex education into higher education, discuss sex as a controversial subject, describe two examples of student backlash and my reflections about them, examine instructor disclosure in the classroom, explore issues that come up in these discussions, and make recommendations on how to mitigate risk.

The Benefits of Sex Education

Philosophically and ethically, I think it is important, particularly in professional programs and the helping professions, that we transition from either ignoring sexuality completely or speaking primarily about sexual risk and violence (Jeyasingham, 2008) and instead (re)introduce topics of desire, pleasure, sexual liberation, and sexual rights into the classroom, and recognize these topics as important and legitimate (Fahs, Plante, & McClelland, 2018; Williams, Prior, & Wegner, 2013). Incorporating positive sexuality into higher education provides students with accurate basic information about sex, breaks the silence, interrogates heteronormativity, and smashes taboos (Johnson, 2009; Williams, Prior, & Wegner, 2013). Frank sex talk in the classroom also sets up conditions to encourage students to better understand their own attitudes and beliefs; desensitize to frank sexual talk, diverse content, and terms; reflect on their own sexualities, identities, attitudes, fears, desires, beliefs, and behaviours; deepen their understandings of the dynamic, intersectional, and diverse nature of sexuality; for some, feel more comfortable and less alone; and speak about private and sometimes uncomfortable things (e.g., masturbation, fellatio, cunnilingus, bisexuality, polyamoury, and anal sex) (Fahs, Plante, & McClelland, 2018; Hicks, S., 2008; Oswalt, Wagner, Eastmann-Mueller, & Nevers, 2014; Satterly & Dyson, 1998).

In terms of social work practice, the provision of quality sex education also teaches students how to develop nonjudgemental attitudes and skills; identify scope of practice and know when to make referrals and to whom; work with sexual assault survivors; feel more comfortable hearing language that some service users use, especially in terms of abuse investigations (e.g., cunt, fuck, pussy, and cock); do a proper sexual assessment and take a sex history; prepare to do individual, family, and couple counselling; and practice necessary skills (for more on these topics, please see Chapter 18.

Even though I believe that sex education is very important, I do acknowledge that these types of discussions can be fraught with intense emotional baggage or triggers (Hillock, 2021a). Indeed, as Stayton (1998) notes, "anxiety, moralizing, and emotionality surround the field of sexuality" (p. 26). I also recognize that because most of my particular students have tended to participate in heteronormative monogamous relationships and are predominantly white, straight, middle-class, Judeo-Christian females, my positive and open sex talk must seem quite shocking. Even though I make assumptions that they are adults, probably sexual, and may have experienced some form of sexual behaviour or activity in their lifetimes, I know that they also bring with them a variety of sexual, cultural, and religious beliefs, experiences, and histories. Moreover, helping professions, geared to providing support and care to others, tend to attract students with trauma histories, including sexual violence, addiction, and mental health issues (i.e., wounded healers) (Ashenberg Straussner, Senreich, & Steen, 2018).

Part of the difficulty, and perhaps the crux of the issue, is that in these neoconservative times, teaching controversial subjects like sex education is so different from what many have experienced in the K–12 system, as well as college and university traditional lecture-didactic formats, that students experience a sort of culture shock when they are asked to learn in different ways, deconstruct their attitudes/beliefs, and explore alternative content. This can be difficult for students (and instructors) and may also lead to backlash, poor evaluations, and student complaints (Hillock, 2021a). However, even though teaching about sex is difficult, that is no reason to stop doing it. This context is important to consider as it impacts how students receive, understand, and respond to what some might call "controversial" subjects in the classroom.

Controversy in the Classroom: Teaching to Transgress

This notion of controversy in the classroom needs further examination. From my perspective, much of what is treated as controversial in today's classrooms is surprisingly not that different from the educational controversies of the 1960s and 1970s (Abramowitz, 1971). These include topics such as abortion, reproductive rights, infidelity, sexual dysfunction, sexually transmitted infections (STIs), homosexuality and trans/nonbinary sexuality(ies), and unwanted pregnancy (Dodd & Tolman, 2017; Wineberg, 2015). Given that we are living in a world where we are constantly exposed across all social media to sexual messages and content, including freely and widely available pornography, one might expect that in 2021, students would no longer find discussions of sex and sexuality and related issues controversial. That is not the case.

Instructor Self-disclosure

When we teach about sex, we dare to transgress (Fahs, Plante, & McClelland, 2018; hooks, 1994). What do I mean by transgressing? As a structural feminist, I live by the mantra that the personal is political (Hanisch, 2009; Levine, 1982). Thus, as a role model, I try to be as open as possible about my locations and identities – a middle-class, white settler, bisexual, polyamorous, and cisgender female.

Additionally, research has repeatedly demonstrated that openness about sexuality, and improved outcomes in terms of sexual health, wellness, and self-esteem, are all connected (Fahs, Plante, & McClelland, 2018; Jeyasingham, 2008; Williams, Prior, & Wegner, 2013). So, to teach this content, I make disclosures about my coming-out stories, sexuality/identity changes over my lifetime, gendered experiences of violence/body shame/empowerment, and life within the polyamoury community (where people choose consensual intimate relationships with more than one partner). I believe that sharing who I am sets the stage for students to feel more comfortable in my classrooms and with their own sexuality(ies) and identity(ies). Accordingly, the use of instructor self-disclosure is consistent with feminist teaching related to topics of identity and sexuality (Hillock, 2021b; Barker & Reavey, 2009). As a teaching tool, it has also been shown to

> decrease power and status differential ... creates an environment of mutuality and nurtures a partnership in learning that allows students to join the instructor in risk-taking disclosure and challenges their personal beliefs. (Cain, 1996, pp. 56–57, as cited in Satterly & Dyson, 1998)

However, despite its benefits, I recognize that instructor disclosure does not come without risks. Furthermore, depending on our administration, colleagues, and students' openness and support (or lack thereof), faculty who occupy vulnerable social locations (e.g., racialized, disabled, or queer) and/or also have more tenuous employment (e.g., new scholars/tenure-track faculty/sessional instructors) may face more backlash and harsher judgement from others. Later on, in this chapter, I make recommendations on how one might go about mitigating these risks.

Sex Positivity

Additionally, I encourage a litany of sex-positive discourse (Dodd & Tolman, 2017; Williams, Prior, & Wegner, 2013) about a variety of sex topics, including orgasm, sexual rights, reproductive choice, inequality/liberation, freedom/consent, masturbation, sex toys, pleasure, desire, fetishism, BDSM (bondage, discipline, dominance, submission, and sadomasochism), and so on. In addition, I try to use humour to share my very human flaws and foibles to demonstrate understanding and acceptance of our bodies and sexuality(ies). However, not every everyone gets my sense of humour and not all students respond well to sex education.

Teaching Sexuality(ies): Two Examples of Student Backlash

Below, are two examples that describe negative student responses to my frank and open classroom discussions of sexuality(ies), sexual diversity, orientation, and identity.

The First Incident

Years ago, I used to facilitate an exercise called "The Precious Jewels Exercise." Before starting, I informed students that this was a sexuality exercise that they must take seriously. I explained that they might feel some anxiety and asked them to trust me enough to complete the exercise. Then, I asked them to describe their most recent sexual experience on a piece of paper. I clarified that it could be solo or with partners. I cautioned them to not pick a sexual experience that was negative or traumatizing. I directed them to describe their experience in erotic detail – all of the smells, the tastes, the sounds, people/objects present, behaviours, and feelings. I gave them about 10 minutes to complete this task.

After they stopped writing, I asked them to quietly fold the paper into a small square and hold the paper. Many students felt uneasy at this point, their anxiety increased, and some giggled. I asked them not to discuss anything with their neighbours. I directed them to very carefully follow the next instructions. I asked them to slowly hand the folded paper to their nearest neighbour. A lot of people looked nervous, but most did as I asked. Next, I told the people receiving the paper not to open it or read it. I let the group sit silently with their anxiety for a few minutes.

While they waited, I asked a series of reflection questions. "How do you feel about this person holding your sexual description?" I invited them to make the empathic leap to "How do you think service users feel when we ask for very private intimate personal details about their lives, sexual behaviours, sexual orientation, sexual violence, or trauma that they have experienced?" I also asked them, "Did you censor yourself? Did you lie, minimize, or exaggerate because you were not sure who might read it"? I encouraged them to think about documentation practices, where and how we store people's valuable information (i.e., precious jewels), as well as how to ensure confidentiality. Students were given plenty of time to share their answers to these questions and give feedback about the exercise. Reactions ranged from people feeling very happy to some having what they describe as "aha" moments, to others wanting to share every intimate detail about their sexuality, to some students refusing to write anything down or hand their papers over.

This exercise had several goals: starting the process of desensitization related to the topic of sexuality(ies); teaching students empathy for what life is like for service users when they are forced to disclose private confidential material; and illustrating clear ethical guidelines around how we treat confidentiality, as well as how to confidentially document and store information. For the most part, the majority of students found this exercise to be an invaluable part of their learning.

One time, I had a female student who refused to do the exercise. As soon as I mentioned sex, she became very upset, challenged me heatedly in class, and refused to participate. She sat on her own and actually left the classroom in the middle of the exercise. I do understand that for some students, this exercise can bring up sexual assault, intensify feelings of body shame, or create feelings of stress and anxiety. So I contacted this student after class, checked to see if she was okay, and tried to help her see the value of the experiential exercise. I was not successful. Instead, she made a complaint to a non–social work, straight white male dean about me, "asking students to tell me about their sex lives." I ended up having to formally explain/defend my teaching content and methods to him.

The Second Incident

As a queer-identified faculty member, I choose to be publicly out in my work and in my classrooms because I think it is important for me to be a role model for students and colleagues who might never have met or worked with someone who is openly queer, who may have questions about their own sexuality/identity, or who may have experienced oppression and discrimination because of their sexual identity, behaviour, or desires. This time, at another institution, as equity chair of a faculty association, I organized a massive campaign to #QueerTheCampus. I worked very closely with students, staff, and faculty to build and implement strategies to warm up campus climates, increase inclusion, and foster equity. As part of this campaign, the owner of a sex shop offered to do a free workshop on the history of sex toys. I thought it was a fascinating topic and would be very popular with students. We immediately included it in our event schedule. As part of public relations and getting the word out about this campaign, and as an example of effective social action, I had discussed the campaign in all of my social work classrooms. Several students had even volunteered to work on the campaign. Unfortunately, at the end of the term, I received notice from my dean (again, another non–social work, straight white male) about a complaint from a student that had to be investigated. Her major complaint was that I had "spoken inappropriately about sex in the classroom." When the dean had asked her for an example, she had brought up the example of the sex-toy workshop. Again, I had to defend myself and provide a rationale for talking about sex in my classroom.

Reflection on Teaching Sex: A Risky Business

In terms of my areas of expertise (i.e., social work education, anti-oppressive practice, queer theory, feminism, and activism), I think that what I tried to teach in the two examples above was congruent with my social work Code of Ethics (CASW, 2005) and absolutely legitimate as subjects for critical analysis and discussion. However, although the majority of students appreciated the content, I still ended up formally defending myself to deans because two students (out of hundreds of students) did not like my teaching choices. Looking back now, I realize that the students' complaints were never about the specific sexual content or my methods, but were instead more about the fact that *I* dared say these things out loud, as a female and a queer-identified person. Indeed, just by existing, surviving traditional institutions such as academia, and daring to be open about our identities and realities, we (the marginalized) disrupt traditional classroom spaces and teaching methods.

Knowing this, it is especially frustrating that both deans, who had several options for how they could handle these complaints, including supporting my academic freedom and dismissing these spurious allegations, still chose the punitive investigative route. For me, these unsupportive institutional responses and processes – which also felt to me like voyeurism and salaciousness – represented both lateral and vertical misogyny and homophobia, and in effect were meant to silence and shame me. Additionally, although I was completely exonerated of any wrongdoing in both cases, these meetings took a heavy emotional toll on me. Because of this backlash, I never taught the Precious Jewels exercise again and still often feel, when I am teaching, that I have to be in defence mode, forever anticipating the next unprovoked attack. As a result, similar to Sloane (2014), I find myself now approaching "the topic with reluctance even though I feel strongly that denying people [basic information about sexuality *sic*] sexual pleasure is a human rights violation" (p. 456).

Thus, the reality is that teaching sexual content is a risky endeavour, especially as we try to implement new modes of teaching, create new landscapes of inquiry, and disrupt heteronormative discourse in traditional university settings. Clearly, teaching about sex threatens dominant spaces and discourses in the academy. In response, others feel compelled to control what we say or do; therefore, those of us who teach about sex are continually at risk of receiving backlash from students, administrators, and/or colleagues. Additionally, on the one hand, disrupting norms is laudable, as it opens up possibilities for some really interesting and creative teaching/learning moments, but on the other hand, it can also be a very risky business, especially for vulnerable instructors. As mentioned previously, this means that based on social location and employment stability, some instructors will face more backlash for teaching about sex than others.

These hostile responses perpetuate the status quo and operate as moral chastity belts: enforcing social norms and regulating our sexuality (Myerson, Crawley, Anstey, Kessler, & Okopny, 2007). As a result, instructors, academics, and researchers are, in many ways, disembodied, metaphorically neutered, and therefore forced, in our writing, teaching, and scholarship, to act as if "we don't fuck" (Rowntree, 2014, p. 2). Most especially, there exists a covert rule and understanding to, at minimum, never let our students know that we do indeed fuck. In other words, similar to the American military and its treatment of same-sex desires and relationships (Burrelli, 2010), as well as much of North American culture (Tepper, 2000), when it comes to instructors, there exists an academic culture of "don't ask/don't tell." And I would argue that there also exists an even greater burden on female, queer, differently abled, and racialized instructors, as well as stricter dictates and mores about what we are allowed to say and how we are expected to behave.

Mitigating Risk: What Can We Do?

Although the literature often speaks about students' safety, trigger warnings, and how to be aware of and minimize power imbalances in the classroom, it rarely addresses instructors' safety; especially the safety of those who are untenured, sessional, or dare to teach from diverse perspectives, social locations, and identities (Hillock, 2021b; Jeyapal & Grigg, 2021). Back to my original question: How safe are we, then, those of us who teach from the margins, to disclose our social locations and identities? And given the fact that there are very real consequences for those of us who teach to transgress, if we choose to share those parts of ourselves for a variety of reasons (e.g., role modelling, desensitization, and transparency), how do we mitigate these risks and what can we do to protect ourselves?

Walking a Fine Line

Obviously, none of us deliberately plan to make students feel badly. However, as I have just explained, we do not always have control over student responses to our teaching. As I teach difficult and controversial topics, even though I am trying to cultivate an open, trusting, and safe learning environment, it is impossible to have strong trusting relationships with every student or to know everyone's background, triggers, or trauma histories. I can not possibly know what is happening within every student's interior landscape nor can I control what other students may say, how they interact with each other in the spur of the moment, or their responses to what happens in class. So I often find myself walking a fine line between helping students expand their thinking (i.e., getting them to reflect on and expand their normal ways of thinking and being, including their biases, attitudes, and world views) and not pushing them so hard that they become so upset that their learning capacity shuts down (i.e., providing a soft place for them to fall). As a consequence, I have learned that sex education in higher education requires a delicate balancing act. One solution that has been suggested to help maintain that balance and prepare students for controversial content is trigger warnings (Ceci, Lilienfeld, & Williams, 2018; Nietzel, 2019).

Trigger Warnings

Currently, universities seem to be grappling with the following question: "Should they prioritize defending free speech or helping students feel emotionally safe" (Ceci, Lilienfeld, & Williams, 2018, para. 1)? From my point of view, in this era of corporatization and a "bums in seats and retention at all costs" mentality (Jamdar, 2018), they tend to land heavily on the side of avoiding upsetting students, no matter what the cost. So, these days on campus, there is a great deal of discussion about, and training opportunities on, trigger warnings. Unfortunately, workshops that I have attended have been mainly geared to other disciplines and focused solely on managing singular unique topics or exceptional moments that might come up. Recommendations have included putting trigger warnings on PowerPoint slides and giving students a week's notice before teaching any difficult or controversial subjects. In contrast, faculty in professional programs and the helping professions have to continually deal – on an almost a daily basis – with teaching painful topics and managing anxious students, while also helping them develop critical self-awareness and reflection skills and ensuring they have the competencies to be safe and effective future practitioners. As well, in concurrence with Ceci, Lilienfeld, and Williams (2018), I am also concerned "that warnings may be counterproductive because they may inadvertently encourage avoidance behavior, which can fuel pre-existing anxiety" (para. 13).

Although the research is mixed on their effectiveness (Nietzel, 2019), I do give a broad trigger warning at the beginning of each semester (Ceci, Lilienfeld, & Williams, 2018) and explain that because of the nature of social work practice, almost everything they hear and everything we do in the social work classroom may be triggering to some students. Accordingly, I speak to them about being aware of their own triggers, seeking counselling help if they require it, and how these might impact their future social work practice with vulnerable service users. In their careers, social workers regularly face people, conditions, opinions, situations, and topics that are uncomfortable, if not downright horrific (e.g., child abuse and sexual assault). Trigger warnings will not change this reality. Unlike the student examples mentioned earlier, if certain difficult topics come up in practice, they will not be permitted to refuse certain work tasks or abandon counselling sessions without facing serious consequences. As Ceci, Lilienfeld, and Williams (2018) explain,

> Warnings do not prepare students for this reality outside the classroom where warnings are not given to brace oneself; instead, warnings may inadvertently make it more challenging for students to cope with this reality by shielding them from anxiety-provoking information. Compared with media representations, the classroom lecture would seem to offer an opportunity to learn coping skills that will prove useful in confronting the inevitable stressors of life. (para. 10)

Setting the Stage and Assessing Each Cohort

In terms of setting the stage, I agree that we need to take preliminary steps in terms of explaining to students – in very clear language, with lots of advance warning (a week may not be enough) – the content of upcoming lectures/discussions and include this information in our course outlines and introductions, especially related to so-called controversial subjects (I am not sure how to deal here with the relentless issue of students choosing not to read course outlines or any written materials). This process is dynamic; thus, it needs to be revisited regularly over the semester. In addition, across the course, we need to think carefully about our own safety, be mindful of why and what we are disclosing (Barker & Reavey, 2009; Satterly & Dyson, 1998), and determine whether or not our self-disclosure is worth the backlash we may encounter (and sometimes, to be honest, it is not).

Although challenging, I think we also have to carefully weigh the maturity of each of the cohorts we teach. This may mean restructuring some of the curriculum and course content, as well as the timing of certain subjects. By weighing the maturity and readiness of the group, in addition to the level of trust in the group, we might more effectively anticipate strong reactions to certain materials. Of course, one cannot predict each semester which student may be upset about what particular discussion or topic, so the setting up and weighing processes are obviously difficult and "fraught with guesswork" (Ceci, Lilienfeld, & Williams, 2018, para. 9). Moreover, there is little evidence-informed research on best practices in this area so further research is needed. Accordingly, we need to explore the best ways to support students through difficult content. One suggestion, borrowed from medicine, is that we adopt the PLISSIT model to assess the readiness of students to receive sexual content (Gil & Hough, 2007; Montgomery, Marshall, Sanders, Phillips, Cline, & Snowden, 2018). For more on recommended models, please see Chapter 18.

Building Alliances

Building alliances is one way to manage the previously mentioned balancing act, mitigate risk, and decrease isolation, as we can often feel as if we are the only ones teaching about sex (Johnson, 2009). We need to recruit our colleagues and administrators to support us in our efforts to teach from the margins, to utilize alternative teaching methods, and to teach difficult subjects such as knowledge/content about sexuality(ies). How can we align our colleagues with us? Within our different faculties, disciplines, and committees, we need to advocate for the inclusion of sex education and examine where and how sexuality is already being taught, and where it should be introduced across the curriculum. Faculty should also discuss whether sex education content should be taught in specific required courses; situated solely as part of elective offerings; infused across all courses; or held in stand-alone sexuality, sexual health, and sexual wellness courses. In addition, we need to explore what methods and topics are best suited for undergraduate versus graduate education.

In terms of social work, we need to determine what sex education knowledge, attitudinal shifts, and skill development are necessary for good social work practice. For example, how do we make sexuality an integral part of our bio-psycho-social assessments and what is the best way to do a sexuality assessment? How can we best teach students to complete a thorough sexual history? For more on this, please see Chapter 18 and Appendix C. We also need to explore where our professional boundaries start and stop, when and to whom do we refer, and what the differences are between generalist practice and sex therapy.

Provincial and National Organizing

More broadly, we need to organize provincially and nationally to promote more avenues for research and publication. We need to push our national and provincial congresses and conferences to include sexuality(ies) as a regular topic and to feature sexuality as a main theme of some conferences. We need to develop national and international sexuality-educator websites, linkages, and listservs so that like-minded educators and groups can communicate and support each other. Additionally, we can take on leadership roles in our institutions by becoming mentors and experts on teaching about sex in our departments, universities, and local communities. We can advocate for ourselves and provide information about sex education teaching to our administrators so that they can better support us and more fully understand the context of some student complaints. We can network with our colleagues and ensure that tenure, promotion, and merit committees understand and value the importance and contributions of sexuality research and education. We can also develop interdisciplinary faculty working groups who want to teach about and research sexuality. For example, we could work together to develop an interdisciplinary curriculum to infuse into different programs, create sexuality specializations at bachelor, master, or doctoral levels, and provide continuing sex education courses and summer institutes for local professionals.

Conclusion

In this chapter, I discussed sex education as a controversial subject and shared two different examples of student backlash, related to teaching sexuality(ies). I discussed the importance of being transparent in terms of our sexuality(ies) and sexual identity(ies). I also examined issues related to instructor disclosure, instructor safety in the classroom, and trigger warnings, and analysed the risks that sex education instructors take, knowing that we tread where no one else may be willing to go. I discussed how we have to maintain a delicate balance between encouraging students to expand their understanding and knowledge while avoiding ratcheting up the anxiety too high for them to learn. I have also explored how building alliances can help manage that balance and mitigate the associated risks. Finally, silence on these topics is not serving our students or society and is certainly not helping to promote effective and ethical social work practice. Sex is and will remain an important human subject. How we teach it, develop best practices, and support each other is up to us.

REFERENCES

Abramowitz, N. R. (1971). Human sexuality in the social work classroom. *The Family Coordinator, 20*(4), 349–354. https://doi.org/10.2307/582165

Ashenberg Straussner, S. L., Senreich, E., & Steen. J. T. (2018). Wounded healers: A multistate study of licensed social workers' behavioral health problems. *Social Work, 63*(20), 125–133. https://doi.org/10.1093/sw/swy012

Barker, M., & Reavey, P. (2009). IV. Self-disclosure in teaching sexuality courses. *Feminism & Psychology, 19*(2), 194–198. https://doi.org/10.1177/0959353509102197

Burrelli, D. F. (2010). "Don't ask, don't tell": The law and military policy on same-sex behaviour. *Congressional Research Service: CRS Report for Congress.* 1–22. https://fas.org/sgp/crs/misc/R40782.pdf

Canadian Association of Social Work (CASW). (2005). *Code of Ethics.* https://www.casw-acts.ca/en/what-social-work/casw-code-ethics/code-ethics

Ceci, S. J., Lilienfeld, S.O., & Williams, W. M. (2018). The one-time-only trigger warning. *Modernizing the Workforce Webcast: Inside Higher Ed.* https://www.insidehighered.com/views/2018/10/18/way-handle-trigger-warnings-develop-one-time-only-one-opinion

Collins, P. H. (1991). *Black feminist thought.* New York: Routledge.

Collins, P. H. (2000). *Black feminist thought: Knowledge, consciousness, and the politics of empowerment* (2nd ed.). New York: Routledge.

Dodd, S. J., & Tolman, D. (2017). Receiving a positive discourse on sexuality within social work. *National Association of Social Workers,* 227–234. https://doi.org/10.1093/sw/swx016

Fahs, B., Plante, R. F., & McClelland, S. I. (2018). Working at the crossroads of pleasure and danger: Feminist perspectives on doing critical sexuality studies. *Sexualities, 21*(4), 503–519. https://doi.org/10.1177/1363460717713743

Gil, K. M., & Hough, S. (2007). Sexuality training, education and therapy in the healthcare environment: Taboo, avoidance, discomfort or ignorance? *Sex and Disability, 25,* 73–76. https://doi.org/10.1007/s11195-007-9033-0

Hanisch, C. (2009). The personal is political: The women's liberation movement classic with a new explanatory chapter. Retrieved from: http://www.carolhanisch.org/CHwritings/PIP.html

Hicks, S. (2008). Thinking through sexuality. *Journal of Social Work, 8*(1), 65–82. https://doi.org/10.1177/1468017307084740

Hillock, S. (2011). *Conceptualizing oppression: Resistance narratives for social work.* Doctoral thesis. St. John's: Memorial University of Newfoundland.

Hillock, S. (2021a). Femagogy: Centring feminist knowledge and methods in social work teaching. In R. Csiernik & S. Hillock (Eds.), *Teaching social work: Reflections on pedagogy and practice.* Toronto: University of Toronto Press.

Hillock, S. (2021b). Teaching from the margins: No good deed goes unpunished. In R. Csiernik & S. Hillock (Eds.), *Teaching social work: Reflections on pedagogy and practice*. Toronto: University of Toronto Press.

Hillock, S., & Mulé, N. J. (Eds.). (2016). *Queering social work education*. Vancouver: UBC Press.

hooks, b. (1994). *Teaching to transgress: Education as a practice of freedom*. New York: Routledge.

Jamdar, S. (2018). Universities want "bums on seats" because you created a market, minister. *The Guardian*. https://www.theguardian.com/profile /smita-jamdar

Jeyapal, D., & Grigg, L. (2021). The crying white woman and the politics of emotion in anti-oppressive social work education. In R. Csiernik & S. Hillock (Eds.), *Teaching social work: Reflections on pedagogy and practice*. Toronto: University of Toronto Press.

Jeyasingham, D. (2008). Knowledge/ignorance and the construction of sexuality in social work education. *Social Work Education, 27*(2), 138–151. https://doi.org/10.1080/02615470701709469

Johnson, S. (2009). II. Between a rock and a hard place. *Feminism & Psychology, 19*(2), 186–189. https://doi.org/10.1177/0959353509102195

Keating, F. (2000). Anti-racist perspectives: What are the gains for social work? *Social Work Education, 19*(1), 77–87. https://doi.org/10.1080/026154700114676

Levine, H. (1982). The personal is political: Feminism and the helping professions. In G. Finn and A. Miles (Eds.), *Feminism in Canada: From pressure to politics* (175–209). Toronto: Black Rose Books.

Montgomery, B. E. E., Marshall, S. A., Sanders, S. E., Phillips, M. M., Cline, M., & Snowden, M. (2018). Stakeholder identification of barriers and facilitators to sexual health education for female survivors of violence: A mixed methods study. *American Journal of Sexuality Education, 13*(10), 18–39. https://doi.org /10.1080/15546128.2017.1410870

Myerson, M., Crawley, S. L., Anstey, E. H., Kessler, J., & Okopny, C. (2007). Who's zoomin who? A feminist, queer content analysis of "interdisciplinary" human sexuality textbooks. *Hypatia, 22*(1), 92–113. https://doi.org/10.1353 /hyp.2006.0071

Nietzel, M. T. (2019). Colleges, don't be so quick on the trigger warnings. They may misfire. *Forbes Magazine*. https://www.forbes.com/sites/michaeltnietzel /2019/03/22/colleges-dont-be-so-quick-on-the-trigger-warnings-they-may-misfire /#7ddd8c995653

Oswalt, S. B., Wagner, L.M., Eastmann-Mueller, H. P., & Nevers, M. (2014). Pedagogy and content in sexuality education course in US colleges and universities. *Sex Education, 15*(2), 172–187. https://doi.org/10.1080 /14681811.2014.991958

Rowntree, M. R. (2014). Making sexuality visible in Australian social work education. *Social Work Education: The International Journal, 33*(3), 1–21. https://doi.org/10.1080/02615479.2013.834885

Satterly, B. A., & Dyson, D.A. (1998). The use of self-disclosure as an educational intervention in the graduate social work human sexuality classroom. *Journal of Sex Education and Therapy, 23*(1), 55–61. https://doi.org/10.1080/01614576.1998.11074207

Sloane, H. M. (2014). Tales of a reluctant sex radical: Barriers to teaching the importance of pleasure for well-being. *Sex and Disability, 32*, 453–467. https://doi.org/10.1007/s11195-014-9381-5

Stayton, W. (1998). A curriculum for training professional in human sexuality using the sexual attitude restructuring (SAR) model. *Journal of Sex Education and Therapy, 23*(1), 26–32. https://doi.org/10.1080/01614576.1998.11074203

Tepper, M. (2000). Sexuality and disability: The missing discourse of pleasure. *Sexuality and Disability, 18*(4), 283–290. https://doi.org/10.1023/a:1005698311392

Williams, D. J., Prior, E., & Wegner, J. (2013). Resolving social problems associated with sexuality: Can a "sex-positive" approach help? *Social Work.* https://doi.org/10.1093/sw/swt024

Wineberg, H. R. (2015). Social work and human sexuality: An examination of the country's top 25-CWSE ranked MSW curricula. *Theses, Dissertations, and Projects.* 663. 1–43. http://scholarworks.smith.edu/theses/663

2 Restoring Indigenous Sexuality

CARRIE BOURASSA, BETTY MCKENNA, MIRANDA KEEWATIN,
SADIE ANDERSON, MARLIN LEGARE, MIKAYLA HAGEL,
DANETTE STARBLANKET, JENNIFER LANGAN,
AND CARI MCILDUFF

To start, discussions of Indigenous Peoples, their gender status, and understandings related to sexuality(ies) must first acknowledge that the binary of male/female is a colonial construct that was forced on Indigenous Peoples at the time of contact and colonization. This colonial construct continues to exist today in many forms. Prior to contact, Indigenous Peoples in North America recognized many genders and sexualities, with a large part of the population having terms or words for those who were neither male nor female (Hunt, 2016). In some nations such as the Ojibwe (Saulteaux), traditional storytelling reflects this reality and further does not differentiate between male and female, as the pronouns s/he are loosely used. Discussing sexuality then becomes many faceted, as lacking a strong duality or binarism allows Indigenous Peoples to be more community minded and holistic in all their approaches. Thus, as part of holistic health, Indigenous Peoples consider sexuality as an important aspect of maintaining wellness (Bourassa, Bendig, Ozog, & Oleson, 2016).

Historically, colonization diminished and limited Indigenous Ways of Knowing, including teachings related to sexuality(ies) and gender. However, more recently, Eurocentric beliefs regarding sexuality are being systematically deconstructed in an attempt to reclaim Indigenous Knowledges and empower decolonization in relation to sexual health. To accomplish this, Knowledge Keepers have started to (re)introduce the Traditional teachings related to gender and sexual representation. The absence of the male/female binary roles in Indigenous societies can help to bring back those Traditional teachings. However, there still remains a lot of work to be done in this area. In terms of teaching sex in higher education, this chapter presents key teachings, explains progressive Indigenous understandings of gender status and sexual identity(ies), examines contemporary issues of which all educators should be aware when teaching about sexuality(ies), and recommends culturally relevant approaches.

Indigenous Peoples' Teachings

Indigenous Peoples' teachings, including that of the "Medicine Wheel," utilize a circle to represent all peoples and the interconnectedness of life (Stark, 2013). Women who are capable of giving and nurturing life are traditionally located at the centre of this wheel. Our Elders' knowledge regarding the importance of going back to our teachings is extremely relevant:

> We are like trees. Our roots are put down very deep. And we take things from the four directions and we take them into our lives. And if you pull us up by the roots, we are lost. We have to go back and find those roots, find those beginnings that are strong so that we can live a good life. (McKenna, as cited in Bourassa, 2010, pp. 75–76)

Many Elders and Knowledge Keepers are reconnecting with the Traditional teachings, including those about gender status and sexuality(ies), to share them with the people.

Indigenous Peoples also widely use the term Two-spirit, which encompasses many aspects of gender status and sexual identity (Thomas, 1997). This term replaces the previously used term "Berdache"; a term placed on Two-spirit people by the Spaniards in early contact, which was later adopted by academics who were not a part of the community. The term Two-spirit was coined in the 1990s in Canada and spread throughout Indigenous communities and has been much more widely accepted and recognized (Slater & Yarbrough, 2011). Renaming and reclaiming terms for Indigenous genders and sexualities were integral steps in regaining Indigenous autonomy, while showcasing our resiliency. Decolonizing how gender and sexuality within Indigenous communities are viewed is critical to reverting to the Traditional teachings that exist within the Nations. Therefore, in terms of education, the focus has now returned to the Traditional Knowledges, as passed down through Knowledge Keepers and Elders.

While colonization sought to create the gender/sex binary of male/female for Indigenous Peoples, and succeeded to a certain extent, the teachings of Knowledge Keepers and Elders inform Indigenous youth today about the absence of this binary in Traditional roles. In fact, Traditional views on Indigenous gender and sexuality(ies) were far more progressive in comparison to their Western counterparts. In most Indigenous societies, a minimum of 4 genders existed, and in some societies, there were 8 genders, while others had up to 16 genders. Indigenous gender status was fluid, giving individuals the freedom to cross between genders within their lifetime (ibid.). Two-spirit individuals were highly regarded as having significant connections to spirit and the spirit world and, in some societies, were considered integral in times of war. While different people had different roles to play within the community, the community itself was not set up along a gendered or sexual divide as colonial practices were; it was understood that people could be born many times and throughout their multiple lives, be both male and female, and carry this spiritual knowledge with them (Slater, 2011).

Indeed, kinship ties and clan memberships were more important than gender or sex, and there was no dichotomy of gendered power until contact. Europeans impacted those systems by introducing Western gender norms as part of Canadian policy and practice (Acoose-Miswonige-esikokwe, 2016). These norms were followed by stereotypes related to Indigenous female sexuality (e.g., "Indian princess" or "savage squaw"). The gendered bias that exists, when depicting Indigenous gender and sexuality, is still prevalent in literature today, as most of what was written in history about Indigenous Peoples was written by European males and inevitably conveyed racial and gendered bias. This bias is illustrated in the way in which colonizers engaged with Indigenous Peoples; for example, having groups elect male chiefs with whom the colonial powers had to deal, rather than the Traditional matriarchs. Various forms of colonial assimilation and, later, government legislation ensured the adoption of gender differentiation among Indigenous Peoples. The Indian Act solidified a sexual and gender divide for Indigenous Peoples in Canada, setting out rules to govern men and women differently, while not acknowledging any other sex/gender (Stark, 2013).

Furthermore, the Indian Act continues to enfranchise certain cohorts of First Nations Peoples over others. For instance, if a status Indian male were to marry a non-status female, children have treaty rights; whereas if a status Indian female were to marry a non-status male, she and her children lose all entitlement to treaty rights. Even after Bill C-31 was introduced in 1985, status Indian women continue to be unable to pass down status to their children. This is also true in the cases in which status Indian women register their children without identifying the father of the child, and then the Department of Indian Affairs assumes the father is thereby not a status Indian male. This is not ancient Canadian history, as it continues today, in more subtle forms (e.g., public health services have limitations on how many times Indigenous Peoples access certain services and programs). Through the Indian Act, the Residential

School system further emphasized gender differentiation with the separation of boys and girls outside the classroom. With colonization and through legislation, the gender binary of male/female was introduced and gradually adopted by Indigenous Peoples. The ways in which Indigenous Peoples viewed gender and sexuality were changed for generations to follow. Today, Two-spirit individuals, Elders, and Knowledge Keepers are helping to restore some of our understanding and teachings about sexuality(ies) and building acceptance of all genders' and their uniqueness. However, the impacts of the Western value and belief system, which severely interrupted Indigenous gender and sexuality, have led to numerous contemporary issues.

Contemporary Issues

The historical trauma of colonization and the resulting racism is one of the causes of health disparities among Indigenous populations, but cultures, Knowledges, and traditions remain at the heart of their resiliency. Moreover, Indigenous Peoples in Canada frequently have to overcome barriers in terms of accessing healthcare services and information (Bourassa, 2011). Some challenges that Indigenous communities face are the recruitment and retention of healthcare resources and clinicians, limited access to healthcare information, and physical barriers to accessing healthcare centres, such as geographical location. These are all barriers that remote communities face but are most often experienced by the most remote and Northern locations, such as in the boreal forest or the Canadian territories.

Negative Sexual Health Outcomes

Barriers to healthcare exacerbate negative sexual health outcomes for Indigenous Peoples. Negative sexual health outcomes for any population may include unplanned pregnancies and the spread of sexually transmitted infections (Ivankovich et al., 2013). In order to avoid these outcomes, populations need to have adequate access to sexual health information and preventive measures, including contraceptives and sexual education, while retaining individual reproductive rights. This particularly applies to Indigenous populations in Canada and the need to reduce human immunodeficiency virus (HIV) infection and transmission. While First Nations, Inuit, and Métis Peoples represent only 4.9% of the Canadian population, it was estimated in 2016 that this group accounted for 11.3% of new HIV infections (Public Health Agency of Canada, 2018). These statistics emphasize the imperative need for Indigenous Peoples to have culturally safe access to sexual health information and preventive measures. According to Bourassa, McElhaney, and Oleson (2016),

> cultural safety analyzes power imbalances (throughout society and throughout healthcare practice); addresses institutional discrimination, colonization, and relationships with colonizers, as they apply to health care; requires an examination of how personal biases, authority, privilege and territorial history can influence the relationships between health care providers and Indigenous [P]eople[s]; and relies on both self-reflection and critical reflection. (p. 1)

An excellent example of culturally safe programming is the All Nations Hope Network (ANHN), located in Regina, Saskatchewan, where individuals are able to access services within their community and through a network that serves their specific needs. Indigenous organizations such as ANHN also continue to work on strengthening different cultural healthcare models by Indigenizing them within communities, so that Elders and Knowledge Keepers are better informed to support community members (e.g., Indigenous perspectives on concerns such as COVID-19 and culturally safe health-support programs).

Social Policy and Legislation Inequalities

Existing government policies, legislation, and agreements that delegate responsibility between federal, provincial, municipal, and Indigenous governments continue to create inequality for parts of the country. For instance, the First Nations Inuit Health Branch (FNIHB) administers several programs for community, but it does not have the benefits to cover expenses that are not covered by provincial healthcare plans, creating barriers to equitable access to healthcare and services for Indigenous Peoples within Indigenous communities (National Collaborating Centre for Aboriginal Health, 2013). This exemplifies how governmental policies have created barriers for Indigenous Peoples living with chronic illness such as HIV and AIDS. Because of these reasons, individuals have to leave their communities to access healthcare resources in urban settings.

Lack of Access to Healthcare

As the effects of European colonialism are ongoing, it is important to acknowledge contemporary issues that act as barriers that Indigenous Peoples consistently have to overcome to seek information or care regarding their health and, more specifically, their sexual health. Although there are barriers to achieving better health outcomes for Indigenous Peoples in Canada, protective factors such as cultures, languages, and traditions aid in their continued resilience, despite adversity. One of the most impactful barriers in achieving holistic health is access to health-care as a social determinant of health (Horrill, McMillan, Schultz, & Thompson, 2018). Physical access to healthcare may be affected by deficits in the Canadian healthcare system, such as the availability and retention of healthcare providers on reserves, long wait lists, geographi-cal barriers or distance, and limited availability to pertinent screening and preventive measures (National Collaborating Centre for Aboriginal Health, 2013). The cost of transportation, especially for those living in remote areas, can become cumbersome and impede a person's access to necessary healthcare. Other reported barriers that Indigenous Peoples identify in regard to accessing healthcare are negative experiences such as racism or negligence when interacting with healthcare professionals, long wait lists, limited screening services, and the cost of transportation for those living in rural and remote areas (Horrill, McMillan, Schultz, & Thompson, 2018). However, within these obvious obstacles, the fact remains that it is the invisible barriers, as described below, that have most impeded access.

Racism, Discrimination, and Lack of Cultural Safety

While geographical or physical access to healthcare is often thought of in terms of equitable access, Indigenous Peoples face much more than just geographical or physical barriers to access; they also face racism, oppression, discrimination, stigma, sexism, and bias (Bourassa, 2018). Particularly, racism has been identified as a major factor in creating and reinforcing all these disparities (Allan & Smylie 2015; Lavallee et al. 2014), especially since much of the racism is systemic in nature. Partici-pants from a recent study of 80 Indigenous women across Canada noted that the combination of racism and sexism produces unsafe access to services (Bourassa et al., 2015). One participant in this study expressed, "Get rid of the stereotypes and treat people with dignity and respect. The healthcare practitioners need to listen and hear what people are saying to them. They need to be respectful of other ways of being and doing things" (cited in Bourassa et al., 2015, p. 11). This particular statement demonstrates the way many Indigenous Peoples feel when accessing healthcare. Thus, the need for respect and dignity is even more impera-tive within the field of sexual health.

Another barrier related to inequality of healthcare is the lack of cul-turally appropriate healthcare for Indigenous Peoples. Fortunately, this barrier is being dismantled by the implementation of innovative Indigenous healthcare models. As mentioned earlier, one of the models that have found international success in healthcare systems is the concept of cultural safety, as developed by Māori nurses in New Zealand. This concept was developed specifically to assist healthcare practitioners in the creation of more culturally relevant and inclusive environments for Indigenous Peoples. While this concept was originally developed for Polynesian and Māori Peoples in 1989, the practice has since been adopted by many countries, including Canada, and attempts have been made to integrate it into their healthcare systems (Papps & Ramsden, 1996).

Gendered and Racialized Violence

The universal phenomenon of violence against women is widely known, and certain races of women are at greater risk for victimization (Bourassa et al., 2017; Kubik, Bourassa, & Hampton, 2009; Perreault, 2015). Gendered and racialized violence have their roots in many of the contemporary issues facing Indigenous Peoples today, particularly the issues facing Indigenous women (Bourassa et al., 2017; Kubik, Bourassa, & Hampton, 2009). The Missing and Murdered Indigenous Women and Girls (MMIWG) crisis in Canada and the United States demonstrates that there are indeed threats faced by Indigenous women based on race. Indigenous women are devalued in contemporary society, and this has resulted in violence against them, to the degree that national inquiries are held to search for solutions (National Inquiry into Missing and Murdered Indigenous Women and Girls, 2019). Influences from Christianity and Western patriarchal societies also contribute to the cases of violence against Indigenous women (Acoose-Miswonigeesikokwe, 2016). These tragedies take place inside and outside Indigenous communities, and often the media portrays the cases in a negative light, as a means of victim blaming and shaming. For instance, the way the cases of Pamela George and so many more women have been (mis)represented is typical (ibid.).

Furthermore, governmental jurisdictions, at all levels, have not responded with a coordinated approach to examine the root cause(s) of this ongoing issue. Part of the solution is to understand the past and its contemporary effects. It is relevant to consider the fact that Indigenous women have been hypersexualized throughout history (e.g., women considered as either pochohontas, princesses, or squaws; affiliation of MMIW with sex workers or drug addicts; victim blaming, etc.). This continues to follow them into contemporary society (Acoose-Miswonigeesikokwe, 2016; Bourassa et al., 2017; Kubik, Bourassa, & Hampton, 2009). Drawing on the need for culturally relevant solutions to address the crisis we face today in regards to the hypersexualization of Indigenous women and victim blaming of Missing and Murdered Indigenous Women and Girls, it is clear that colonization and its lasting effects still impact current Indigenous gender and sexuality(ies). Bourassa et al. (2017) note, "The tragically high rates of violent victimization of Indigenous women demand that discussions of this issue occur within the context of the systemic and intergenerational roots of the epidemic of violence in all its forms" (p. 48).

Colonial violence intersects with gender inequity for Indigenous women in a way that creates unique risk factors for this population. The rate of violent victimization experienced by Indigenous women is more than three times higher than the rate for their non-Indigenous counterparts (Perreault, 2015). Bourassa et al. (2017) explain why attention to the history of colonial violence is needed: "We focus on Indigenous women because despite being incredibly resilient and being the life-givers in our communities – the ones who were traditionally considered the sacred and honoured mothers, grandmothers, daughters, aunties, and sisters in our communities – we are instead often seen as the most vulnerable, marginalized, and at-risk population in Canada" (pp. 47–48). The statistics are alarming throughout Canada and are especially high in certain provinces. In Saskatchewan alone, 60% of missing women are Indigenous, though they make up only 6% of the province's population (Amnesty International, 2014). Although Indigenous women self-report violent victimization at a rate of almost three times higher than that of their non-Indigenous counterparts, more than three quarters of non-spousal violent incidents involving Indigenous women are not reported to any formal support service (Perreault, 2015). Instead, most Indigenous women choose to confide in informal sources, within their own support networks. With only a glimpse of the overwhelming data demonstrating that Indigenous women are vastly overrepresented when it comes to violent victimization (both sexual and physical in nature), the necessity for culturally appropriate and safe sexual health becomes even more imperative. Sadly, Indigenous activists and feminists have highlighted these issues for a long time but were ignored. It is only in recent years that these issues have become more mainstream, through media and political communication. While this is a significant step, it is essential to ensure that this coverage continues and does not treat this issue as a "one-off" (Bourassa et al., 2017).

Systemic and Intergenerational Roots

The exceedingly high rates of violent victimization of Indigenous women demand that discussions of this issue occur within the context of systemic and intergenerational roots. The roots of oppressions facing Indigenous women can be traced back to colonialism and assimilation and the related representations of Indigenous women (Bourassa et al., 2017; Kubik, Bourassa, & Hampton, 2009). Traditionally, Indigenous women were granted great authority and respect and were highly honoured as the givers of life. When the patriarchal models of governance were imposed on Indigenous communities, these same women were sexualized and demoralized, reduced to bodies to be categorized; a physical beauty to behold ("Indian princess"), worthless ("savage squaw"), abused, or disregarded. This demoralization and sexualization of Indigenous women continues today, as we are still often treated as second-class citizens.

The experience of living in societies that do not value our lives is obscured by ongoing discriminatory narratives, such as those in the media that perpetuate colonial categorizations (Razack, 2002). Even the Royal Canadian Mounted Police's report on MMIW (2014) continues this discrimination in their listing of the risk factors for Indigenous women (e.g., employment status, use of intoxicants, and involvement in the sex trade) while failing to report on the historical colonial context behind their findings. Without this acknowledgment of context, the report does great injustice to MMIW and takes attention away from the societal norms that provide perpetrators with the justification that these women are "lesser than." Indigenous women continue to be seen as second-class, passive citizens whose power in Canadian society is insubstantial (Kubik, Bourassa, & Hampton, 2009). This reality speaks to the great need for sexual health to be culturally appropriate and safe, to support these women to move beyond these stereotypes with education and knowledge in this area that empowers them.

How Sexuality and Rates of HIV Are Understood

Increased rates of HIV in Saskatchewan have largely been driven by increased use of intravenous drugs (Vogel, 2015). Although the driving force of increased rates may be related to drug use and issues of addiction, in society today HIV connotes sex and sexuality. Implying HIV is solely attached to sexual activity is harmful to Indigenous sexuality as rates of HIV are shown to be higher within Indigenous communities (Public Health Agency of Canada, 2018). The stigma resulting from the conflation of Indigenous HIV rates with sex and sexuality creates a shameful and demeaning environment for testing (Vogel, 2015). The distress of receiving HIV testing alone can deter people from accessing necessary services as people may fear being blamed with personal irresponsibility or moral fault for an HIV diagnosis (e.g., slut shaming and/or homophobia). As rates of HIV continue to rise in Canada (Public Health Agency of Canada, 2018), an Indigenous patient-centred approach must be undertaken to remain culturally safe and relevant when providing HIV care and follow-up services. Rather than taking a top-down approach, a more upstream initiative must be taken to reduce the stigma related to testing for HIV to effectively improve the quality of life and address Indigenous social determinants affecting access to healthcare. Rural and remote Indigenous communities are especially susceptible as there are inadequate supports in place to reduce barriers. To affect positive change, Indigenous-oriented care must be determined to address said inequities.

Research findings by Tarasuk et al. (2014) agree with previous literature about findings that suggest Indigenous Peoples disproportionately represent a large number of newly diagnosed HIV cases in Saskatchewan. With only 66.7% of positive HIV cases reporting that they had at some time taken prescription drugs for their illness, this statistic provides evidence that Indigenous populations are less likely to seek essential treatment. Although this statistic is critical to understand, what is more important are the greater external forces that influence a person's access to necessary healthcare. To address Indigenous social determinants of health, further investigation is needed to determine the effectiveness and accessibility of Indigenous-centred HIV healthcare to avoid further perpetuating health disparities between Indigenous and non-Indigenous populations. Acknowledging the greater external factors that influence a person's ability to achieve sexual health could help to further inform service development, leading to culturally safe interventions that contextualize environments of risk and resilience, which, in turn, could influence behaviors in accessing healthcare (ibid.).

Restoring Health in Individuals and Communities: Key Teachings

Many traditional territories across Canada are made up of diverse Indigenous communities, with customary laws and cultural protocols that are critical for the preservation, use, development, and transmission of Indigenous Traditional Knowledges. A consideration of customary laws and cultural protocols of each unique community helps reclaim Indigenous traditional wellness and aids in the restoration of individual and community health. The utilization of Indigenous culture and Knowledge translation is essential to the development of Indigenous persons, as it is the practice and outcomes of culture and ceremonies that deliver essential messages of growth and development. These cultural practices, such as the rights of passage, coming of age, and moon lodge ceremonies, also help to sustain healthy well-being through the crucial development from childhood to adulthood. Within these teachings, the lifelong process of learning and growth is encompassed (Knight & Musqua, 2001).

It is also very important to acknowledge that there are recognized guides, wisdom, and Knowledge Keepers in Indigenous communities and that communities themselves hold the teachings that are being implemented in the wellness and restoration of individual and community health. For instance, Bear Clan teachings taught by the Musqua Family, explain that the development and growth of an individual are guided by the Bear clan practices throughout the relationships one builds with one's teachers (ibid.). Within these relationships are told stories of the lessons and key concepts necessary for the healthy development of individuals. Additionally, one should consider the teachings of Indigenous Traditional Knowledges and history as they deliver information and perspectives on existence, medicines, songs, stories, and respect for the interconnectedness to all beings (ibid.). Moreover, Indigenous Traditional Knowledges are transferred through individuals, families, or groups of people throughout the community. Indigenous Traditional Knowledges from different Indigenous nations are practiced for the use or benefit of the community and might be exchanged and developed between communities and migrated from community to community by marriage, trade, and warfare between nations or tribes. It is this history that develops the teachings throughout our oral history, in which remains the connection to our Traditional teachings. These vital pieces/processes of information sharing and storytelling are important and considered "teachable moments" about history, nations, communities, and oneself.

Furthermore, the protection of Traditional Knowledges for Indigenous Peoples and the importance of practice within the communities are necessary for the well-being and development of all Indigenous Peoples and families as systems. Many Indigenous organizations implement and practice these methods, through programming and research projects, to restore the natural laws of life through cultural intervention practices (Anderson, 2011; Knight & Musqua, 2001). These organizations and research projects have identified that Indigenous Traditional Knowledges are a key concept to restoring the relationship between Indigenous Peoples, cultural practices, and gender responsibility. The Tribal Councils in Saskatchewan have also begun to undertake some of this work.

Positive Sexuality and Sexual Health

Restoring Indigenous Peoples' sexual health through culture, language, and resilience also promotes positive, self-determined understandings of sexuality and sexual health (Bourassa, McKenna, & Juschka, 2017). In many Indigenous communities, the body, including sex and sexuality, was considered a natural, sacred, positive construction for both men and women (Anderson, 2000). Indigenous women, including mothers, aunties, and grandmothers, all played a vital role in the development of a child's understanding of sexuality and reproduction (Anderson, 2011; Bourassa, McKenna, & Juschka, 2017; Wilson, 2004). Many Indigenous communities also had an understanding of women's menstruation as a powerful, sacred time (Anderson, 2000; Bourassa, McKenna, & Juschka, 2017). Women's sexual authority included the fact that they exhibited control over their own reproductive cycles and sexuality (Acoose-Miswonigeesikokwe, 2016; Anderson, 2000). Anderson (2000) concludes, "Aboriginal women must work with our girls to create an understanding that there is a place for sex, a place for intimacy and a place or love in their lives and that they have choices to make about how it all takes place" (p. 200). Indigenous Traditional Knowledges and cultural practices can contribute to the self-determination of Indigenous sexuality by reclaiming sacred teachings and having ownership of sexuality and sexual health.

Conclusion

Indigenous sexuality is returning to its Traditional understandings. Eurocentric beliefs regarding sexuality are being deconstructed in an attempt to reclaim Indigenous Knowledges and empower decolonization in relation to sexual health. Colonization diminished and limited Indigenous Ways of Knowing, including teachings surrounding sexuality and gender. As health is considered holistic, sexuality is an important aspect of maintaining wellness (Bourassa, Bendig, Ozog, & Oleson, 2016). In order to affect positive change, upstream solutions such as culturally relevant patient-centred care must be considered to fully address the social determinants of health affecting Indigenous health (Bourassa, McKay-McNabb, & Hampton, 2004).

In the midst of facing adversity, as a result of inequitable access to healthcare and ongoing colonization, Indigenous cultures remain resilient with many protective factors such as Traditional Knowledges, cultures, and ceremonies. These factors can contribute to Indigenous autonomy and showcase the diversity and fluidity of Indigenous identities, especially in regard to gender and sexuality. Traditional Indigenous worldviews on sexuality clash with and challenge Western gender norms, as Indigenous worldviews on sexuality are nonbinary and much more dynamic in regard to Two-spirit Peoples. By connecting to Traditional cultural teachings, Indigenous Peoples continue to restore sexuality and sexual health (Kubik, Bourassa, & Hampton, 2009). Indigenous Peoples are strong and resilient and therefore are able to meaningfully contribute to the innovation and development of autonomous practices and understandings of health and well-being, and in particular, sexuality and sexual health.

REFERENCES

Acoose-Miswonigeesikokwe, J. (2016). *Iskeweak Kah'ki yaw ni Wahkomakanak: Neither Indian princesses nor easy squaws.* 2nd Ed. Vancouver, BC: Canadian Scholars Press.

Allan, B., & Smylie, J. (2015). *First peoples, second class treatment: The role of racism in the health and well-being of Indigenous peoples in Canada.* Discussion Paper: Wellesley Institute. Canadian Electronic Library & Wellesley Institute.

Amnesty International. (2014). *Violence against Indigenous women and girls in Canada: A summary of Amnesty International's concerns and call to action.* Retrieved from https://www.amnesty.ca/sites/amnesty/files/iwfa_submission_amnesty _international_february_2014_-_final.pdf

Anderson, K. (2000). *A recognition of being: Reconstructing Native womanhood.* Toronto, ON: Second Story Press.

Anderson, K. (2011). *Life stages and Native women: Memory, teachings, and story medicine.* Winnipeg, MB: University of Manitoba Press.

Bourassa, C. (2010). The construction of Aboriginal identity: A healing journey. In B. Anderson, W. Kubick, & M. Hampton (Eds.) *Torn from our midst: Voices of grief, healing and action from the Missing Indigenous Women Conference* (pp. 75–85). Regina, SK: CPRC Press.

Bourassa, C. (2011). *Métis health: The invisible problem.* Vernon, BC: J Charleton Ltd.

Bourassa, C. (2018). Addressing the duality of access to healthcare for Indigenous communities: Racism and geographical barriers to safe care. *Healthcare Papers, 17*(3), 6–10. https://doi.org/10.12927/hcpap.2018.25507

Bourassa, C., Bendig, M., Oleson, E., Ozog, C., Billan, J., Owl, N., & Ross-Hopley, K. (2017). Campus violence, Indigenous women, and the policy void. In E. Quinlan, A. Quinlan, C. Fogel, G. Taylor (Eds.), *Sexual violence at Canadian universities: Activism, institutional responses, and strategies for change* (pp. 45–60). Waterloo, ON: Wilfrid Laurier Press.

Bourassa, C., Bendig, M., Ozog, C., & Oleson, E. (2016). Health as a feminist issue. In N. Mandell & J. Johnson (Eds.), *Feminist issues: Race, class, and sexuality* (pp. 311–335). Prentice-Hall, Canada: Pearson.

Bourassa, C., Blind, M., Dietrich, D., & Oleson, E. (2015). Understanding the intergenerational effects of colonization: Aboriginal women with neurological conditions – Their reality and resilience. *International Journal of Indigenous Health, 10*(2), 3–20. https://doi.org/10.18357/ijih.102201515113

Bourassa, C., McElhaney, J., & Oleson, E. (2016). *Cultural safety.* Queen's University. Available at: https://www.queensu.ca/sps/sites/webpublish .queensu.ca.spswww/files/files/Events/Conferences/RCAP/Papers /Bourassa_RCAP_conceptsOct2016.pdf

Bourassa, C., McKay-McNabb, K., & Hampton, M. (2004). Racism, sexism and colonialism: The impact on the health of Aboriginal women in Canada. *Canadian Woman Studies, 24*(1), 23–29.

Bourassa, C., McKenna, B., & Juschka, D. (2017). *Listening to the beat of our drum: Indigenous parenting in contemporary society.* Bradford, ON: Demeter Press.

Horrill, T., McMillan, D., Schultz, A., & Thompson, G. (2018). Understanding access to healthcare among Indigenous peoples: A comparative analysis of biomedical and postcolonial perspectives. *Nursing Inquiry, 25*(3). doi: https://doi.org/10.1111/nin.12237

Hunt, S., & Canadian Electronic Library. (2016). *An introduction to the health of Two-spirit People: Historical, contemporary and emergent issues* (Documents Collection). DesLibris.

Ivankovich, M., Fenton, K., & Douglas, J. (2013). Considerations for national public health leadership in advancing sexual health. *Public Health Reports, 128*, 102–110. https://doi.org/10.1177/00333549131282S112

Knight, D., & Musqua, Dan. (2001). *The seven fires: Teachings of the Bear Clan as recounted by Dan Musqua: Knowledge of human growth and learning practiced in the old world of the Nacowaninawuk (Saulteaux).* Muskoday, S. K.: Many Worlds Publisher.

Kubik, W., Bourassa, C., & Hampton, M. (2009). Stolen sisters, second class citizens, poor health: The legacy of colonization in Canada. *Humanity & Society, 33*(1–2), 18–34. https://doi.org/10.1177/016059760903300103

Lavallee, B., Diffey, L., Dignan, T., & Tomascik, P. (2014 January). Is cultural safety enough? Confronting racism to address inequities in Indigenous health [Paper]. Challenging Health Inequities, Indigenous Health Conference, Toronto ON. https://www.researchgate.net/publication/275043268_Is _cultural_safety_enough_Confronting_racism_to_address_inequities_in _ Indignous_health

McKenna, B., Hampton, M., Bourassa, C., McKay-McNabb, & Baysala, A. (2010). Voices from the Moon Lodge. In Geissler, S., Loutxenhiser, L., Praud, J., & Streifler, L. (Eds.), *Mothering Canada: Interdisciplinary voices* (pp. 231–240). Bradford, ON: Demeter Press.

National Collaborating Centre for Aboriginal Health. (2013). *An overview of Aboriginal health in Canada.* : http://www.nccah-ccnsa.ca/Publications/Lists /Publications/Attachments/101/abororiginal_health_web.pdf

National Inquiry into Missing and Murdered Indigenous Women and Girls. (2019). *Reclaiming power and place: The final report of the National Inquiry into Missing and Murdered Indigenous Women and Girls.* https://www.mmiwg-ffada .ca/wp-content/uploads/2019/06/Final_Report_Vol_1a-1.pdf

Papps, E., & Ramsden, I. (1996). Cultural safety in nursing: The New Zealand experience. *International Journal for Quality in Health Care, 8*(5), 491–497. doi: https://doi.org/10.1093/intqhc/8.5.491

Perreault, S. (2015). Criminal victimization in Canada, 2014. *Juristat: Canadian Centre for Justice Statistics* (Statistics Canada Catalogue no. 85–002-X). http:// www.statcan.gc.ca/pub/85-002-x/2015001/article/14241-eng.pdf

Public Health Agency of Canada. (2018). *Summary: Estimates of HIV incidence, prevalence and Canada's progression on meeting the 90–90–90 HIV targets, 2016.* https://www.canada.ca/content/dam/phac-aspc/documents/services /publications/diseases-conditions/summary-estimates-hiv-incidence -prevalence-canadas-progress-90-90-90/pub-eng.pdf

Razack, S. H. (2002). Gendered racial violence and spatialized justice: The murder of Pamela George. In S. H. Razack (Ed.), *Race, space, and the law: Unmapping a white settler society* (pp. 121–278). Toronto, ON: Between the Lines.

Royal Canadian Mounted Police. (2014). *Missing and murdered Aboriginal women: A national operational overview.* https://www.rcmp-grc.gc.ca/en/missing-and -murdered-aboriginal-women-national-operational-overview

Slater, S. (2011). Nought but women: Constructions of masculinities and modes of emasculation in the New World. In *Gender and sexuality in Indigenous North America, 1400–1850* (p. 30). Columbia, South Carolina: University of South Carolina Press.

Slater, S., & Yarbrough, F. (2011). *Gender and sexuality in Indigenous North America, 1400–1850.* Columbia, South Carolina: University of South Carolina Press.

Stark, J. (2013). Unequal communities: Exploring the relationship between colonialism, patriarchy and the marginalization of Aboriginal women. *Footnotes, 6*(May). https://journal.lib.uoguelph.ca/index.php/footnotes /article/view/2383

Tarasuk, J., Ogunnaike-Cooke, S., Archibald, C., Poitras, M., Hennink, M., Lloyd, K., et al. (2014). A pilot behavioural and biological surveillance survey for HIV and other bloodborne infections among Aboriginal people in Regina, Saskatchewan. *Canada Communicable Disease Report, 40*(18), 388–396. doi: https://doi.org/10.14745/ccdr.v40i18a04

Thomas, W. (1997). Navajo cultural constructions of gender and sexuality. In S-E. Jacobs, W. Thomas, & S. Lang (Eds.), *Two-spirit People: Native American gender identity, sexuality, and spirituality* (pp. 156–173). Urbana: University of Illinois Press.

Vogel, L. (2015). HIV in Saskatchewan merits urgent response. *Canadian Medical Association Journal, 187*(11), 793–794. doi: https://doi.org/10.1503/cmaj.109-5105

Wilson, A. (2004). Living well: Aboriginal women, cultural identity and wellness. *Centres of Excellence for Women's Health Research Bulletin, 4*(2), 6–8.

Wilson, D., de la Ronde, S., Brascoupé, S., Apale, A. N., Barney, L., Guthrie, B., et al. (2013). Health professionals working with First Nations, Inuit, and Métis consensus guideline. *Journal of Obstetrics and Gynaecology Canada, 35*(6), 1–4. doi: https://doi.org/10.1016/S1701-2163(15)30699-X

3 Teaching Sexual Consent

TERRY HUMPHREYS

With all the sexuality topics available to teach to college and university undergraduates, why prioritize sexual consent? The World Health Organization defines sexual health, in part, as requiring "a positive and respectful approach to sexuality and sexual relationships, as well as the possibility of having pleasurable and safe sexual experiences, free of coercion" (WHO, 2006, p. 5). In their 2014 Declaration of Sexual Rights, the World Association for Sexual Health (WAS) affirms that "everyone has the right to control and decide freely on matters related to their sexuality and their body. This includes the choice of sexual behaviours, practices, partners and relationships with due regard to the rights of others" (WAS, 2014, p. 2). This point speaks to bodily integrity, an important component of sexual consent. In 2019, the Sex Information and Education Council of Canada (SIECCAN) released its revised *Canadian Guidelines for Sexual Health Education.* Under the core principle of promoting gender equality and prevention of sexual and gender-based violence, the guidelines indicate that "sexual health education programs should assert the right of everyone to: (1) set boundaries communicated verbally or non-verbally, understanding that consent can be with withdrawn at any time and (2) clearly ask for and communicate affirmative consent (e.g., saying yes)" (SIECCAN, 2019, p. 26). These leading organizations, as well as many others, recognize that a focus on sexual consent is key to preventing sexual violence as well as improving personal sexual well-being and pleasure.

Despite these global declarations, sexual assault prevalence rates suggest that adolescent girls and young women in their early 20s are the most at-risk population (Black et al., 2011; Tjaden & Thoennes, 2000), with approximately one in five women experiencing sexual assault (broadly defined) during their time in college or university (Muehlenhard,

Peterson, Humphreys, & Jozkowski, 2017).[1] Comparable rates for men are difficult to ascertain. Studies conducted with men in postsecondary institutions find lifetime rates ranging from 2 to 27%, depending on definitions and methods (Peterson, Voller, Polusny, & Murdoch, 2011). In addition, a review of the literature from 2000 to 2017 by Anderson and colleagues (2019) found the rate of sexual perpetration (ranging from unwanted sexual contact to rape) by men in college is approximately 29%. Given these high rates of victimization and perpetration within the college and university system, education about sexual consent is warranted.

Accordingly, this chapter brings conceptual considerations and empirical research together to inform the teaching of sexual consent. At the postsecondary level, connections between teaching and research are abundant. Most notably, teachers routinely review the research literature to ensure the content that they present reflects the most accurate and up-to-date knowledge on a given subject. Students also have opportunities to interact with research through writing papers and participating in research studies. This is particularly relevant in the sexuality field, where much of our knowledge about consent attitudes and behaviours, as well as sexual assault prevalence rates, is developed through survey-based research conducted with undergraduate students. Further, research tools and findings can be utilized in the classroom to enhance engagement and make the material come to life. Specific examples of such applications will be interspersed in the text and addressed more globally at the end of this chapter.

Understanding the Context

Like many aspects of sexuality, teaching sexual consent requires an understanding of the research that has been conducted on the topic, including definitions, gender and sexual orientation issues, attitudes, and behavioural norms.

Definitions

Hickman and Muehlenhard (1999) were the first to conceptualize and define sexual consent for the research community. Sexual consent was defined as "the freely given verbal or nonverbal communication of a

---

1 The most recent review of the literature suggests that sexual assault rates between student and nonstudent populations in the same age group do not differ (Muehlenhard et al., 2017).

feeling of willingness" (p. 259) to engage in sexual activity. Although seemingly straightforward, there is a good deal of complexity in this definition. First, the definition includes an internal, agreeable private decision to have sex (i.e., a feeling of willingness), as well as a way to demonstrate that private decision to a partner(s) (i.e., communication). Both mental and physical aspects of the consent process are required. Second, because people can signal their own consent or ask for consent from a partner in a variety of ways, nonverbal and verbal behaviours need to be included. As an example, the introduction of a condom into a sexual encounter can be perceived as a way of asking for a partner's consent and giving one's own, all without ever saying a word. Third, the entire definition is predicated on the requirement that consent is "freely given." This aspect of the definition speaks to personal agency for sexual decision-making and raises contextual considerations such as coercion, alcohol, drugs, or incapacitation. In legal terms, Canada's *Criminal Code* (section 273.1(1)) defines consent as "the voluntary agreement ... to engage in the sexual activity in question" (Department of Justice, 2015). Canadian law uses affirmative consent language, asserting that "silence or lack of resistance cannot be interpreted as consent; instead, nonconsent must be assumed until consent is actively communicated" (Muehlenhard, Humphreys, Jozkowski, & Peterson, 2016, p. 464).

Gender and Sexual Orientation

As with most topics in the field of sexuality, gender and sexual orientation need special consideration. Most of the research on sexual consent has been conducted on heterosexuals, partly because it has been framed in terms of sexual assault prevention (specifically, male perpetrators and female survivors), partly because of the relative ease of accessing large heterosexual samples for quantitative analyses, but also because the field is generally heterocentric. Given this heteronormative focus, one of the most commonly used theories to discuss consent is sexual-script theory because it highlights the gendered nature of sexual communication and behaviour.

"Sexual scripts are cognitive frameworks, learned through socialization, that describe how people are expected to behave (as well as the sequencing of behaviours) in sexual situations" (Humphreys, 2000, p. 15). Scripts are organized and communicated via the culture and, once adopted at the individual level, decrease uncertainty by "providing direction on how to feel, think, and behave in particular situations" (Wiederman, 2005, p. 496). Sexual-script theory posits that men and women have been socialized with overlapping but somewhat different messages about their sexuality from birth. As a consequence, women and men have differing gender roles that they enact when negotiating consent. Traditionally, men are supposed to have sexual knowledge and therefore fulfil the initiator role, orchestrating sexual activity. In terms of sexual consent, this means that males use more direct – but nonverbal – approaches to obtaining consent (e.g., initiating a kiss, instead of asking). Women, however, are socialized to show restraint and personal control, acting as gatekeepers of their sexual reputation. In terms of sexual consent, this means they frequently engage in more indirect and nonverbal approaches to sexual activity, unless they are refusing a sexual advance. Women's refusal skills are an indelible part of traditional sexual scripts (and many sexual assault prevention campaigns), often at the expense of the development of agentic skills to request what is desired (Fine, 1988). Everyone needs to know how to say "yes" as well as "no." Sanchez, Fetterolf, and Rudman (2012) support the harmful effects of traditional sexual scripts for both women and men, specifically in terms of genuine sexual expression, but also see the female submissive role as particularly debilitating (p. 168). A thorough review of scripting theory is beyond the scope of this chapter (see Gagnon, 1990; Gagnon & Simon, 1973); however, it can be a very useful teaching tool to discuss traditional gender roles in the context of sexual consent negotiations. Challenging traditional gender roles helps students approach sexual consent with greater sexual agency, equity, and personal responsibility. This also merits a larger discussion of patriarchal culture and gender inequality.

The other deleterious influence of a heterocentric focus on sexual consent is that we know very little about the consent attitudes or behaviours of LGBTQ* communities. Does sexual orientation influence how individuals think about sexual consent? Would a lesbian couple negotiate consent any differently than a heterosexual couple? And if there are differences, do they arise because of orientation or gender? Very few studies have examined sexual consent with LGBTQ* samples. Using a sample of 257 individuals in same-sex relationships, Beres, Herold, and Maitland (2004) found that nonverbal behaviours were used most often to ask for and to indicate consent to a same-sex partner. When responding to sexual initiations, men who have sex with men (MSM) and women who have sex with women (WSW) continue to use "no resistance" as their primary response. Beres and colleagues (2004) also found no difference between the initiating behaviours used by MSM and WSW. This study seems to indicate more similarities than differences between heterosexual and LGBTQ* relationships. McKie, Skakoon-Sparling, Levere, Sezlik, and Humphreys (2020) examined the consent behaviours of MSM in Canada, the United States of America, and Western Europe. Their findings revealed some rather concerning behaviours between MSM in some contexts, such as gay bars, dark rooms, and sex clubs, where the pressures to fit in and be hypersexual, combined with alcohol and drugs, negated the ability to negotiate consent.

If we look to groups or communities who have a more formalized or structured approach to negotiating sexual consent, bondage, discipline, sadism, and masochism (BDSM) communities could offer helpful insights to the broader society. It is the norm within consensual BDSM practice that explicit negotiations (i.e., a contract) take place for a range of behaviours (i.e., type of play, body parts involved, boundaries, and safewords) before a "scene" occurs (Kaak, 2016). Safety concerns and explicit communication are of paramount importance given that many of the practices induce pain for pleasure or play with power dynamics (Barker, 2013; Beckmann, 2004). If the mainstream culture adopted these same skillful pre-sex discussions, a number of positive outcomes might be possible, including better sexual communication, comfort, and pleasure. More research is needed to explore the structure of consent negotiations within the BDSM context to provide insights into how they might apply to non-BDSM communities.

Attitudes

A sizable portion of the sexuality literature focuses on attitudinal research, including young adults' attitudes toward sexual consent. Researchers have used both qualitative and quantitative methodological tools such as focus groups, interviews, attitude scales and hypothetical vignettes. When asked in focus groups about their general understanding of sexual consent, university students tend to provide answers that match up fairly well with established research and legal definitions. Students talk about mutual understanding, notions of willingness or approval, agreeing on sexual behaviours, and a mind unclouded by excessive alcohol or drugs (Humphreys, 2004; Jozkowski, Sanders, Peterson, Dennis, & Reece, 2014). A minority of students still refer to consent in gendered terms; for example, "not resisting" as a typical female consent behaviour. In contrast, another minority of students talk about consent in more progressive terms, discussing how consent is a process, not a one-time event.

These qualitative studies have led to the development of scaled measures that help to assess different aspects of consent with much larger samples. Humphreys and Brousseau (2010) created the Sexual Consent Scale–Revised (SCS–R), which examines (1) attitudes about the importance of consent in different contexts; (2) whether individuals believe they have the skills and comfort to negotiate consent; and (3) consent norms within their peer group. Jozkowski and colleagues (2014) developed "dual measures of consent" (p. 437), assessing internal feelings of willingness (i.e., arousal, safety, and readiness) and external behaviours indicative of willingness (i.e., behavioural signals or verbal communication). This scale is based on the original ideas of the dual nature of sexual consent by Muehlenhard (1995–1996). In addition, Beres and colleagues (2004) developed the Same-Sex Sexual Consent Scale (SSSCS) to examine consent signals in same-sex sexual encounters. Specifically, this scale asked how individuals ask for and give consent for different types of sexual activity.

Numerous consent studies also use scenarios or vignettes to explore variables that may influence perception. Understanding perception is key to assessing underlying beliefs and potentially predicting behaviours. For example, Humphreys (2007) examined whether the length of the relationship or previous sexual history of a couple would influence perceptions of consent. Vignettes were developed featuring "Kevin" and "Lisa" watching a movie together after dinner. During the movie, Kevin initiates sexual behaviour; however, all of the behaviours portrayed in the scenarios are nonverbal and Lisa's consent is left as ambiguous. Humphreys (2007) manipulated both the length of the relationship as well as their past sexual history together to see if these variables influenced perceptions of sexual consent. Spoiler alert: they do. The gender of the participant also influences perceptions of consent. Men tend to see these ambiguous scenarios as more appropriate and consensual than women do (Humphreys, 2007).

With respect to a general understanding of sexual consent, the research suggests that students "get it." They understand what consent is and that they should obtain it prior to engaging in sex. Postsecondary students are exposed to the messaging about consent through poster campaigns, frosh-week orientations, and the like, creating greater awareness about consent than elsewhere in society. It is not surprising that students can mimic the key concepts of consent back to inquiring researchers. However, the true test of any good prevention or intervention campaign is whether the messaging translates into changes in actual behaviour.

Behaviours

Grounding the discussion of consent in current behavioural norms is critical for it to resonate with students. How do older adolescents and young adults currently negotiate their sexual encounters? Not surprisingly, sexual consent is rarely *formally* negotiated. Hickman and Muehlenhard (1999) asked participants to list the behaviours that they used to communicate sexual consent. The researchers categorized all the reported behaviours along two continua: verbal – nonverbal and direct – indirect. As an example, asking partners if they would like to "come upstairs for coffee" would be a verbal, but indirect, way to ask for consent to sexual activity. Overall, Hickman and Muehlenhard (1999) concluded that both women and men demonstrated their own consent to intercourse most often by making no response (i.e., not resisting). This is an unnerving finding, although researchers note that multiple signals likely occur leading up to the immediate situation that may not get repeated "in-the-moment" (Muehlenhard et al., 2016; Shumlich & Fisher, 2018). Keep in mind, consent needs to be understood as a process, not a one-time event. Even so, researchers have concluded that nonverbal forms of consent communication are much more common than verbal approaches (Beres et al., 2004; Hall, 1998; Hickman & Muehlenhard, 1999). There is also evidence that the type of sexual behaviour being contemplated may influence the consent communication. Hall (1998) and Humphreys (2007) found that undergraduate students believed that consent communication should be more explicit for oral or penile-vaginal intercourse than it is for kissing or fondling. In addition, Humphreys (2007) also found that students believe consent communication should be more explicit for new relationships in comparison to established relationships. Although it is clear that university students draw these distinctions when reporting what "should" happen, examining actual behaviours is a different matter. There is good support for the counterintuitive finding that students in committed relationships are more likely to use verbal consent cues than those in casual relationships (Marcantonio et al., 2018; Shumlich & Fisher, 2018; Willis, et al., 2019). This is opposite to what students report "should" occur (Humphreys, 2007; Muehlenhard et al., 2016). Hickman and Muehlenhard (1999) found that the signals most highly rated as indicators of consent are direct nonverbal and direct verbal signals, followed by indirect verbal signals, and then indirect nonverbal signals. A lack of response was listed as the least indicative of consent. The paradox is that when asked how often they use these signals in real life, students reported the signals in the inverse order. In other words, the cues least indicative of consent were those most often used.

The disconnect between students' attitudes toward sexual consent (which are generally quite progressive) and their reported behaviour is so great that Shumlich and Fisher (2018) provided a blunt appraisal of the situation, stating that "clear, unambiguous, and verbal sexual consent is rare, and veiled or coded means to infer consent are usually employed.

This pattern … is strikingly discordant with emerging normative requirements for affirmative sexual consent" (p. 258).

A Contributing Factor: Our Sex-Negative Culture

North America tends to be ambivalent about sexuality in general and, some would argue, is sex negative (Gabosch, 2014; Glickman, 2000; Irvine, 2004; Jorgensen, 2016). Our media coverage of issues relating to sexuality has never been as explicit as it is now, yet explicitness is not the same as sex positivity. Mass media tends to perpetuate highly stereotyped messages about sexuality and young people. Most of the messages are warnings, particularly aimed at girls and young women, about the dangers of sexuality, including unplanned pregnancies, sin, sexual assault, sexually transmitted infections, reputation, regret, and broken hearts. As noted earlier, gender stereotypes also permeate the culture, teaching, for example, that men should initiate sexual encounters and continue even in the face of resistance.

A number of researchers and therapists have suggested that talking is limited during sex because people believe it violates current sexual scripts and carries with it the risk of embarrassment and awkwardness (Blunt-Vinti, Jozkowski, & Hunt, 2019; MacNeil & Byers, 2009). Mass media, particularly movies and television, reifies these belief systems by portraying most scenes of sexuality as spontaneous, torrid moments of frantic breathless kissing, fondling, and the removal of clothes, followed by a cutaway scene the next morning with the couple smiling in bed; words are rarely uttered in any of these scenes. Jozkowski and colleagues (2019) coded the sexual consent signals used in the 50 most popular mainstream movies geared toward adult audiences in 2013. They found that approximately 75% of the coded cues used to communicate consent were nonverbal. This recurrent theme in movies is likely reinforcing the cultural notion that explicit or verbal consent is, by default, the antithesis of sexy (Beres, 2010).

With respect to sexuality education, the American approach has predominately been one of abstinence only (Fox, Himmelstein, Khalid, & Howell, 2019), even in the face of clear and substantiated evidence that, not only does it not work, it actually contributes to negative outcomes (Kirby, 2000; Kirby, 2008). Canada has generally been more progressive, teaching comprehensive sexuality education at best and abstinence plus at worst; however, there is substantial variability in Canada given that education is the jurisdiction of the provinces.

The culture's malaise toward sex combined with a sexual health curriculum that is quite varied leads to the limitation of our sexual language and sexual communication skills. Without the tools to communicate clearly and comfortably, people struggle to find the words to articulate their sexual wants and desires. In addition, young adults do not always know specifically what they want to engage in before sexual activity starts. They tend to *feel their way* through the process – passively consenting to specific behaviours as the event progresses. This is not necessarily a problem; however, many sexual consent campaigns dictate that consent should be established *prior* to the start of sexual activity.

Teaching Sexual Consent in Higher Education

How does the preceding discussion of consent attitudes and behaviours and the influence of current sexual scripts, gender and orientation, and our sex-negative culture inform teaching about sexual consent? First and foremost, it is important to acknowledge that many of the education/prevention campaigns regarding sexual consent require, either subtly or not so subtly, a very substantial departure from normative sexual scripts.

Building Sexual Communication Skills

Instead of trying to teach students the subtle (but ultimately futile) art of reading sexual cues or how to enthusiastically consent with a partner, I suggest stepping back and focusing on general sexual communication skills. The stumbling block for many students (and adults alike) is simply getting comfortable talking to a partner about sex in the first place. It is ironic that people are more uncomfortable talking about sex than having it, and this can be an ideal starting point for the discussion.

To introduce the discussion of consent in the classroom, an activity similar to that which has been undertaken in research studies to unpack the definition of sexual consent could be conducted to make students understand the various elements and why they are important. Similarly, the reverse process could be undertaken, whereby individuals or groups of students are asked to develop their own definition of sexual consent. A larger class discussion can follow to highlight the three key aspects of the definition, as noted earlier in this chapter.

Further, as teachers, we need to be aware of the heterocentric bias of the literature and make a conscious effort to discuss sexual consent as an inclusive communication skill, beneficial for all. Thus, be sure to include queer, straight, and kink stories/vignettes/examples in any classroom activity. Modelling safety and inclusivity in the classroom may require deliberate and direct discussions about sexual orientation and sexual consent – even when we do not have all the answers.

Teaching students how to get more comfortable talking about sex is not only about making sure young people exchange information about sexually transmitted infections and contraception, but also requires that students spend time thinking about their own sexual desires and how to satisfy them. Learning how to ask for what they want and to decline activities that do not fit within their personal boundaries are two types of assertiveness skills that need to be developed (Bouchard & Humphreys, 2019). When teaching about sex, acknowledging that this set of skills feels awkward at first and may come with the risk of rejection or being labelled as promiscuous increases the authenticity and realism of the ensuing class discussion. Ultimately, having the skills to comfortably talk about sex before, during, and after an encounter, as well as at times other than when sex is imminent, will vastly improve our clarity around sexual consent. Key messages to emphasize are that consent is a process, decision-making is ongoing, and consent can be given or rescinded at any time.

Surveys and Scales

Scales that assess general attitudes or preferences about consent can be drawn from research studies and incorporated as a classroom activity. The purpose here is not to collect data, which, of course, would be unethical, but simply to get students to think more deeply about the issues. Starting classes with a scale assessing consent attitudes is a good way to introduce the topic. Using student-response systems, attitudinal scale items could be incorporated into interactive and anonymous classroom polling so students get immediate feedback on their classmates' responses. These are very teachable moments in which to introduce Canadian consent law, research definitions, or discuss contextual factors that may influence the responses to specific survey items. Many research scales are freely available for educational use. See the *Handbook of Sexuality-Related Measures* (Milhausen, Sakaluk, Fisher, Davis, & Yarber, 2020) for an excellent compendium of scales related to consent and many other sexuality issues.

Vignettes and Scenarios

The use of vignettes or scenarios can be an effective technique to introduce many of the nuances and complexities of sexual consent to a classroom setting and to encourage students to consider their values, beliefs, and potential behaviours in a safe environment. When developing vignettes to use in the classroom, it is important to ensure that diversity in gender, orientation, ethnicity, and ability are reflected in the scenarios.

The use of vignettes also enables the teacher to highlight the complexities of consent, through emphasizing or modifying variables such as gender stereotypes, relationship status, sexual precedence, and alcohol/drug use. One scenario-based activity used by this author involves designating one wall in the classroom as "completely consensual" and the opposite wall as "completely nonconsensual." Students are then presented with a brief scenario describing a sexual encounter, similar to the "Kevin and Lisa" scenario described earlier in this chapter, and are invited to physically move to the location in the classroom that fits their perspective of consent, in the scenario presented. Students can position themselves at one wall or the other, or anywhere in between. They are then invited to comment on why they chose to stand where they did. This allows students to physically see the diversity of perspectives among their peer group and to learn from each other.

Critical Analysis of Consent Policies and Education Programs

Reviewing, analysing, and discussing actual consent policies and programs enable students to work with real-world examples; apply critical-thinking skills; put recently acquired skills and knowledge to use, and reflect on their own reactions to such policies, programs, or prevention campaigns at local colleges/universities (e.g., yes means yes, consent is sexy, don't be that guy, and enthusiastic consent). These can also be specifically critiqued in terms of the behaviours being promoted, terminated, or changed, and how realistic students think the requests are – for self and others. The exercise of critiquing existing programs allows class conversations to become more nuanced in terms of student concerns, the sexual and gender norms under scrutiny, and the way programming may need to change to resonate better with young adults. For an example of this approach in the research, see Humphreys and Herold (2003).

Conclusion

Teaching sexual consent to college and university students requires a comprehensive approach. Being cognizant of the social context in which one's teaching exists is important. Designing activities, exercises, or discussions that include aspects of cultural and gender norms, sexual-script theory, legal issues, and sexual orientation will make lesson plans more inclusive and realistic. Any approach that does not recognize the cultural backdrop of entrenched sex negativity, as well as sexual and gendered norms, is bound to be ineffective because it will not resonate with the lived experience of those we are trying to educate. Sexual communication skills are the foundation of consent education. Teaching students about the challenges inherent in verbalizing sexual wants and desires to their partners and working to break down the discomfort, shame, traditional norms, and media messages that impede a sex-positive approach to teaching sexual consent are essential.

REFERENCES

Anderson, R. E., Silver, K. E., Ciampaglia, A. M., Vitale, A. M., & Delahanty, D. L. (2019). The frequency of sexual perpetration in college men: A systematic review of reported prevalence rates from 2000 to 2017. *Trauma, Violence, and Abuse*, 1–15. https://doi.org/10.1177/1524838019860619

Barker, M. (2013). Consent is a grey area? A comparison of understandings of consent in *Fifty Shades of Grey* and on the BDSM blogosphere. *Sexualities*, 16, 896–914. https://doi.org/10.1177/1363460713508881

Beckmann, A. (2004). "Sexual rights" and "sexual responsibilities" within consensual "S/M" practice. In M. Cowling & P. Reynolds (Eds.), *Making sense of sexual consent* (pp. 195–208). Aldershot, England: Ashgate.

Beres, M. A. (2010). Sexual miscommunication? Untangling assumptions about sexual communication between casual sex partners. *Culture, Health and Sexuality, 12*, 1–14. https://doi.org/10.1080/13691050903075226

Beres, M. A., Herold, E., & Maitland, S. B. (2004). Sexual consent behaviors in same-sex relationships. *Archives of Sexual Behavior, 33*, 475–486. https://doi.org/10.1023/b:aseb.0000037428.41757.10

Black, M. C., Basile, K. C., Breiding, M. J., Smith, S. G., Walters, M. L., Merrick, M. T., … Stevens, M. R. (2011). *National intimate partner and sexual violence survey: 2010 summary report*. Atlanta, GA: Centers for Disease Control and Prevention. Retrieved from http://www.cdc.gov/ViolencePrevention/pdf/NISVS_Report2010-a.pdf

Blunt-Vinti, H., Jozkowski, K. N., & Hunt, M. (2019). Show or tell? Does verbal and/or nonverbal sexual communication matter for sexual satisfaction? *Journal of Sex and Marital Therapy, 45*, 206–217. https://doi.org/10.1080/0092623x.2018.1501446

Bouchard, L., & Humphreys, T. P. (2019). Asserting sexual (dis)interest: How do women's capabilities differ? *Canadian Journal of Human Sexuality, 28*, 226–241. https://doi.org/10.3138/cjhs.2019-0012

Department of Justice (2015). A definition of consent to sexual activity. Retrieved from the Government of Canada website: https://www.justice.gc.ca/eng/cj-jp/victims-victimes/def.html

Fine, M. (1988). Sexuality, schooling, and adolescent females: The missing discourse of desire. *Harvard Educational Review, 58*, 29–53. https://doi.org/10.17763/haer.58.1.u0468k1v2n2n8242

Fox, A. M., Himmelstein, G., Khalid, H., & Howell, E. A. (2019). Funding for abstinence-only education and adolescent pregnancy prevention: Does state ideology affect outcomes? *American Journal of Public Health, 109*, 497–504. https://doi.org/10.2105/ajph.2018.304896

Gabosch, A. (2014). *A Sex Positive Renaissance*. Retrieved from https://allenagabosch.wordpress.com/2014/12/08/a-sex-positive-renaissance/

Gagnon, J. H. (1990). The explicit and implicit use of the scripting perspective in sex research. *Annual Review of Sex Research, 1*, 1–43.

Gagnon, J. H., & Simon, W. (1973). *Sexual conduct: The social sources of human sexuality*. Chicago: Aldine.

Glickman, C. (2000). The language of positive sexuality. *The Electronic Journal of Human Sexuality, 3*. Retrieved http://www.ejhs.org/volume3/sexpositive.htm

Hall, D. S. (1998). Consent for sexual behavior in a college student population. *Electronic Journal of Human Sexuality, 1*. Retrieved from http://www.ejhs.org/volume1/consent1.htm

Hickman, S. E., & Muehlenhard, C. L. (1999). "By the semi-mystical appearance of a condom": How young women and men communicate sexual consent in heterosexual situations. *Journal of Sex Research, 36*, 258–272. https://doi.org/10.1080/00224499909551996

Humphreys, T. P. (2000). Sexual consent in heterosexual dating relationships: Attitudes and behaviours of university students, *Dissertation Abstracts International: Section B: The Sciences and Engineering, 61*(12-B), 6760.

Humphreys, T. P. (2004). Understanding sexual consent: An empirical investigation of the normative script for young heterosexual adults. In M. Cowling & P. Reynolds (Eds.), *Making sense of sexual consent* (pp. 209–225). Aldershot, England: Ashgate.

Humphreys, T. P. (2007). Perceptions of sexual consent: The impact of relationship history and gender. *Journal of Sex Research, 44*, 307–315. https://doi.org/10.1080/00224490701586706

Humphreys, T.P., & Brousseau, M. (2010) The Sexual Consent Scale–Revised: Development, reliability, and preliminary validity. *Journal of Sex Research, 47*, 420–428. https://doi.org/10.1080/00224490903151358

Humphreys, T. P., & Herold, E. (2003). Should universities and colleges mandate sexual behavior? Student perceptions of Antioch College's Consent Policy. *Journal of Psychology and Human Sexuality, 15*, 35–51. https://doi.org/10.1300/j056v15n01_04

Irvine, J. (2004). *Talk about sex: The battles over sex education in the United States*. California: University of California Press.

Jorgensen, J. (2016). The sex-negativity mindset in academe. *Inside Higher Ed*. Retrieved https://www.insidehighered.com/print/advice/2016/08/12/sex-negativity-mind-set-academe-essay

Jozkowski, K. N., Marcantonio, T. L., Rhoads, K. E., Canan, S., Hunt, M. E., & Willis, M. (2019). A content analysis of sexual consent and refusal communication in mainstream films. *Journal of Sex Research, 56,* 754–765. https://doi.org/10.1080/00224499.2019.1595503

Jozkowski, K. N., Sanders, S., Peterson, Z. D., Dennis, B., Reece, M. (2014). Consenting to sexual activity: The development and psychometric assessment of dual measures of consent. *Archives of Sexual Behavior, 43,* 437–450. https://doi.org/10.1007/s10508-013-0225-7

Kaak, A. (2016). Conversational phrases in BDSM pre-scene negotiations. *Journal of Positive Sexuality, 2,* 47–52.

Kirby, D. B. (2000). What does the research say about sexuality education. *Educational Leadership, 58*(2), 72–76.

Kirby, D. B. (2008). The impact of abstinence and comprehensive sex and STD/HIV education programs on adolescent sexual behaviour. *Sexuality Research and Social Policy, 5,* 18–27. https://doi.org/10.1525/srsp.2008.5.3.18

MacNeil, S., & Byers, E. S. (2009). Role of sexual self-disclosure in the sexual satisfaction of long-term heterosexual couples. *Journal of Sex Research, 46,* 3–14. https://doi.org/10.1080/00224490802398399

Marcantonio, T., Jozkowski, K. N., & Wiersma-Mosley, J. (2018). The influence of partner status and sexual behavior on college women's consent communication and feelings. *Journal of Sex & Marital Therapy, 44,* 776–786. https://doi.org/10.1080/0092623x.2018.1474410

McKie, R. M., Skakoon-Sparling, S., Levere, D., Sezlik, S., & Humphreys, T. P. (2020). *Is there space for our stories? An examination of North American and Western European gay, bi, and other men who have sex with men's non-consensual sexual experiences. Journal of Sex Research,* 57, 1014-1025. https://doi.org/10.1080/00224499.2020.1767023

Milhausen, R. R., Sakaluk, J. K., Fisher, T. D., Davis, C. M., & Yarber, W. L. (Eds.). (2020). *Handbook of sexuality-related measures* (4th ed.). New York: Routledge.

Muehlenhard, C. L. (1995–1996). The complexities of sexual consent. *SIECUS Report, 24,* 4–7. Retrieved from https://siecus.org/wp-content/uploads/2015/07/24-2.pdf

Muehlenhard, C. L., Humphreys, T.P., Jozkowski, K., & Peterson, Z. (2016). The complexities of sexual consent among college students: A conceptual and empirical review. *Journal of Sex Research, 53,* 457–487. https://doi.org/10.1080/00224499.2016.1146651

Muehlenhard, C. L., Peterson, Z. D., Humphreys, T. P., & Jozkowski, K. N. (2017). Evaluating the one-in-five statistic: Women's risk of sexual assault while in college. *Journal of Sex Research, 54,* 549–576. https://doi.org/10.1080/00224499.2017.1295014

Peterson, Z. D., Voller, E. K., Polusny, M. A., & Murdoch, M. (2011). Prevalence and consequences of adult sexual assault of men: Review of empirical findings and state of the literature. *Clinical Psychology Review, 31*, 1–24. https://doi.org/10.1016/j.cpr.2010.08.006

Sanchez, D. T., Fetterolf, J. C., & Rudman, L. A. (2012). Eroticizing inequality in the United States: The consequences and determinants of traditional gender role adherence in intimate relationships. *Journal of Sex Research, 49*, 168–183. https://doi.org/10.1080/00224499.2011.653699

Sex Information and Education Council of Canada (SIECCAN). (2019). *Canadian guidelines for sexual health education.* Retrieved from http://sieccan.org/wp-content/uploads/2019/08/Canadian-Guidelines-for-Sexual-Health-Education.pdf

Shumlich, E. J., & Fisher, W. A. (2018). Affirmative sexual consent? Direct and unambiguous consent is rarely included in discussions of recent sexual interactions. *Canadian Journal of Human Sexuality, 27*, 248–260. https://doi.org/10.3138/cjhs.2017-0040

Tjaden, P., & Thoennes, N. (2000). *Full report of the prevalence, incidence, and consequences of violence against women (NCJ 183781).* Washington, DC: Department of Justice. Retrieved from https://www.ncjrs.gov/pdffiles1/nij/183781.pdf

Wiederman, M. W. (2005). The gendered nature of sexual scripts. *The Family Journal: Counseling and Therapy for Couples and Families, 13*, 496–502. https://doi.org/10.1177/1066480705278729

Willis, M., Hunt, M., Wodika, A., Rhodes, D. L., Goodman, J., & Jozkowski, K. N. (2019). Explicit verbal sexual consent communication: Effects of gender, relationship status, and type of sexual behavior. *International Journal of Sexual Health, 31*, 60–70. https://doi.org/10.1080/19317611.2019.1565793

World Association for Sexual Health (2014). Declaration of sexual rights. Retrieved from https://worldsexualhealth.net/wp-content/uploads/2013/08/Declaration-of-Sexual-Rights-2014-plain-text.pdf

World Health Organization (2006). *Defining sexual health: Report of a technical consultation on sexual health, 28–31 January 2002, Geneva.* Retrieved from https://www.who.int/reproductivehealth/publications/sexual_health/defining_sh/en/

4 What about the Boys? University Students Learning about Sexual Consent Talk from Youth in Northeastern Ontario

JENNIFER L. JOHNSON

This chapter queries how sexual violence and consent are discussed in some feminist postsecondary classrooms and how these discussions can benefit from the inclusion of men's and boys' perspectives. As evidence, I examine curriculum that was developed collaboratively for 12- and 13-year-old boys and their youth mentors at an annual conference in Northeastern Ontario about consent, sexual violence, and masculinity. In turn, I explore how this experience transformed the work I do with postsecondary students who are predominantly cisgender, queer, and trans women who are studying the liberal arts and sciences, and/or located in professional programs for Indigenous social work and social work, teacher education, and midwifery. I argue that by acknowledging the vulnerabilities of men and boys and the uncertainties or awkwardness they face while developing their own healthy relationships, new and productive discussions about gender-based and sexual violence are enhanced within postsecondary education.

How Are Sexual Violence and Consent Discussed in Feminist Classrooms?

As a field, women's and gender studies – and feminist classrooms more broadly – are locations within academia where adult learners openly discuss sexual violence, sexuality education, and antiviolence. Feminist scholarship within specific disciplines and professional studies, as well as within the interdisciplinary field of women's and gender studies (WGS), document the dramatic shift in the past four decades of feminist teaching about sexual consent and antiviolence (Calixte, Motapanyane, & Johnson, 2016; McKenna, 2016; Sheehy, 2012). The shift in question is one in which public acknowledgment of the existence of gender-based sexual violence in North American society (i.e., men typically the perpetrators and women/children usually the survivors) has expanded to query how this violence can be understood as a systemic problem and challenged effectively (Close, 2005; Connolly & Josephson, 2007; Cramer, Ross, McLeod, & Jones, 2015; McLeod, Jones, & Cramer, 2015; Greig & Pollard, 2016). Feminist scholars use a complex understanding of gendered sexual violence as located at the intersections of sexism and racism, leading to robust fields of study that cover legal, political, social, and intimate settings in which sexual violence occurs or is perpetuated (Bruckert & Law, 2018; Cho, Crenshaw, & McCall, 2013). Importantly, observations and theories about challenging sexual assault within the context of Indigenous women's experiences in Northern Ontario have given rise to a growing argument for resistance strategies as a continuum of effort of which sexuality education is certainly a part (Hrynyk, 2018) rather than a full-stop solution.

There are two major sources for data on sexual assault in Canada. The first is the General Social Survey (GSS) that gathers self-reported data once every four years. In the 2014 data cycle, 636,000 incidents of sexual assault were reported. The second source is the Uniform Crime Reporting (UCR) Survey, which in 2014 collected records of just over 21,000 sexual assaults. It is important to note that the UCR Survey only includes reports from police services across Canada and that the stark difference in numbers of reports between the two sources illustrates how many social and legal barriers limit talk about sexual assault. Both databases define a "victim" as a person who has experienced sexual assault.

Incidences of sexual assault in Canada remain relatively constant, with self-reported assaults being highly differentiated by gender, age, student status, as well as sexual and Indigenous identity, among other important variables. In their analysis of the GSS Statistics Canada data, Conroy and Cotter (2014) demonstrate that women and girls continue to experience the highest rates of sexual assault. Of 555,000 incidents of sexual assault reported in 2014, "the vast majority (87%) were committed against women," while the perpetrators are mostly male-identified (p. 6). For the purpose of understanding why the topic of this chapter and, indeed, this entire book is so critical, the age range during which many people experience postsecondary education is also frequently the age range when young women are assaulted: "Of all sexual assault incidents, nearly half (47%) were committed against women aged 15 to 24." While sexual assault is perpetuated against women for the duration of their lives, adolescence and young adulthood appear to be critical moments for the formation of expectations about sexuality and bodily integrity and autonomy.

The rates of assault against girls and young women overlap significantly with other variables. One in five First Nations, Métis, and Inuit women and girls ages 15 to 24 experienced sexual assault in 2014, making age, Indigenous identity, and student status a significant intersection to which postsecondary educators should pay attention. Individuals identified as homosexual or bisexual in the GSS survey, of any gender, were six times more likely than heterosexuals to have experienced sexual assault in this same year. And, significantly, 80% of assailants are friends and family of the survivor (Conroy & Cotter, 2014), suggesting that sexual assault continues to be a problem located within new and established intimate and family relationships.

In Ontario, when it comes to university and college students, the provincial Ministry of Training, Colleges and Universities reports that within their first few semesters of study, 63% of women-identified undergraduates at university and nearly 50% in college will have experienced some form of sexual harassment (CCI Research, 2019, p. 12). The same study found that in those first few semesters, "23% of Ontario university students and 17.2% of college students will have had a non-consensual sexual experience" (p. 19). The Canadian Federation of Students argues that there can be no more compelling reason to extend education on sexual health, relationships, and sexual violence as soon and as effectively as possible (Canadian Federation of Students, 2017; CCI Research, 2019). In what follows, I trace what I have learned about how to teach about the prevalence of sexual assault by working with material from critical masculinity studies in feminist classrooms to working with quite young male-identified children, and then back to the university classroom again.

Critical Masculinity Studies in Feminist Classrooms and the Community

No matter the sensitivity and nuance with which it is delivered, the subtext that some learners take away from the conversation about sexual violence in feminist classrooms, when it is presented roughly in the way I have just outlined, is very grim. Learners infer that the role prescribed to women and girls is to hope that sex is safe and fulfilling for them one day, but that statistically they are doomed to suffer in the meantime (Antle, Sullivan, Dryden, Karam, & Barbee, 2011). Though intended to be objective, the language of victimhood used in the quantitative research reflects the diminished confidence many young women experience as a result of sexual assault. It also ignores the significant roles men play in this violence, as well as the construction of masculine violence as a social norm, both of which I will examine later (Katz, 2006; Katz & Earp, 1999). But for male-identified learners, their subject position is even less clear. How do these learners relate to the 13% of boys and men in the 2014 GSS who reported an experience of sexual violence? I suggest that these problems are related and stem from the persistent pleasure/danger dichotomy in sexuality education (Cameron-Lewis, 2016). The language of victim-hood or danger comes to be associated with femininity, while the invis-ibility of men and boys in these statistics leaves a big question mark for learners. In this invisible dialogue about sexual assault of men and boys, learners are able to fill in the blanks with the assumption that men are all potential rapists and/or people who get to enjoy sex, while women are always potential victims or people who must protect themselves from sex. Feminist scholarship did not invent this dichotomy; it is one of the unarticulated discourses in Western views of sexuality that persist over time (Kimmell, 2007; Mallet & Herbe, 2011). Research in a range of cultural milieus suggests that adolescence is a time in which aggression and violence do increase in the context of dating, and as such, it is an important time for very direct messaging about sexual consent and the negotiation skills in equitable sexual relationships (Guidi, Magnatta, & Meringolo, 2012; SIECAN, 2019). There are gender-based differences in youth experiences of violence. Boys do tend to engage in sexual aggres-sion, while girls tend to engage in physical and emotional aggression (O'Leary & Smith Slep, 2012). But overall, boys more than girls tend to engage in gender-based violence and sexual harassment at the hands of one another, as well as imposing it on girls (Hokoda, Del Campo, & Ulloa, 2012; Taylor, Stein, & Burden, 2010).

Men's antiviolence organizing, inspired by feminism and decoloniz-ing movements in North America, provides arguments to help dislodge some of these attitudes. Scholar activists dedicated to antiviolence pro-duce curriculum and programs that focus on the experiences of different groups of boys and men. Some of these programs begin with dismantling sexual and gender stereotypes that are toxic to all women and especially to racialized women and girls. See, for example, the Mentors in Violence Prevention model (Katz, Heisterkamp, & Fleming, 2011); Teach One Reach One (Ritchwood, 2015); My Strength Is Not for Hurting (2019) and Masters' (2010) comments on the development of this program; as well as the White Ribbon Campaign (2019). In Canada, White Ribbon (2019) is notable for including material on the links between homo- and trans-phobia and men's violence toward other men, and Petering, Wen-zel, and Winetrobe (2014) discuss effective programming with youth who are homeless, an important consideration when we consider that many queer and trans+ youth are disproportionately subject to homelessness.

While these programs centrally build on feminist campaigns to recognize women's personhood, they also problematize common beliefs about the links between sexual dominance over women and other men as a tenet of "true" manhood in Western societies (Grimmett, Conley, Foster, & Clark, 2018). Very successful programs, such as My Masculinity Helps (Grimmett, Conley, Foster, & Clark, 2018) and I Am a Kind Man (2019), aimed at racialized and Indigenous men and boys, take a different approach. They work to reclaim values associated with manhood that have been suppressed through colonial practices of excluding Black and Indigenous men from political, legal, and education systems (Grimmett et al., 2018). These programs variously suggest that by reclaiming identities and responsibilities, lost through the intergenerational impacts of slavery, genocide, colonialism, and ongoing systemic disadvantages incurred through poverty, men and boys can come to respect themselves and, by extension, the women and girls in their communities. In all these antiviolence programs aimed at men and boys, the goal is to restore respect for one's self as a foundation for the respectful treatment of women and girls.

Regardless of whether the approach is to reclaim and ground boys in their identities, or to deconstruct the most toxic aspects of Western manhood, it has been demonstrated that just one significant instance of critical discussion with youth aged 12 to 14 about these topics can decrease the risk of their participating in a violent act, or accepting the consequences of one, within the context of an intimate relationship (Foshee et al., 2004). Adolescence is a time where people consider dating or generally become more aware of intimate relationships. This age group, in Canada, is also on the cusp of being able to consent legally to sexual activity, making it an important time to provide antiviolence sexual education.

The Voices of 12- and 13-Year-Old Boys in Antiviolence Education: A Community Example

In 2012, local agencies and community educators began collaborating on an annual conference about consent, sexual violence, and masculinity for young boy/male-identified youth in the English-language public education system in Sudbury, Ontario. For nearly 10 years previous, the lead agency ran a conference for girls focused on empowerment, positive body image, and introductions to feminism, with approximately 200+ girl-identified students in attendance each year. The lead organization for this conference always focused on girls' empowerment because of its own larger policy mandate, but for a variety of reasons began to ask,

What about the boys? In my contributions to other events and policies related to this agency, I had been vocal about the need to account for men's antiviolence work and trans-inclusiveness, which is possibly what afforded me an invitation to join in curriculum development.

Context, Process, and Outcomes

Participants in the conference are 12- and 13-year-old boy/male-identified youth, who are accompanied by 16- to 24-year-old peer mentors. The mentors can be of any gender but are typically young cis or trans men; in other programs, organizers have said that mentors are an untapped resource but their involvement in general has proven to be beneficial for both the youth and the peer mentors themselves (Cramer et al., 2015; Kernsmith & Hernandez-Jozefowicz, 2011). As of 2020, nearly 1,000 youth in Northeastern Ontario will have experienced the conference. Between 120 and 170 students from several different public schools attend each year. The participants and their teachers are predominantly white and cisgender and include Indigenous youth and youth of colour and/or openly queer and trans+ youth. Attendees frequently include boys with disabilities who attend with a support person. It is this diverse group of boys that has come to inform what I think about when I plan discussions about sexual violence and consent in my postsecondary classrooms.

In addition to at least one full-time career antiviolence educator and activist, the conference facilitators are all involved in the direct delivery of service in the community. They include sexual assault counsellors, shelter workers, a police officer or civilian police employee with specific training about sexual assault and intimate-partner violence, and youth-group leaders who represent a variety of organizations. Following the lead of the most experienced among us, we have adopted the policy of overtly asking the boys to "bring their best, most mature selves" to the table, and for most of the time, they do. Their goodwill is reinforced with pizza, bottles of water, new pens, swag bags stuffed with goodies and free samples, and snacks.

While the material in the very first offering of the conference was largely produced by facilitators who came with ready content, the curation and order of the workshops was directed by an organizing committee. Over the past four years, the group has come to agree that there are three components that prompt positive feedback from the participants and seem to be in step with the existing antiviolence literature. The first workshop addresses dominant constructions of masculinity and the ways in which racism, homophobia, and privilege undermine the development of boys' well-being. The facilitator makes the argument that dominant expectations of men's behaviour and accomplishments in North American society are frequently toxic to them and to those around them. After a multimedia presentation, the facilitator then asks the boys to articulate and deconstruct stereotypes about masculinity. In a second workshop, on healthy relationships and sexual consent, the participants focus first on sexting and online spaces where they are invited to think of themselves as potentially vulnerable to sexual exploitation and bullying. These themes segue to a discussion of healthy relationships and how people relate to one another equitably versus one person being treated as instrumental or as an object for another person to control. They are given the legal definition of sexual consent, and a discussion about the varying ages of sexual consent in Canada follows. In the third and final part of the conference, they are provided with an opportunity to synthesize and fact check what they have learned. They are provided with a concise handout that includes statistics on gendered violence and sexual assault in Canada and locally in Sudbury. The information includes statistics on violence against Indigenous women, as well as women and girls with disabilities. Their main task is to analyse one of four cases studies. Their original solutions are validated or redirected and refined with the help of the youth mentors and the facilitators. In what follows, I shift focus to explore how these conferences changed my curriculum choices when teaching about sexual violence, and how I now present this information to predominantly adult cis female, queer, and trans+ identified university students.

Recommendations for the University Classroom

Teaching about sexual violence and consent in feminist postsecondary classrooms benefits in several ways specifically from the perspectives of men and boys. Most importantly, the 12- and 13-year-old boys at the conferences position themselves as supporters on equal footing with girls of their age. Statistically, their experiences of violence will have diverged significantly by the time they reach age 18, and the boys largely express dismay when they are presented with this fact. So while at ages 12 and 13, boys see girls as their peers, girls will on average experience sexual assault more often than boys before the age of 18. Given that youth experiences of violence can be differentiated by sex, racialization, gender identity, poverty, and disability, there is much to discuss (Conroy & Cotter, 2014; Cotter, 2018; Violence Against Women Learning Network, 2018). Based on a preliminary analysis of their completed exit surveys over the past four years, and in their candid discussions with their mentors, they say things such as "I would like to help"; "I don't like the way people treat some girls"; and so on. These statements indicate a strong empathy in response to the workshop material. I do not read the boys' expressions of interest in responding to sexual violence against girls and women as patronizing or facetious, or even just as aiming for adult approval. No one is hovering when they fill out the evaluations, which are anonymous and are analyzed by the lead organization after the conference. Instead, I think this expression of empathy could lend itself to a kind of solidarity that must still be negotiated through further work with boys as they mature and should complement education with older youth in high school and postsecondary education.

Since working with this conference, I have redoubled messaging about how important it is for university students to speak with male-identified family members to discover and compare their knowledge about sexual consent and violence. I have not adopted this approach because I think that women and girls are wholly responsible for educating men about sexual violence. Rather, I have come to the understanding that some men's and boys' relationship to sexual and other violence as survivors, and young boys' propensity for empathy, mean they are an important resource for adult women who want to address this issue in their own families and relationships. I have begun to include the same discussion strategies we use with 12- and 13-year-olds in these university classes. For example, one of the greatest predictors of an intervention program's effect on sexual violence is young men's ability to communicate sexually, or what has been called "sexual communication assertiveness," which is associated with consent-related attitudes, intentions, and interpretations (Shafer, Ortiz, Thompson, & Huemmer, 2018). Just as we have done at the boys' conference, I provide university students with jargon-free resources that include definitions or statistics sheets. These are not academic readings that require a lot of analysis to understand: they are meant to be read in a few minutes and left on a kitchen table or open on a screen for parents, siblings, and roommates to read. University students add to these resources with videos, memes, and news stories, which we share within our classroom.

Perhaps the most significant shift I have made in my teaching since being involved with the conferences is to critically interrogate how and why discussions about violence and sexuality are so separate in my own syllabi. After the first two years of the boys' conference and observing their responses to the curriculum, I began to reconsider how the topic of sexual violence punctuates my first-year WGS class in particular. I noted that while material on intimate-partner violence, gender, and race-based violence are presented throughout the course, material on sexuality and sex-positive feminism was hived off into separate lectures and readings.

Without intending to, I had recreated the pleasure/danger dichotomy that Cameron-Lewis (2016) argue organizes some sexuality education. Reflecting on the teaching strategies we used with 12- to 13-year-old boys, I noted that our attempts to engage them involved humour. I began to think about what might change if I invited this strategy into the classroom with predominantly young adult women.

One of the resources we have used at the conferences is a short video called "Internetseks," in which a teenager who is coded as masculine nearly sends a naked picture of himself to someone online (Sense, 2019). The exchange of images between the teens is interrupted by a parent. A few moments later at the breakfast table, the teenager recognizes his sister's clothing from the neck-down image he was just watching online. They both realize they had been about to send sexually explicit images of themselves to one another. The video brings about tremendous peals of laughter from the conference participants. The boys indicate serious engagement with the dilemma (to hit send or not) by asking a lot of questions. They share so many stories in response to this video that we frequently have to force them to move on. The goal of the workshop prompts the participants to think about what is safe for them and what is not. Thus, regardless of the extent of their personal experiences, the boys are recognized as the experts in their own lives and in the subject matter of sexting, which we also later discuss in relation to healthy relationships and sexual consent.

Humour is a really important part of challenging the dichotomy of sex as a risk for girls or sexual exploration for boys, and actually, given the right context and presentation, humour can work with everyone, including postsecondary students. Admittedly, we used humour during the creation of the curriculum for the boys' conference because we were concerned that the boys might not be able to sit still without this type of engagement. The assumption demonstrated sexual stereotyping and inexperience on our part, but the boys' positive and engaged reactions to it made me immediately return to my own syllabus to ask, When did humour exit my classroom? In an effort to handle the very serious and real problem of learning about sexual assault and placing it in its historical and contemporary contexts through coursework, I realized that I was inadvertently separating it from all of the silly, funny, and strange things that can happen as we learn about sexuality (Carmody, 2005). Of course, the experiences of survivors deserve thoughtful and respectful consideration. But I had come to carefully separate talking about sexual empowerment and sex-positive creativity from the existence of intimate-partner violence (Carmody & Ovenden, 2013). When I looked at what had been accomplished in the boys' curriculum, I realized that we were offering the boys the luxury – or perhaps the necessity – of confronting sexual danger with humour. It is important to note that the feminine-coded character in the short video is similarly engaged in the (near) act of sharing a sexually explicit image, and in this instance, neither character demonstrates feeling coerced. I believe that an appropriate use of humour was successful for the boys because it positions them as peers to the two characters in the video. They are provided with an opportunity to think through a dilemma together and thus have a chance to diversify their own skill set for talking about sexuality. Confronting sexual danger with humour works in this feminist classroom because it allows young adults to confront the idea of sex as risk that is too often imposed on women and girls.

It is the organizers' hope to eventually expand the conference to reach specific groups of learners, including young people with disabilities and queer and trans+ youth who may be underserved in our community and are underserved by this conference in its present form. In the meantime, the group aims for inclusiveness while recognizing that knowledge about sexuality directed at cisgender boys is a specific deterrent to their support of rape culture (Mallet & Herbe, 2011). Feminist researchers have shown that even a brief intervention of only 45 minutes of interaction and information about the topic, delivered in culturally appropriate ways, can make a measurable difference in whether or not boys will be tolerant of rape culture (Smith & Welchans, 2000). If this is true, then should we not be opening our classrooms to the significant others of our students, regardless of their gender identify or sexual orientation? Since beginning work on the boys' conference, the partners, younger siblings, and friends of my students have been invited to join and participate in conversation in my Introduction to Women's and Gender Studies course on any day, but especially in the moments when we talk about masculinity.

Finally, the perspectives of 12- and 13-year-old boys require attention in university classrooms because they could be subject to violence themselves. If in Sudbury in 2018 there were more than 3,000 cases of intimate-partner violence reported to the police, and an additional 217 sexual assaults, there will have been conference participants directly affected by gendered violence, possibly within their own families (GSPS, 2018). Additionally, we acknowledge that on average, 13% of those who experience sexual assault in calendar year in Canada are male-identified (Conroy & Cotter, 2014). Material about their lives can be included in any university learning about sexuality and antiviolence education in order to ground men's connection to sexual assault. Sun, Miu, Wong, Tucker, and Wong (2018) as well as Weisz and Black (2010) also suggest that older peers such as college and university students aged 18 to 25 are an important but untapped resource for helping younger people engage with sexuality and consent education. A lot more in-depth work with youth mentors could be done with those who are age 12 and up, the age when sexual violence is most prevalent in early high school. Could university students in my classes provide this kind of mentorship to someone else? By being open to discussing the risks that men and boys face in relation to sexual violence, their fragility in the face of understanding what sexual consent is, and how to communicate it for themselves, we will be educating people for this important dialogue.

Conclusion

Teaching about sexual violence and consent in feminist post-secondary classrooms requires acknowledging the creative potential of diverse men and boys to challenge toxic masculinity. Sexuality education about consent and violence must include many ways of becoming emotionally literate and must begin to draw on the voices of those who would like to challenge gender-based violence but may not be seen as typically knowledgeable about this experience. In my work with both predominantly university-aged and female-identified learners and 12- to 13-year-old boys, I have found that both groups have creative insights about sexual assault and consent. They are indeed "talking about the same thing" when asked to learn about sexuality, consent, and violence, albeit from different perspectives that inform one another.

I have argued here that direct interventions in discourses of toxic masculinity at the age of 12 to 13 is not only a promising intervention for adolescents, but that there is also an important connection to what should be done in university classrooms. What would happen to the statistics on sexual assault in Ontario universities if more 12- and 13-year-olds had access to knowledgeable peer mentors and trained facilitators talking about sexual assault? Programs that directly challenge the idea that suppressing women in sexual relationships is endemic of what it is to be a man have been shown to have profound success in changing the attitudes of men and boys (Grimmett et al., 2018). For vulnerable groups such as youth with intellectual disabilities, these direct conversations about sex and relationships are essential to their well-being (Gougeon, 2009). Feminist and other educators might ask themselves how postsecondary education can collaborate on and support this type of learning in the elementary and high school systems. The literature suggests that there are benefits for youth as well as for their university-aged learners.

REFERENCES

Antle, B. F., Sullivan, D. J., Dryden, A., Karam, E. A., & Barbee, A. P. (2011). Healthy relationship education for dating violence prevention among high-risk youth. *Children and Youth Services Review, 33*(1), 173–179. https://doi.org/10.1016/j.childyouth.2010.08.031

Bruckert, C., & Law, T. (2018). *Women and gendered violence in Canada: An intersectional approach.* University of Toronto Press.

Calixte, S., Johnson, J. L., & Motapanyane, M. (2016). Theorizing women's oppression and social change. In N. Mandell & J. L. Johnson (Eds.), *Feminist issues: Race, class, and sexuality,* 6th ed. (pp. 1–27). Toronto: Pearson Canada.

Cameron-Lewis, V. (2016). Escaping oppositional thinking in the teaching of pleasure and danger in sexuality education. *Gender and Education, 28*(4), 491–509. https://doi.org/10.1080/09540253.2016.1171297

Canadian Federation of Students. (2017). Fact sheet on sexual assault. Retrieved from https://cfsontario.ca/wp-content/uploads/2017/07/Factsheet-SexualAssault.pdf

Carmody, M. (2005). Ethical erotics: Reconceptualizing anti-rape education. *Sexualities, 8*(4), 465–480. https://doi.org/10.1177/1363460705056621

Carmody, M., & Ovenden, G. (2013). Putting ethical sex into practice: Sexual negotiation, gender and citizenship in the lives of young women and men. *Journal of Youth Studies, 16* (6), 792–807. https://doi.org/10.1080/13676261.2013.763916

CCI Research Inc. (2019). *Summary report of the Student Voices on Sexual Violence Survey.* Ministry of Training, Colleges and Universities (MTCU), Province of Ontario.

Cho, S., Crenshaw, K. W., & McCall, L. (2013). Toward a field of intersectionality studies: Theory, applications, and praxis. *Signs: The Journal of Women in Culture and Society, 38*(4), 785–810. https://doi.org/10.1086/669608

Close, S. M. (2005). Dating violence prevention in middle school and high school youth. *Journal of Child and Adolescent Psychiatric Nursing, 18*(1), 2–9. https://doi.org/10.1111/j.1744-6171.2005.00003.x

Connolly, J., & Josephson, W. (2007). Aggression in adolescent dating relationships: Predictors and prevention. *The Prevention Researcher, 14*(5), 3–6. https://doi.org/10.1037/e400292008-002

Conroy, S., and Cotter, A. Self-reported sexual assault in Canada, 2014. *Juristat.* Statistics Canada. Catalogue no. 85–002-X.

Cotter, A. (2018). Violent victimization of women with disabilities, 2014. Canadian Centre for Justice Statistics. Catalogue no. 85–002-X.

Cramer, E. P., Ross, A. I., McLeod, D. A., & Jones, R. (2015). The impact on peer facilitators of facilitating a school-based healthy relationship program for teens. *School Social Work Journal, 40*(1), 23–41.

Foshee, V. A., Bauman, K. E., Ennett, S. T., Linder, G. F., Benefield, T., & Suchindran, C. (2004). Assessing the long-term effects of the Safe Dates program and a booster in preventing and reducing adolescent dating violence victimization and perpetration. *American Journal of Public Health, 94*(4), 619–624. https://doi.org/10.2105/ajph.94.4.619

Gougeon, N. A. (2009). Sexuality education for students with intellectual disabilities, a critical pedagogical approach: outing the ignored curriculum. *Sex Education, 9*(3), 277–291. https://doi.org/10.1080/14681810903059094

Greater Sudbury Police Services (GSPS). (2018). *Annual/quarterly reports on domestic violence.* Sudbury, ON: Greater Sudbury Police Services.

Greig, C. J., & Pollard, B. (2016). Men, masculinities, and feminism. In N. Mandell & J. Johnson (Eds.), *Feminist Issues* (pp. 175–200). Toronto: Pearson Canada.

Grimmett, M. A., Conley, A. H., Foster, D., & Clark, C. W. (2018). A thematic analysis of the impact of My Masculinity Helps as a tool for sexual violence prevention. *Journal of Interpersonal Violence,* 1–19. https://doi.org/10.1177/0886260518772106

Guidi, E., Magnatta, G., and Meringolo, P. (2012). Teen dating violence: The need for early prevention. *Interdisciplinary Journal of Family Studies, 17*(1).

Hokoda, A., Del Campo, M. A. M., & Ulloa, E. C. (2012). Age and gender differences in teen relationship violence. *Journal of Aggression, Maltreatment & Trauma, 21*(3), 351–364. https://doi.org/10.1080/10926771.2012.659799

Hrynyk, M. M. (2018). *Towards the development of a culturally sensitive, empowerment-based sexual assault resistance model for Anishinaabe women* (Doctoral dissertation). Laurentian University of Sudbury).

I Am a Kind Man/Kizhaay Anishinaabe Niin Ojibway. (2019). *I Am a Kind Man.* Retrieved from: www.iamakindman.ca

Katz, J. (2006). *The macho paradox.* Naperville, IL: Sourcebooks.

Katz, J., & Earp, J. (1999). *Tough guise: Violence, media & the crises in masculinity.*

Katz, J., Heisterkamp, H. A., & Fleming, W. M. (2011). The social justice roots of the mentors in violence prevention model and its application in a high school setting. *Violence Against Women, 17*(6), 684–702. https://doi.org/10.1177/1077801211409725

Kernsmith, Poco D., & Hernandez-Jozefowicz, D.M. (2011). A gender-sensitive peer education program for sexual assault prevention in the schools. *Children & Schools, 33*(3), 146–157. https://doi.org/10.1093/cs/33.3.146

Kimmell, M. S. (2007). Masculinity as homophobia: Fear, shame and silence in the construction of gender identity. In N. Cook (Ed.), *Gender relations in global perspective: Essential readings* (pp. 73–82). Toronto: Canadian Scholars' Press.

Mallet, P., & Herbe, D. (2011) Does knowledge about sexuality prevent adolescents from developing rape-supportive beliefs? *Journal of Sex Research, 48*(4), 372–380. https://doi.org/10.1080/00224491003794048

Masters, T. (2010). "My Strength Is Not for Hurting": Men's anti-rape websites and their construction of masculinity and male sexuality. *Sexualities, 13*(1), 33–46. https://doi.org/10.1177/1363460709346115

McKenna, K. J. (2016). Violence against women in Canada. In N. Mandell & J. Johnson (Eds.), *Feminist Issues* (pp. 201–228). Toronto: Pearson Canada.

McLeod, D. A., Jones, R., & Cramer, E. P. (2015). An evaluation of a school-based, peer-facilitated, healthy relationship program for at-risk adolescents. *Children & Schools, 37*(2), 108–116. https://doi.org/10.1093/cs/cdv006

My Strength Is Not for Hurting. (2019). *My Strength Is Not for Hurting.* Retrieved from www.mystrength.org.

O'Leary, K. D., & Smith Slep, A. M. (2012). Prevention of partner violence by focusing on behaviors of both young males and females. *Prevention Science, 13*(4), 329–339. https://doi.org/10.1007/s11121-011-0237-2

Petering, R., Wenzel, S., & Winetrobe, H. (2014). Systematic review of current intimate partner violence prevention programs and applicability to homeless youth. *Journal of the Society for Social Work and Research, 5*(1), 107–135. https://doi.org/10.1086/675851

Ritchwood, Tiarney D., et al. (2015). The effect of Teach One Reach One (TORO) on youth acceptance of couple violence. *Journal of Child and Family Studies, 24*(12), 3805–3815. https://doi.org/10.1007/s10826-015-0188-5

Sense, Netherlands. (2019). *Internetseks.* Retrieved from https://sense.info /nl/werkstukinformatie/onderwerpen/internetseks

Shafer, A., Ortiz, R. R., Thompson, B., & Huemmer, J. (2018). The role of hypermasculinity, token resistance, rape myth, and assertive sexual consent communication among college men. *Journal of Adolescent Health, 62*(3), S44–S5.0. https://doi.org/10.1016/j.jadohealth.2017.10.015

Sheehy, E. (Ed.). (2012). *Sexual assault in Canada: Law, legal practice and women's activism.* Ottawa: University of Ottawa Press.

SIECCAN (Sex Information & Education Council of Canada). (2019). *Canadian guidelines for sexual health education.* Toronto, ON: SIECCAN. www.sieccan.org

Smith, P., & Welchans, S. (2000). Peer education: Does focusing on male responsibility change sexual assault attitudes? *Violence against Women, 6*(11), 1255–1268. https://doi.org/10.1177/10778010022183622

Sun, W. H., Miu, H. Y. H., Wong, C. K. H., Tucker, J. D., & Wong, W. C. W. (2018). Assessing participation and effectiveness of the peer-led approach in youth sexual health education: Systematic review and meta-analysis in more developed countries. *The Journal of Sex Research, 55*(1), 31–44. https://doi.org /10.1080/00224499.2016.1247779

Taylor, B. G., Stein, N, & Burden, F. F. (2010). Exploring gender differences in dating violence/harassment prevention programming in middle schools: Results from a randomized experiment. *Journal of Experimental Criminology, 6*(4), 419–445. https://doi.org/10.1007/s11292-010-9103-7

Violence Against Women Learning Network. (2018). *Violence against women with disabilities and deaf women.* Retrieved from http://www.vawlearningnetwork.ca/our-work/infographics/index.html

Weisz, A. N., & Black, B. M. (2010). Peer education and leadership in dating violence prevention: Strengths and challenges. *Journal of Aggression, Maltreatment & Trauma, 19*(6), 641–660. https://doi.org/10.1080/10926771.2010.502089

White Ribbon. (2019). *The White Ribbon Campaign.* Retrieved from http://www.whiteribbon.ca

5 The Down Low on Getting Down: Reframing Problem-Focused Narratives by Focusing on Sex-Positivity and Desire-Based Education

AMIE KROES

We live in a society that overtly sexualizes bodies in the name of capitalist marketing, yet openly shames persons for participating in, talking about, or learning about acts of sexuality. This discrepancy is in part responsible for uninformed sexual exploration that often leads to miscommunicated expectations, entitlement, and sexual violence. Due to political and moral disagreements about what is "appropriate" in earlier school years, it is often the case that 18- to 24-year-olds hear comprehensive information related to sexuality and sexual violence for the first time in postsecondary workshops. Typically, this is *after* they have had at least one sexual experience in their lives. Though students may not be getting comprehensive education before coming to postsecondary, this time of independence and experimentation is an ideal time to focus on both the dangers and the pleasures related to sex and sexuality(ies).

One of the most commonly discussed dangers related to sexuality is the topic of sexual violence. According to a recent survey completed at most postsecondary institutions in Ontario, 63% (university), 50% (college), and 30% (private career college) of students experienced at least once incident of sexual harassment in the past academic year (CCI Research, 2019). The same survey identified that 23% (university), 17% (college), and 10% (private career college) of students had experienced at least one nonconsensual sexual experience during the same time frame. Though efforts have been made to decrease rates of sexual violence, the occurrences remain largely unchanged over the last number of decades (Conroy & Cotter, 2017).

The provincial government in Ontario presented *It's Never Okay: Action Plan to Stop Sexual Violence and Harassment* (Bill 132, 2015), which was ratified and enacted in 2016 (Ontario, 2015). This legislative document highlighted several commitments, one of which mandated all colleges and universities to have sexual violence prevention programming. However, no direction was provided about best practice for prevention. The purpose of this chapter is to identify how postsecondary institutions have attempted to educate students in an effort to decrease the prevalence of sexual violence, and to make recommendations for future practice.

Locating Myself in the Work

At the beginning of my career as a social worker, I was working with a group of youth aged 14 to 18 years in a community setting. I provided programming and asked the group of young women what they wanted to learn about. I was quickly bombarded by questions such as if "queefing" was normal; how do you know when you have had an orgasm; and how to most effectively pleasure a man with your mouth. Though comfort level clearly varied within the group, their curiosity was evident. As I engaged in this conversation, I learned that these young women had (often incorrect) information, acquired from friends, the internet, and pornography, but no reliable, safe place to get accurate information. The experiences of these youth are not unique (Rye, Mashinter, Meaney, Wood, & Gentile, 2015), and unsurprisingly, I am asked many of the same questions in the postsecondary context. These experiences have reinforced for me that current prevention approaches, though encouraging, are not enough.

Current Prevention Strategies

A few main trends have emerged in addressing the prevention of sexual violence on campus. Newlands and O'Donohue (2016) suggest that "prevention programs with men, risk-reduction programs with women, ... and community-level programs (such as bystander-prevention/social-norms campaigns)" (p. 3) are the most effective. I will include psycho-education in this list as a recognized stand-alone intervention strategy. A review of the research below demonstrates that each type of prevention has its own benefits and challenges.

Psycho-Educational Approaches

Psycho-educational approaches to the topic of sexual violence, as popularized by Anderson, Hogarty, and Reiss (1980), often include material on the topics of consent, how to seek support after an experience of sexual harm, and how to help a friend who may have experienced sexual harm. Psycho-education can take the form of posters, pamphlets, digital marketing, online modules, and in-person workshops. All options demonstrate positive attitude change (Jouriles, Krauss, Vu, Banyard, & McDonald, 2018). There is also evidence to support the idea that most students have an awareness of the main issues and concepts related to sexual violence (Walsh, Banyard, Moynihan, Ward, & Cohn, 2010). However, many students lack knowledge about how to understand and apply the material they learn to their own lives. As an example, many students still believe that most sexual assaults are perpetrated by strangers (Hayes-Smith & Levett, 2010) and that perpetrators often target "pretty," white, cisgender, heterosexual women (Hockett, Saucier, & Badke, 2016). Although having an informed community is a legitimate goal, information needs to be presented in a way that not only identifies issues but also stimulates critical thinking and allows for application of knowledge. Without critical thought and application of knowledge, there is a missing link between awareness and behaviour change. Although attitudes may have changed, there is no evidence to support that attitude changes directly connect with decreasing incidents of sexual violence (DeGue et al., 2014).

Risk Reduction and Resistance Training for Women

Historically, sexual assault prevention involved safety tips for women on how to avoid sexual assault such as "Try not to walk alone at night but if you do, be alert" (CTV Ottawa, 2014, para. 7), and, "It's not just about keeping an eye on your drink but on how much you drink" (Weiss, 2017, para. 2). These safety techniques are heavily criticized as perpetuating myths and victim-blaming narratives (Femifesto, 2014, July; Grinberg, 2013, February 26). Programs have adapted to focus on empowerment and actively work against the problematic sexual assault myths (see Orchowski & Gidycz, 2018 for a review). In terms of resistance, there are examples of rigorously evaluated programs, such as Enhanced Access, Acknowledge and Act (Senn et al., 2015), Empowerment Self-Defense classes (Hollander, 2014, 2016), and the Ohio University Sexual Assault Risk Reduction Project (Gidycz et al., 2001).

Research about the effectiveness of resistance training for women has been mixed. While some programs found no differences in sexual victimization between those in the research and control groups (Gidycz et al., 2001; Gidycz et al., 2015), others found that women experienced fewer completed and attempted situations of sexual assault after participating in resistance training in comparison with women who engaged only with psycho-education (Senn et al., 2017). Further, multiple studies found that women who participated in resistance programs had more self-confidence and were less likely to believe myths about self-blame should an assault occur (Gidycz et al., 2015; Senn et al., 2015; Senn et al., 2017). Though sexual violence is still taking place, and programs need to target men and the deconstruction of male violence as a social norm (see Katz, 1995, 2018), lessening the negative impacts of harm is a positive finding.

Prevention with Men

Men are more likely to perpetrate sexual harm, regardless of the gender of their target (Conroy & Cotter, 2017), yet fewer than one third of prevention programs target male audiences (DeGue et al., 2014). Though women's movements have been highlighting the issue of male violence for decades, with the recent explosion of the #MeToo and the subsequent #TimesUp movement, working directly with men has been reignited as a mainstream priority. Given the relative infancy of programs directed toward men, there are few rigorously evaluated programs, and little is known about the impact of certain programs on men's behaviour. Of the programs that have been evaluated, such as the Mentors in Violence Prevention program (Katz, 1995), the Men's Program (Foubert, Newberry, & Tatum, 2007), and the Men's Workshop (Gidycz, Orchowski, & Berkowitz, 2011), some show promise for changing attitudes related to common risk factors of violence, but few have researched the impact on behaviour change. Furthermore, rebound effects have been found, in which change is identified shortly after the intervention but then participants slowly revert to old attitudes and behaviours (Gidycz et al., 2011; Newlands & O'Donohue, 2016). Sadly, there are no known programs specifically for men that discuss healthy sexuality explicitly.

Bystander Programs

Bystander-intervention programs are typically a mix between skill building and social-norm evaluations. From a skills-based perspective, bystander intervention is often grounded in the situational model of bystander behaviour (Burn, 2009; Latané & Darley, 1970) and is meant to help people identify possibly risky situations and the types of interventions that can mitigate risks. However, social-norm theory uses social-norm evaluation, a concept based on the hypothesis that if students believe that their peers agree with a specific behaviour, they are more likely to engage in said behaviour (Perkins & Berkowitz, 1986). Applied to sexual violence, if there is the perception – it does not need to be reality – that a peer group approves of coercive, aggressive sexual behaviours, social-norm theory would suggest that people are likely to act in accordance with that behaviour because of their desire to be a part of the group. The hope of these programs is to reframe social norms to highlight consent and mutual respect.

Although there are some programs that demonstrate positive effects on bystander behaviour, such as recognizing possibly risky situations and feeling capable of intervening should such a situation arise, few studies on bystander intervention specifically measure whether bystander intervention impacts perpetration of sexual assault (Jouriles et al., 2018; Katz & Moore, 2013). Therefore, more research is needed to identify if bystander intervention can impact the rates of sexual assault perpetration.

Critiquing Common Themes: Risk and Harm

Whether we are discussing psycho-education, risk-reduction strategies, programs for men, or bystander intervention, one common theme among all program types is the focus on risk and harm as they relate to sex and sexuality. Thus, most psycho-educational programs focus on identifying risks and behaviours to respond to such risks. Programs such as Don't Be That Guy (Sexual Assault Voices of Calgary, 2019), Who Will You Help (Ministry of the Status of Women, 2016, November 25), and Draw-the-Line (Draw The Line, 2019) are examples of psycho-educational approaches that highlight popular victim-blaming myths and problematic situations, and then challenge people to act in less harmful ways. There is value in risk identification and risk mitigation; however, risk is not the only narrative that should be applied to education and programming related to sexuality.

Likewise, risk-reduction and resistance strategies alone may empower women and provide defence skills that can reduce the likelihood of reoccurring sexual violence. Though this may limit available opportunities for perpetrators of harm, it may mean that sexual violence is still occurring, just with other targets. Also, risk-reduction programs for female-identified people can reinforce the stereotype that only women experience sexual harm and that their behaviours and choices can control whether they experience a sexual assault. Though risk-reduction and resistance strategies are demonstrating some positive outcomes, they would not be effective as a stand-alone prevention solution.

One criticism that arises in evaluating risk reduction in bystander intervention is that participants often do not evaluate situations between known parties as risky, even though this is the most likely situation they will encounter (Koelsch, Brown, & Boisen, 2012). People are often not looking for risks among their friends, roommates, family members, or partners. Alternatively, the riskiness of a situation is often based on external factors, such as how much alcohol a possible target of violence – typically a female – has consumed. Therefore, a person may act in good faith based on the information they learned in a bystander-intervention program by stopping a woman from sexually engaging with a potential partner because of her alcohol consumption. If the bystander is incorrect on the state of the woman's sobriety, intervening will mean taking the agency of her sexuality out of her hands. Bystander-intervention programs often discuss techniques such as deflection, distraction, telling an authority, or using groups to intervene; rarely do modules provide strategies on how to stop the potential perpetrator.

This focus on risk reduction in sexuality is not limited only to sexual violence. Other topics that are often stigmatized, such as contraception options, family planning, sexual health, and various forms of relationships outside of heterosexual monogamy, are often met with abstinence-type "education" (Ingham, 2005). The highest level of risk for most dangers related to sexuality is found in typical college-age demographics (Oulman, Kim, Yunis, & Tamim, 2015; Public Health Agency of Canada, 2017), so it is understandable that conscientious educators want to help young people avoid the challenges that come along with situations such as unplanned pregnancy and/or sexually transmitted infections. However, we do see examples of people knowingly disregarding risks (such as choosing not to use condoms) in the name of chasing pleasure. This has led to health-promotion programs opting for a harm-reduction approach by eroticizing safer sex (Philpott, Knerr, & Boydell, 2006).

The reality is that students have questions about their sexuality and few factually informative sources of information. Teaching students only about abstinence and risk does not speak to their lived experience. Strategies that attempt to bring attention to the prevalence of dangers and possible harm may be inadvertently promoting judgment-laden and shame-inducing messages about sexuality. When students hear messages that are incongruent with their own lived experience of sex, they may be less likely to engage. Engaging in sex-positive conversations, conversations where pleasure and desire are discussed openly and without judgment, while embracing diversity and simultaneously emphasizing the importance of consent and safety, is how we can meet the needs of the students and their inquisitive desire-based questions, while also fulfilling mandates to educate students about how to prevent risks.

Sex-Positive and Pleasure-Based Education

Focusing on desire is not a new idea but has not seemed to gain traction in mainstream prevention work. Fine (1988) has identified three main discourses in education as they relate to female sexuality:

specifically, "*sexuality as violence*," "*sexuality as victimization*," and "*sexuality as individual morality*" (pp. 31–32). Fine argues that we need to discontinue these narratives and instead focus on what she has coined as "*the discourse of desire*" (p. 33). Fine argues that if young women were encouraged to experiment with what feels good and desirable, then they would be better able to communicate those desires with their partners and negotiate needs and limits. More recently, researchers are finding that students want more information related to navigating sexual relationships and sexual pleasure (Hirst, 2013). By highlighting and celebrating sexual pleasure, we are teaching students that they are deserving of sexual pleasure. If students feel that desire and pleasure are normative sexual experiences, regardless of gender, they may be more able and willing to identify what they desire, to communicate these desires to their partners, and to feel justified in declining pressure or attempts at coercion (Cameron-Lewis & Allen, 2013; Hirst, 2013; Tolman, 2012).

Though it would be ideal to encourage assertive communication, social norms and social expectations based on gender roles make it difficult. When delivering programming to a group of female students, few identified that they can communicate their desires to their partners, due to a lack of confidence, feeling that they may hurt their partners' feelings, or concern that they will be perceived as "slutty" if they speak about their desires. Yet these same female workshop participants often say that good communication is a mandatory trait of a healthy relationship, with researchers agreeing that "extraordinary communication … [is] crucial for the experience of great sex" (Kleinplatz et al., 2009, p. 6).

Ways to Incorporate Sex Positivity

Some of the ways that community-based programs are having conversations about healthy sexuality, with both a sex-positive focus and a recognition of risk, is by highlighting the components of great sex and not being afraid to talk about a variety of diverse topics. Diverse topics can include themes such as using sex toys, kink culture, queer sex, and sex and disability (Jolly, 2016). It is important to normalize and make space for sex-positive conversation about multiple types of sex. For education to be socially relevant, whether it be in the classroom of any academic discipline, it must speak to the lived experiences of multiple social identities.

Another strategy employed is the use of humour and engaging the audience. A program targeting younger teens uses musical and dramatic art to engage the topic of sexuality and sexual violence, often having humour at the centre of the conversation (Gordon & Gere, 2016). Engaging the audience means straying from the traditional lecture-style workshop toward facilitated conversations in which activities help students interact with the material in a way that stimulates critical thinking and self-reflection (Jolly, 2016; Katz, 2018; Rich, 2010). Katz (2018) identifies this as "a supportive context to *experience* a new way of thinking" (p. 1767).

As demonstrated by the success of some resistance and bystander programs discussed earlier in this chapter, skill building is also a useful tool. As an example, a notable finding from resistance programs for women is the increase in self-efficacy: not only feeling confident in their physical self-defence strategies, but also in having the confidence to use assertive communication when feeling uncomfortable (Hollander, 2014). By including sex-positive topics, we can reframe the types of skills we want the audience to learn. Researchers studied the necessary components for "great sex" and found many themes that can all be linked to the ability to communicate assertively, negotiate boundaries, and connect in an authentic and respectful way (Kleinplatz et al., 2009). Knowing this, engaging audiences in skill-building workshops that focus on healthy communication of boundaries and respectful interactions with partners could be a useful strategy. We can also connect these same skills to those required to respectfully communicate boundaries in bystander situations or resistance situations, expanding content to include both sex-positive and risk-reduction conversations.

Sex Positive while Maintaining Safe Spaces

While we should strive to make prevention more engaging for students, it is also important to ensure that all content is delivered through a trauma-informed lens. Bearing in mind prevalence statistics, it is very likely that there are multiple survivors in the room. Being able to present material in a way that is safe(r) and empowering, while also recognizing resilience, is ideal. It is important to recognize that healthy sexual experiences are possible regardless of previous experiences of violence (Fava & Bay-Cheng, 2013). Therefore, sexualities education cannot be solely about risks or solely about pleasure. Sexuality education must also include information on how to negotiate needs with an understanding that one sexual situation may include both positive and negative experiences. It provides agency to students by communicating an unbiased, informative, and accurate portrayal of sex and sexuality (Cameron-Lewis & Allen, 2013; Pound et al., 2017).

Facilitator Choices and Facilitation Format

Evidence suggests that the most important aspect of facilitators is their comfort with the material. Through a global review of research, researchers found that "good sex educators enjoy teaching SRE [Sex and relationship education], have experiential knowledge and are comfortable with their own sexuality. They are professional, confident, unembarrassed, straightforward, experienced in talking about sex and use everyday language" (Pound et al., 2017, p. 6). Some programs prefer to use peer educators, or near-to-peer educators, while others prefer in-house or external experts. A review of multiple program outcomes found that the type of facilitator did not change the impact of program interventions (Jouriles et al., 2018). However, I would argue that using "in-group" facilitators – facilitators that best represent the demographic of the population being taught – would be an asset; for example, having male facilitators for men's groups (Katz, 2018), members of the LGBTQ+ community speaking to groups from the LGBTQ+ population (Jolly, 2016), or having an ex-athlete speak to a professional athletics club (Albury, Carmody, Evers, & Lumby, 2011). Diversity is often underrepresented in traditional conversations about sexuality and sexual violence prevention, and it can add credibility to facilitators if they have a good understanding of their audience.

Whether groups should be all gender or single gender is not consistently agreed (Jouriles et al., 2018). Although a review of programs showed no difference for bystander intervention programs by group composition (Jouriles et al., 2018), resistance programs and men's programs tend to be single gender. Katz (2018) has argued for a dual approach, recognizing the benefit of having mixed groups in which students get to hear from members of different genders, but then break out into single-gender groups for more "in-group" conversations. Katz (2018) highlights the importance of single-gender groups by saying,

> If single-gender sexual assault prevention workshops provide the space for men to have frank and unvarnished discussions about sensitive topics, women-only sessions can give women the opportunity to express opinions and share their experiences of sexism in a supportive setting where they do not have to worry about minimizing or defensive reactions from men. (p. 1770)

Accordingly, Katz (2018) is recognizing the need for a feeling of safety, but also recognizes that men and women have different perspectives on the issue of sexual violence. Additionally, educators need to consider how to make groups inclusive as well for trans and nonbinary folks.

The Role of Men: Addressing Patriarchy and Privilege

When analyzing men's programs, it must be noted that it has become the preferred method to engage with men as potential allies and bystanders, with most programs ignoring any discussion of the construction of masculine violence as a social norm. This approach is purposeful, limiting the rhetoric of "all men" as perpetrators and attempting to decrease the likelihood of defensiveness from male audiences (Albury et al., 2011; Gidycz et al., 2011; Katz, 2018). This defensiveness has been identified as "psychological reactance" or the "boomerang effect" (Sensenig & Brehm, 1968), in which outcomes turn out to be opposite to the intended effect of the intervention. Applied to sexual violence prevention, the boomerang effect shows itself when antiviolence campaigns increase, instead of decrease, the acceptance or probability of problematic behaviours. Social media has amplified some of these effects. Reviewing online responses to the #MeToo and #HowIWillChange online movements, PettyJohn, Muzzey, Maas, and McCauley (2018) found that while there were people who engaged in a positive way, others had "indignant resistance to social change" (p. 616) while some had "hostile resistance to social change" (p. 617).

Speaking to men as allies and bystanders may seem to protect against the boomerang effect by inviting men to participate in the conversation through a helping or leadership role (Katz, 2018; Rich, 2010). One of the criticisms of this approach is that speaking to men as only bystanders reinforces gender stereotypes and patriarchal power dynamics by inadvertently saying that women need to be saved, and men are the ones to do the saving. While it is true that we do not want to send the message that all men are perpetrators of violence, it is important to acknowledge that they do all benefit from a society based on patriarchy. Rich (2010) articulates how we can acknowledge possible feelings of discomfort or conflict when discussing complex issues related to privilege and possibly use said conflict to encourage students to be open to change because "conflict can be embraced as a crucial element of transformation" (p. 521). Thus, Katz (2018) and Rich (2010) both strategically place social justice as a main pillar within their intervention strategies to purposefully address the gendered dynamic of sexual violence and the role men need to play in addressing sexual violence. Katz argues that for a program to be effective, it is not just about teaching intervention skills to men, but also about encouraging critical dialogue to examine and "interrupt the enactment of abuses that are often micro manifestations of macro systems of power and control" (p. 1766).

Informed by feminist, intersectional, and antiracist analysis, power is viewed as central to the experience of sexual violence, especially when considering how it has been used historically in Western civilizations. Linder (2018) provides a comprehensive explanation of how social identities, which are given meaning through social construction (e.g., gender, race, sexual orientation, and ability), interact with systems of oppression. Linder goes on to explain how these systems of oppression (e.g., sexism, racism, homophobia, transphobia, and ableism) provide people in dominant groups with more privilege. Additionally, in terms of the importance of intersectional understanding, as a white, pansexual, able-bodied, cisfemale, I recognize that I have multiple privileged identities. I also must recognize the positionality(ies) of the people with whom I work. For instance, once when I was having a group conversation about bystander intervention, students suggested contacting authority figures as a tactic they could use in a harmful situation. In contrast, one of the female participants, who identified her immigrant status, discussed how in her experience, calling the police was not safe. Another racialized female in the room agreed, while many white women in the room could not relate. This example is not uncommon (Bang, Kerrick, & Wuthrich, 2017), demonstrating that the intersection of race and gender creates a different dynamic than just race or gender independently. More importantly, prevalence statistics demonstrate that racialized women, people who are a part of the LGBTQ+ community, and people who have disAbilities, experience sexual violence at higher rates than white, straight, cisgender, and able peers (Conroy & Cotter, 2017; Porter & McQuiller Williams, 2011). People with intersecting marginalized identities experience sexual violence at even higher rates (Coulter et al., 2017). Because power and privilege benefit some identities at the cost of others, it is imperative to address the root causes of sexual violence in our communities (Hong, 2017; Katz, 2018; Linder, 2018).

Bringing It All Together: Recommendations

From common trends, institutions of higher education tend to pick one or two prevention programs and use those as their sole strategy for sexual violence prevention. However, advocates identify that an integrated approach is more appropriate (Linder, 2018; Orchowski et al., 2018; Palacios & Aguilar, 2017). Orchowski et al. (2018) highlight the common foundations, between resistance, bystander, and men's programs – specifically, the aim to increase knowledge and awareness but also to build skills and strategies for the reduction and elimination of sexual violence. Each type of prevention program is unique and works to target a different audience. Program goals are not only to increase the amount of people participating in programs, but also to reinforce messages through a variety of teaching methods, with each new interaction acting like a booster session. This hopefully reduces the possibility of rebound effects. Implementing an integrated and comprehensive approach also means embedding content related to sex-positive healthy sexuality. While each institution may promote its own programming, booster sessions can be made available through classroom conversations by embedding sex and sexuality(ies) into the curriculum of multiple disciplines.

Conversations related to healthy sexuality must stay socioculturally relevant, providing information that students want. A component of being socioculturally relevant includes programs built for a variety of populations. Using a power-conscious social justice lens, it is important to understand for whom programs are meant, and whom they may intentionally or unintentionally exclude. These are good steps in evaluating if programs are accessible to diverse populations. It is important to ensure that all students see themselves represented in awareness-raising campaigns, but also in the action phase of intervention. An example could be ensuring that resistance programs for women are open to cis women and trans women and to people with differing levels of ability. Another is to engage with traditionally marginalized groups to better understand their lived experiences and establish content that speaks to the common dynamics of their lives. This means that content is not only "open" for anyone but also truly accessible and useful for all.

Conclusion

Instead of attempting to create a one-size-fits-all approach, creating multiple different programs targeting different audiences with the ability for overlap is recommended. Prevention strategies can be crafted in a way similar to classroom curriculum design, in which information is presented in thematic modules that scaffold on each other. To ensure diversity, sex positivity, and trauma-informed curriculum design are delivered, educators must reevaluate the learning objectives targeted within their programs. There should be emphasis on empowering students to recognize and critically question the root causes of sexual violence and how they may permit or promote harm, while also being able to identify and participate in desire-based conversations. To create transformational experiences for students, conversations must include both the risks and pleasures associated with sexuality.

REFERENCES

Albury, K., Carmody, M., Evers, C., & Lumby, C. (2011). Playing by the rules: Researching, teaching and learning sexual ethics with young men in the Australian National Rugby League. *Sex Education, 11*(3), 339–351. https://doi.org/10.1080/14681811.2011.590332

Anderson, C. M., Hogarty, G. E., & Reiss, D. J. (1980). Family treatment of adult schizophrenic patients: A psycho-educational approach. *Schizophrenia Bulletin, 6*(3), 490–505. https://doi.org/10.1093/schbul/6.3.490

Bang, A., Kerrick, A., & Wuthrich, C. K. (2017). Examining bystander intervention in the wake of #blacklivesmatter and #translivesmatter. In S. C. Wooten & R. W. Mitchell (Eds.), *Preventing sexual violence on campus: Challenging traditional approaches through program innovation* (pp. 65–85). New York: Routledge.

Burn, S. M. (2009). A situational model of sexual assault prevention through bystander intervention. *Sex Roles: A Journal of Research, 60*(11–12), 779–792. https://doi.org/10.1007/s11199-008-9581-5

Cameron-Lewis, V., & Allen, L. (2013). Teaching pleasure *and* danger in sexuality education. *Sex Education, 13*(2), 121–132. https://doi.org/10.1080/14681811.2012.697440

CCI Research. (2019). Summary report of the student voices on sexual violence survey. Retrieved from https://files.ontario.ca/tcu-summary-report-student-voices-on-sexual-violence-survey-en-2019-03.pdf

Conroy, S., & Cotter, A. (2017). *Self-reported sexual assault in Canada, 2014.* (Catalogue No. 85-002-X). Retrieved from Statistics Canada: https://www150.statcan.gc.ca/n1/en/pub/85-002-x/2017001/article/14842-eng.pdf?st=U__8u-A4

Coulter, R., Mair, C., Miller, E., Blosnich, J., Matthews, D., & McCauley, H. (2017). Prevalence of past-year sexual assault victimization among undergraduate students: Exploring differences by and intersections of gender identity, sexual identity, and race/ethnicity. *Prevention Science, 18*, 1–11. https://doi.org/10.1007/s11121-017-0762-8

CTV Ottawa. (2014, July 14). Ottawa police investigate two sexual assaults in city's west-end. Retrieved from https://ottawa.ctvnews.ca/ottawa-police-investigate-two-sexual-assaults-in-city-s-west-end-1.1914522

DeGue, S., Valle, L. A., Holt, M. K., Massetti, G. M., Matjasko, J. L., & Tharp, A. T. (2014). A systematic review of primary prevention strategies for sexual violence perpetration. *Aggression and Violent Behaviour, 19*, 346–362. https://doi.org/10.1016/j.avb.2014.05.004

Draw the Line. (2019). *Engaging Ontarians in a dialogue about sexual violence.* Retrieved from http://www.draw-the-line.ca/index.html

Fava, N. M., & Bay-Cheng, L. Y. (2013). Trauma-informed sexuality education: Recognizing the rights and resilience of youth. *Sex Education, 13*(4), 383–394. https://doi.org/10.1080/14681811.2012.745808

Femifesto. (2014, July 18). *How to not get raped.* Retrieved from http://www
.femifesto.ca/how-to-not-get-raped/

Fine, M. (1988). Sexuality, schooling, and adolescent females: The missing
discourse of desire. *Harvard Educational Review, 58,* 29–53. https://doi.org
/10.17763/haer.58.1.u0468k1v2n2n8242

Foubert, J. D., Newberry, J. T., & Tatum, J. L. (2007). Behaviour differences seven
months later: Effects of a rape prevention program. *Journal of Student Affairs
Research and Practice, 44*(4), 728–749. https://doi.org/10.2202/1949-6605.1866

Gidycz, C. A., Lynn, S. J., Rich, C. L., Marioni, N. L., Loh, C., Blackwell, L.
M., … Pashdag, J. (2001). The evaluation of a sexual assault risk reduction
program: A multisite investigation. *Journal of Consulting and Clinical Psychology,
69*(6), 1073–1078. https://doi.org/10.1037/0022-006x.69.6.1073

Gidycz, C. A., Orchowski, L. M., & Berkowitz, A. D. (2011). Preventing
sexual aggression among college men: An evaluation of a social norms
and bystander intervention program. *Violence Against Women, 17,* 720–742.
https://doi.org/10.1177/1077801211409727

Gidycz, C. A., Orchowski, L. M., Probst, D. R., Edwards, K. M., Murphy, M., &
Tansill, E. (2015). Concurrent administration of sexual assault prevention
and risk reduction programming: Outcomes for women. *Violence Against
Women, 21*(6), 780–800. https://doi.org/10.1177/1077801215576579

Gordon, R., & Gere, D. (2016). Sex squad: Engaging humour to reinvigorate
sexual health education. *Sex Education, 16*(3), 324–336. https://doi.org
/10.1080/14681811.2015.1120193

Grinberg, E. (2013, February 26). Beyond vomiting, how to prevent rape.
CNN. Retrieved from https://www.cnn.com/2013/02/26/living/colorado
-university-rape-prevention-tips/index.html

Hayes-Smith, R. M., & Levett, L. M. (2010). Student perceptions of sexual
assault resources and prevalence of rape myth attitudes. *Feminist Criminology,
5*(4), 335–354. https://doi.org/10.1177/1557085110387581

Hirst, J. (2013). "It's got to be about enjoying yourself": Young people, sexual
pleasure, and sex and relationships education. *Sex Education, 13*(4), 423–436.
https://doi.org/10.1080/14681811.2012.747433

Hockett, J. M., Saucier, D. A., & Badke, C. (2016). Rape myths, rape scripts,
and common rape experiences of college women: Differences in perceptions
of women who have been raped. *Violence Against Women, 22*(3), 307–323.
https://doi.org/10.1177/1077801215599844

Hollander, J. A. (2014). Does self-defense training prevent sexual violence
against women? *Violence Against Women, 20,* 252–269. https://doi.org/10.1177
/1077801214526046

Hollander, J. A. (2016). The importance of self-defense training for sexual
violence prevention. *Feminism & Psychology, 26,* 207–226. https://doi.org
/10.1177/0959353516637393

Hong, L. (2017). Digging up the roots, rustling up the leaves: A critical consideration of the root causes of sexual violence and why higher education needs more courage. In J. C. Harris & C. Linder (Eds.), *Intersections of identity and sexual violence no campus: Centering minoritized students experiences* (pp. 194–213). Sterling, VA: Stylus Publishing, LLC.

Ingham, R. (2005). "We didn't cover that at school": Education *against* pleasure or education *for* pleasure? *Sex Education, 5*(4), 375–388. https://doi.org/10.1080/14681810500278451

Jolly, S. (2016). Positive approaches to sexuality and new normative frames: Strands of research and action in China and the USA. *Sex Education, 16*(3), 294–307. https://doi.org/10.1080/14681811.2015.1091767

Jouriles, E. N., Krauss, A., Vu, N. L., Banyard, V, L., & McDonald, R. (2018). Bystander programs addressing sexual violence on college campuses: A systematic review and meta-analysis of program outcomes and delivery methods. *Journal of American College Health, 66*(6), 457–466. https://doi.org/10.1080/07448481.2018.1431906

Katz, J. T. (1995). Reconstructing masculinity in the locker room: Mentors in violence prevention. *Harvard Educational Review, 65*, 163–174. https://doi.org/10.17763/haer.65.2.55533188520136u1

Katz, J. T. (2018). Bystander training as leadership training: Notes on the origins, philosophy, and pedagogy of the Mentors in Violence Prevention model. *Violence Against Women, 24*(15), 1755–1776. https://doi.org/10.1177/1077801217753322

Katz, J., & Moore, J. (2013). Bystander education training for campus sexual assault prevention: An initial meta-analysis. *Violence and Victims, 28*, 1057–1067. https://doi.org/10.1891/0886-6708.vv-d-12-00113

Kleinplatz, P. J., Ménard, A. D., Paquet, M-P., Paradis, N., Campbell, M., Zuccarino, D., et al. (2009). The components of optimal sexuality: A portrait of "great sex." *The Canadian Journal of Human Sexuality, 18*, 1–13.

Koelsch, L. E., Brown, A. L., & Boisen, L. (2012). Bystander perceptions: Implications for university sexual assault prevention programs. *Violence and Victims, 27*(4), 563–579. https://doi.org/10.1891/0886-6708.27.4.563

Latané, B., & Darley, J. M. (1970). *The unresponsive bystander: Why doesn't he help.* New York: Appleton Century Crofts.

Linder, C. (2018). *Sexual violence on campus: Power-conscious approaches to awareness, prevention and response.* Bingley UK: Emerald Publishing Ltd.

Ministry of the Status of Women. (2016, November 25). Award winning #whowillyouhelp campaign continues to raise awareness and challenge norms. Retrieved from https://news.ontario.ca/owd/en/2016/11/award-winning-whowillyouhelp-campaign-continues-to-raise-awareness-and-challenge-norms.html

Newlands, R., & O'Donohue, W. (2016). A critical review of sexual violence prevention on college campuses. *Acta Psychopathol, 2*(2), 2–14. https://doi.org/10.4172/2469-6676.100040

Ontario. (2015). *It's never okay: An action plan to stop sexual violence and harassment.* Retrieved from http://docs.files.ontario.ca/documents/4136/mi-2003-svhap -report-en-for-tagging-final-2-up-s.pdf

Orchowski, L. M., Edwards, K. M., Hollander, J. A., Banyard, V. L., Senn, C. Y., & Gidycz, C. A. (2018). Integrating sexual assault resistance, bystander, and men's social norms strategies to prevent sexual violence on college campuses: A call to action. *Trauma, Violence and Abuse.* Advance online publication. https://doi.org/10.1177/1524838018789153

Orchowski, L. M., & Gidycz, C. A. (Eds.). (2018). *Sexual assault risk reduction and resistance: Theory research and practice.* London, UK: Academic Press.

Oulman, E., Kim, T.H.M., Yunis, K., & Tamim, H. (2015). Prevalence and predictors of unintended pregnancy among women: An analysis of the Canadian Maternity Experience Survey. *BioMed Central Pregnancy and Childbirth, 15,* 1–8. https://doi.org/10.1186/s12884-015-0663-4

Palacios, N. C., & Aguilar, K. L. (2017). An empowerment-based model of sexual violence intervention and prevention on campus. In J. C. Harris & C. Linder (Eds.), *Intersections of identity and sexual violence on campus: Centering minoritized students experiences* (pp. 194–213). Sterling, VA: Stylus Publishing, LLC.

Perkins, H. W., & Berkowitz, A. D. (1986). Perceiving the community norms of alcohol use among students: Some research implications for campus alcohol education programming. *International Journal of the Addictions, 21,* 961–976. https://doi.org/10.3109/10826088609077249

PettyJohn, M. E., Muzzey, F. K., Maas, M. K., & McCauley, H. L. (2019). #HowIWillChange: Engaging men and boys in the #MeToo movement. *Psychology of Men & Masculinities, 20*(4), 612–622. https://doi.org/10.1037 /men0000186

Philpott, A., Knerr, W., & Boydell., V. (2006). Pleasure and prevention: When good sex is safer sex. *Reproductive Health Matters, 14*(28), 23–31. https:// doi.org/10.1016/s0968-8080(06)28254-5

Porter J., & McQuiller Williams, L. (2011). Intimate violence among underrepresented groups on a college campus. *Journal of Interpersonal Violence, 26*(16), 3210–3224. https://doi.org/10.1177/0886260510393011

Pound, P., Denford, S., Shucksmith, J., Tanton, C., Johnson, A. M., Owen, J., et al. (2017). What is best practice in sex and relationship education? A synthesis of evidence, including stakeholders' views. *British Medical Journal Open, 7,* 1–11. https://doi.org/10.1136/bmjopen-2016-014791

Public Health Agency of Canada. (2017, May). *Report on sexually transmitted infections in Canada: 2013–2014.* (ISSN: 1923–2977). Retrieved from https:// www.canada.ca/en/public-health/services/publications/diseases-conditions /report-sexually-transmitted-infections-canada-2013-14.html

Rich, M. D. (2010). The interACT model: Considering rape prevention from a performance activism and social justice perspective. *Feminism & Psychology, 20*(4), 511–528. https://doi.org/10.1177/0959353510371366

Rye, B. J., Mashinter, C., Meaney, G. J., Wood, E., & Gentile, S. (2015). Satisfaction with previous sexual health education as a predictor of intentions to pursue further sexual health education. *Sex Education, 15*(1), 93–107. https://doi.org/10.1080/14681811.2014.967389

Senn, C. Y., Eliasziw, M., Barata, P. C., Thurston, W. E., Newby-Clark, I. R., Radtke, H. L., et al. (2015). Efficacy of a sexual assault resistance program for university women. *New England Journal of Medicine, 372*, 2326–2335. https://doi.org/10.1056/nejmsa1411131

Senn, C. Y., Eliasziw, M., Hobden, K. L., Newby-Clark, I. R., Barata, P. C., Radtke, H. L., et al. (2017). Secondary and 2-year outcomes of sexual assault resistance program for university women. *Psychology of Women Quarterly, 41*(2), 147–162. https://doi.org/10.1177/0361684317690119

Sensenig, J., & Brehm, J. W. (1968). Attitude change from an implied threat to attitudinal freedom. *Journal of Personality and Social Psychology, 8*(4), 324–330. https://doi.org/10.1037/h0021241

Sexual Assault Voices of Calgary. (2019). *Don't be that guy*. Retrieved from http://www.savcalgary.ca/

Tolman, D. L. (2012). Female adolescents, sexual empowerment and desire: A missing discourse of gender inequity. *Sex Roles, 66*(11), 746–757. https://doi.org/10.1007/s11199-012-0122-x

Walsh, W. A., Banyard, V. L., Moynihan, M. M., Ward, S., & Cohn, E. S. (2010). Disclosure and service use on a college campus after an unwanted sexual experience. *Journal of Trauma & Dissociation, 11*, 134–151. https://doi.org/10.1080/15299730903502912

Weiss, S. (2017, September 2). College's anti-drinking poster victim-blames sexual assault survivors. *Teen Vogue*. Retrieved from https://www.teenvogue.com/story/victim-blaming-sexual-assault-drinking-posters

6 Transgender Experiences in Healthcare: Addressing Challenges while Teaching Compassion in Higher Education

COLLEEN MCMILLAN, MIKE LEE-POY, AND CARYS MASSARELLA

A multitude of systemic factors converge to make the experience of accessing basic healthcare problematic for transgender individuals. For this chapter, we use the definition transgender, adapted from Dubin et al., 2018), to include people whose gender identity differs from their sex assigned at birth, as well as those known as gender non-binary or gender nonconforming, whose gender identity does not conform to conventional binary gender categories (p. 377). We also acknowledge that definitions vary by geographic region and by individual and are considered fluid and evolving (American College of Obstetricians and Gynecologists, 2011). Being mindful of language, the risk of homogenizing transgender individuals as being the same, and the necessity of recognizing the importance of cultural diversity, we include the term "Two-spirited" as part of our definitions. This term is used by Indigenous peoples in Canada and is a translation of the Anishinaabemowin term *niizh manidoowag* or Two-spirit. Two-spirit people may also use terms akin to their own Indigenous language to describe same-sex attraction or gender variance, such as *winkt* (Lakota) or *nàdleehé* (Dinéh) (Brotman, Ryan, Jalbert, & Rowe, 2002). Please see Box 6.1 for definitions of various terms relevant to working with trans individuals in healthcare, adapted from the Ontario Human Rights Commission (n.d.).

Regardless of the terms used, what transverses all definitions are the multiple and intersecting micro and macro discourses that result in healthcare being experienced as unsafe for some, regardless of practice context. The following is an excerpt of an actual case that took place in Ontario:

Nine months ago, Wesly Heney, near collapse from viral pneumonia, was taken by ambulance to a large teaching hospital near his home in London,

---

Box 6.1: Definitions of Relevance to Healthcare

Cisgender: Applies to individuals whose gender identity is congruent with their sex assigned at birth.

Transgender: Applies to individuals whose gender identity is different than their sex assigned at birth.

Trans: An umbrella term used to describe individuals who do not identify as cisgender. This includes not only those who identify as transgender but also those with identities that fit outside of the male-female binary. These identities include but are not limited to *trans man, trans woman, gender non-conforming, agender, nongendered, genderqueer, nonbinary, two-spirit,* and *third gender.*

Ontario. Paramedics asked whether he took any medications, so Heney disclosed that as a transgender person (female-to-male, or FTM) he was taking injectable testosterone. While he was waiting in the hospital hallway on a gurney, a nurse came over to put on his patient ID bracelet. "She must have heard the paramedics' report," Heney surmises, "because she referred to me as 'it.'" Later, Heney heard two nurses arguing about who would do his blood draw because, "neither of them wanted to touch me." (as cited in Henkel, 2014, p. 1)

Despite such discrimination being well documented in healthcare through the efforts of government-funded programs and community-advocacy groups such as Rainbow Health Ontario, there appears to exist a poor transfer of clinical practice knowledge to curriculum development within higher institutions (Morrison, Wilson, & Smith, 2017). This chapter presents a space to explore the more deeply embedded reasons for ongoing micro-aggressions against this group of individuals, especially given that they have an equal right to compassionate and competently informed healthcare. Two health practice contexts that illuminate the lack of knowledge, inclusive language, and documentation, and where discriminatory altitudes prevail, are the family physician's office and the emergency room. By drawing upon actual case-based examples from these two settings, we hope to narrow the practice-to-curriculum gap by labelling the types of covert and overt prejudicial acts that occur and, more importantly, how such acts can serve as lessons for learners about to enter healthcare as direct-care practitioners and the educators who teach them.

Literature Review

Current literature elucidates the existence of substandard health practices confronting transgender individuals who seek care either from their family physician and/or in their local emergency department, with such practices ranging from overt discrimination, as in refusing to provide care, to more subtle forms of othering, as in using incorrect pronouns. Several recent Canadian studies speak to these occurrences and contextually provide a wider backdrop in order to understand the myriad of barriers this population experiences when seeking healthcare. A phenomenological study of 11 transgender individuals living in Kingston, Ontario, found that all participants experienced some form of discrimination, ranging from a single to multiple episodes, with their family physicians (Bell & Purkey, 2019). The most commonly reported discriminatory acts are misgendering and being refused care by the physician (Bell & Purkey, 2019). While the participants acknowledged that misgendering acts were remedied when pointed out, others believed such acts were malicious or intentional and may have reflected underlying feelings of practitioner transphobia. While transgender individuals routinely tolerate such acts as an expected consequence in order to receive care (Rotzinger, 2018), the known accumulated outcome of these micro-aggressions is anxiety, depression, and emotional distress (Kattari, Walls, Speer, & Kattari, 2016). The discomfort experienced by transgender individuals is supported quantitatively by an Ontario study that explored the patient-physician relationship. In this study trans female individuals reported having three or more negative experiences with their family physicians, as compared to trans male individuals, who reported two such encounters (Bauer, Zong, Scheim, Hammond, & Thind, 2015). The most common negative experience reported was being told by physicians that they did not know enough about trans-related health to provide care. The authors of this study questioned whether this in fact was true, meaning educational training in transgender health was indeed absent, or if providers assumed that trans-specific knowledge was needed to practice competently.

Acts of nuanced hostility toward transgender patients are not just limited to family practice offices. Transgender individuals reported multiple acts of discriminatory behaviour in the emergency department to the degree that urgent care was avoided for fear of judgement and humiliation (Bauer, Scheim, Deutsch, & Massarella, 2014). A study of 433 transgender patients, also in Ontario, found that 29% avoided going to the emergency room when warranted for reasons of fear, ridicule, humiliation, or dismissal, suggesting a burden of unmet need in this population (Bauer, Scheim, Deutsch, & Massarella, 2014). Similarly, a self-report questionnaire distributed to 152 transgender individuals living in 40 American states asked about care received related to their gender identity or presentation (Kosenko, Rintamaki, Raney, & Maness, 2013). The study found insensitive and uninformed care extended beyond the physician to include nurses, allied professionals, and emergency technicians and represented six themes: gender insensitivity; displays of discomfort; denied services; substandard care; verbal abuse; and forced care.

To self-protect against such discriminatory acts from healthcare providers, many individuals resorted to online purchasing of prescription medications. A review of eight clinical cases of individuals who were pursing gender-affirming surgery found the two main reasons medications for the purposes of masculination (testosterone preparations) or feminisation (estradiol preparations) were purchased over the internet were the lack of access to specialists due to discrimination and long wait lists (Metastasio, Negri, Martinotti, & Corazza, 2018). The American College of Obstetricians and Gynecologists estimates more than 50% of persons who identified as transgender have used injected hormones that were obtained illegally or used outside of conventional medical settings (ACOG, 2011). Such risky behaviours were expressed as being more tolerable, despite potentially serious health repercussions (National Center for Transgender Equality, 2016). Hormonal treatment without medical supervision poses significant consequences (Brown & Fu, 2013). Despite the risks, it is estimated 43% of trans individuals are currently using hormones, with 11% obtaining hormones from nonmedical sources, including a friend or relative, the street, strangers, and internet pharmacies (Rotondi et al., 2013). The need to seek medications from unauthorized virtual sites draws attention to the myriad of structural barriers that impede safe and compassionate care.

In addition to using hormonal treatments purchased from nonlegitimate online sites, there also exists the more extreme avenue of individuals performing self-surgery –referred to as DIY assignment – as a result of systemic rejections for gender reassignment surgery (Rotondi et al., 2013). Other systemic barriers, including treatments being deemed ineligible for insurance coverage, inappropriate electronic records, forms, lab references (Cahill & Makadon, 2014), and inclusive clinic facilities (Safer et al., 2016), all converge to become significant emotional, psychological, and logistical impediments for transgender patients. Additionally, social determinants such as adequate housing and poverty-line income reflect ingrained negative societal attitudes regarding transgender persons and their basic human rights (Scheim, Bauer, & Coleman, 2016).

If these acts of clinical and societal discriminatory behaviours are regularly observed and experienced by transgendered individuals in both family practice offices and emergency rooms alike, then the obvious question arises of what is being done about this chronic condition of marginalization of and substandard healthcare for a vulnerable group. To extend this point into the realm of medical education, lauded to be in an era of patient-centered medicine (Rosen & Hoang, 2017), how can exclusion of knowledge about sexuality(ies) be condoned within medical curriculum across medical schools in universities? If partnership is a key tenet of patient-centred care, one questions then, how this translates to a clinical setting, where the transgender patient is expected to assume the role of educator to the physician.

Roter and Hall (2006) state that despite ample evidence of the benefits of enhanced communication skills such as higher patient satisfaction, better treatment partnerships, and heightened clinical outcomes, most medical schools devote little time and attention to communication. When it comes to the ability to speak compassionately, in an informed manner reflective of the diversity of populations seeking healthcare, the curriculum for medical learners is dismal. In medicine, communication skills tend to be taught in a deficient-oriented or problem-based-learning (PBL) way because they are "easier to teach" (Simmenroth-nayda, Weiss, Fischer, & Himmel, 2012, p. 8). The ability to show empathy or respect was found to require a strong influence of innate emotional and cultural sources that not all individuals possess. Such skill development is required if the deeper issue of embedded biases and prejudices toward transgender individuals are to be identified and rooted out within higher institutions of learning.

Unconscious Bias, Assumptions, and Humility
Issues Outside the Classroom

Sukhera and Chahine (2016) argue that traditional pedagogy masks unidentified or unrealized biases, reproducing negative or pejorative perspectives against those patients who are labelled as different. Instead, they promote a concept referred to as "unconscious bias informed education," described as "a systematic approach to address implicit biases in healthcare, through content awareness and understanding in order to improve compassion and empathy" (p. 2). As practicing healthcare professionals, we endorse Sukhera and Chahine's (2016) approach but argue it does not go far enough, as it fails to recognize the unique pedagogical emphasis placed on student fieldwork in healthcare professions such as medicine, pharmacy, nursing, and social work. A cornerstone to these professions is an extensive practicum in which the learner engages in experiential learning with patients under the guidance of a clinical preceptor or supervisor. While teaching about unconscious bias in a classroom is important and establishes a template for understanding when in practice, it is during clinical encounters that unconscious biases and assumptions organically surface and become problematic for transgender individuals. The case presented in Box 6.2 highlights the importance of creating a learning environment within clinical rotations that facilitate discussions within the moment when a rupture has occurred caused by health provider prejudice or assumption.

This case highlights the need for practitioner humility in the moment. The literature on the importance of transparency within the clinical encounter raises an interesting paradox regarding what physicians state is essential when such a mistake occurs versus the corresponding remedial behaviour actually taken. A survey of 149 patients were asked if they felt it was important for their physician to acknowledge a mistake, regardless of how minor, should one occur (Witman, Park, & Hardin, 1996). Virtually all patients (98%) stated that some acknowledgment was needed, regardless of how minor the error was, to avoid the physician-patient relationship being harmed. The same question was also asked of physicians in a study reported by Anwer and Abu-Zaid (2014). When presented with a hypothetical question involving a medical error, 90% of the 538 physicians and medical residents surveyed stated they would disclose and address the mistake with the patient, yet in real-life situations only 41% confirmed actually doing so (Kaldjian et al., 2007). This discrepancy was explored by Anwer and Abu-Zaid (2014), who identified an absence in the curriculum specific to physician mistakes and transparency. They found that in higher institutions, formal instruction regarding mistakes and transparency was "largely negligible and not adequately instructed in the vast majority of undergraduate medical education curricula" (p. 1). This lack of preparedness fosters little confidence in medical students who may feel ill prepared or uncomfortable with disclosing their mistakes in the moment, which requires a willingness to admit wrongdoing as part of professional humility. Without adequate in-class exploration of prejudices and a priori assumptions held by the healthcare provider, the probability of the physician–patient relational rupture described in the case is likely to be repeated, highlighting one reason why many transgender patients state feeling unsafe.

The next case, presented in Box 6.3, highlights the importance of various challenges, and not only for learners. Implicit bias and assumptions left unaddressed inform practice decisions by even the most experienced and compassionate healthcare providers. Experience and knowledge are

Box 6.2: Case 1 – The Importance of Immediacy in Addressing Prejudices within Clinical Encounters

As the primary physician, I had a follow-up appointment with Rosalyn that was noted as "for medication review." I was surprised when I went into the room and she mentioned that she experienced an uncomfortable encounter with my medical student the other week but had hesitated to bring it up with the learner up at the time.

Rosalyn was a 40-year-old trans woman who transitioned later in life. She had experienced significant of transphobia that delayed the timing of her transitioning. For this reason, she was always very eager to be involved in teaching clinics and helping to educate physicians of tomorrow. She has always shown patience and openness with medical learners.

In this particular encounter, Rosalyn was coming in for a visit to update her immunizations. The medical learner took the opportunity to review her chart and discuss other aspects of preventive medicine. Roslyn welcomed this opportunity. During the chart review, the medical student pointed out to Rosalyn that she did not have a pap smear on record. The medical student then continued to review the relevant guidelines and asked Rosalyn if she was sexually active. Rosalyn replied yes, but before she could explain why she did not have a pap the previous year, the medical student began a long narrative about the evidence behind paps. This narrative was based on the assumption that Rosalyn was against preventive screening. Rosalyn eventually interrupted the medical student mid-sentence to mention that she was a trans woman, meaning she did not have a cervix. The medical student appeared flustered, stated she was aware Rosalyn was trans, but then failed to realize why a pap test was unnecessary. Unable to process this information in the moment, the medical student continued listing off a long list of female preventive screening guidelines, including those for cervical cancer, stating the necessity of such guidelines for "normal" for "natural" women.

Rosalyn later expressed she felt demeaned by the language of "normal" and "natural." She had come to accept that she needed to educate medical learners during past clinical encounters but had never felt this demoralized. She did not feel safe challenging the medical learner in that moment. After listening to Rosalyn, I thanked her for this feedback and asked how she would like this situation addressed. She gave permission for me, as the clinical preceptor, to have a conversation with the medical learner.

Box 6.3: Case 2 – The Necessity of Ongoing Critical Reflection as a Practitioner to Identify "Blind Spots"

I had first heard about M from one of the outreach workers who worked at the clinic. M was a young female-assigned-at-birth person, who, according to several sources, was experiencing intense gender dysphoria, with a desire to remove their breasts, unconcerned of possible consequences. M also had a diagnosis of significant intellectual disability. His mental health providers in the community were concerned that he was experiencing a form of delusional disorder with regards to his body and were unwilling to entertain the diagnosis of gender dysphoria.

As a practicing transgender physician, I had, at that time, no experience with a patient with gender dysphoria and intellectual disability. I was reluctant to proceed with care that was heightened by the lack of available literature, or even case reports, regarding gender dysphoria and intellectual disability. During this entire time, the patient continued to be treated with a number of psychiatric medications to attempt to control their gender dysphoria.

The outreach worker continued to advocate for me to see M, which eventually did happen. M, was accompanied by his mother, who was supportive of his wishes. At this point, I had to rethink and re-examine my own biases: specifically, my constructions of why could someone with intellectual disability not also experience gender dysphoria? I had to think: How did informed consent (as I practice the concept) work under these circumstances, and was it safe to proceed with hormone care, and if so, the desired surgery? Could this person manage hormone care and post-op care and understand surgical consent?

By pausing and reflecting on my implicit bias, it became clear to me, along with my colleagues who worked with M, that it was actually easy to separate his gender dysphoria from the intellectual disability. There was no doubt in my mind that M suffered from significant gender distress that would likely be relieved with appropriate treatment, including testosterone and surgical measures such as chest reduction/contour surgery. As a result, we carefully reviewed the informed consent with the patient and his mother, and both parties signed the consent. We prescribed testosterone and referred M to appropriate surgical services.

M has been one of our most compliant and focused patients. M does his blood work without fail, follows prescriptions accurately, and when referred to surgeons has been diligent in following post-op care plans. I speak for the team when I say that it has been a privilege to work with M; we all have been enriched by his presence and have learned a great deal about how assumptions and implicit biases can both inform and impede treatment.

not always sufficient to prevent the emergence of bias that can inter-fere in the provision of care to transgender individuals, as the case demonstrates.

The distinction, in this second case, is between holding extensive knowledge of transgender health issues as being separate and different from that of implicit bias and assumptions. While it is largely accepted that there exists a dearth of curriculum on transgender health within teaching institutions, there is a greater absence of curriculum related to the issues of self-reflectivity on implicit bias, assumptions associated with sexual minorities, and professional humility (Obedin-Maliver et al., 2011). To practice these concepts in the field after graduation requires earlier and deeper coverage to occur during medical school training. A key finding from a study that surveyed 2,533 medical students represent-ing 49 medical schools found that greater visibility of LGBT issues within the curriculum reduced implicit bias toward these patients and, thus, health disparities (Wittlin et al., 2019). As well, the importance of trans-parency and practitioner humility was noted by Rubertson et al. (2016), whose study surveyed 100 primary care physicians and 297 patients. Physician ability to practice humility was ranked as a critical component of the clinical encounter by patients as compared to "shutting out the patient, with their own authority" (p. 1143).

These actual cases highlight that despite best intentions and assump-tions, nuanced bias and the absence of professional humility can still permeate one's lens of practice when working with trans people within healthcare settings. How this links to teaching about sexualities in the higher educational institutions is clear. The core way to approach Sukhera and Chahine's (2016) concept of unconscious bias-informed education is to go beyond teaching "content" and deliberately have learners enter the deeper and more uncomfortable realm of explor-ing the self for not-yet-realized embedded prejudices associated with the transgender population and, at the same time, learn the art and practice of humility when mistakes are made. Explicitly teaching infor-mation related to transgender healthcare practices as students progress through their medical training mitigates the risk of masking internal biases and offers the necessary space to deconstruct belief systems and prejudices toward this group of patients. Mayer et al. (2008) found that simply increasing the hours of curriculum related to transgender health is largely ineffective as a way to improve providers' competence. We agree with this finding and advocate for a shift in pedagogy that sup-ports medical learners in continuously engaging and being guided by lessons in the use of self, humility, reflectiveness and reflexivity. There-fore, we offer the following patient informed recommendations.

Recommendations for Compassionate and Informed Care

Recommendations on how to sensitize future healthcare providers in the classroom do currently exist, but such advice tends to remain at the pedagogical surface and is not absorbed at a deeper level, and thus risks repetition of discriminatory acts during care with a trans patient. A meta-analysis of 1,272 papers related to medical education and trans health (Dubin et al., 2018) identified curriculum barriers, including "limited classroom time, lack of topic-specific competency among faculty, and underwhelming institutional support to support trans health content" (p. 377). The authors attributed the existence of larger health inequities to, in part, the exclusion of transgender-specific health needs from medical school and residency curricula. The authors found that, in the United States, transgender medical education is largely composed of one-time attitude and awareness-based interventions that show significant short-term improvements but not sustainable or longitudinal attitudinal shift. The authors conclude, "There is no consensus on the exact educational interventions that should be used to address transgender health" (p. 379). Bonvicini (2017) extends this sentiment by simply stating, "best practices and acceptable measures of evaluating trainings remain unknown" (p. 2360).

The lack of universal and consistently implemented curriculum across medical schools on transgender health suggests the cultural reproduction of ignorance, referred to as agnotology. In the book *Agnotology: The Making and Unmaking of Ignorance,* Proctor (2008) talks about active versus passive kinds of ignorance and how both contribute to decisions that marginalize certain groups of individuals. Passive ignorance is the awareness of not knowing sufficient information in order to be helpful or competent in the provision of care but deciding to do nothing. This kind of ignorance was widely reported by community-based physicians (Shires, Stroumsa, Jaffe, & Woodford, 2018). It compares to active ignorance, in which the provider holds incorrect information and erroneously guides behaviours and makes decisions, even when such information is challenged (for example, assuming that all trans individuals one encounters in clinical practice want to transition). Medina (2013) takes this one step further, identifying that structural active ignorance is intentional and meant to maintain control over another group through silencing.

We suggest that critiquing both types of ignorance within the teaching realm of sexualities and trans health in higher institutions is a prudent first step. To concretize this suggestion would mean developing curriculum that initially requires educators, followed by students, to embark on their own discoveries of how implicit bias and prejudices toward transgender individuals may compromise care. While an important step, such individual awareness through self-discovery must be supported institutionally as a way to legitimize such learning and instil learner accountability. This latter suggestion equates to an overhaul of current pedagogical practices and how transgender health is still currently taught. Pragmatic ways to address implicit bias, as informed by transgender individuals, are offered in the following clinical and teaching pearls. Within medical education, a "pearl" is defined as "small bits of free standing, clinically relevant information based on experience or observation" (Lorin, Palazzi, Turner, & Ward, 2008, p. 870). Below, we offer the acronym of RIANE, a term we created from our experiences of working with transgender patients and other healthcare providers:

1. *Require* all faculty and learners to engage in critical self-awareness and reflection to mitigate embedded bias on an ongoing basis. Such pedagogy can assume multiple forms and range from individual reflection (as in taking online knowledge tests such as those available through Project Implicit: https://implicit.harvard.edu /implicit/education.html) to trans-persons-involved facilitated discussions and workshops, role plays, simulated office orals, and videotapes of student clinical encounters. Furthermore, we recommend the granting of continuing medical education (CME) credits to both learners and practitioners to take professional development courses in transgender health, as this provides incentive while ensuring accountability. Professional humility as a component of critical self-reflection cannot be overstated.

2. *Incorporate* transgender clinical competencies across the curriculum, instead of teaching LGBTQ content intermittently in condensed lectures for undergraduate medical students, which has been proven to not improve knowledge sustainability. A total of 176 medical schools were surveyed to assess the content related to sexualities, including that of transgender, that were provided to medical learners (Obedin-Maliver et al., 2011). The survey identified that the median time allocated by these higher education institutions to cover LGBTQ content during the entire medical program was 5 hours. A more recent study by Dubin et al. (2018) reinforced this earlier finding and advocated for embedding competencies within their relevant clinical contexts, with emphasis over time, as compared to the "one off" lecture. A longitudinal incorporation of transgender health topics into the standard curriculum would also support its disaggregation from the generalized topic of LGBTQ health. For example:

> this could include discussions of sex organs as opposed to "male and female genitalia" in anatomy, or a discussion of gender identity during

lectures on puberty. Because of the issues discussed here, one-time interventions for transgender education are insufficient to create sustainable learning and clinical improvements (pp. 377–391).

The development of patient-informed competencies specific to transgender patients is a first and necessary step in order for medical learners to be knowledgeable, and comfortable, when addressing the health needs of this population. To date, no comprehensive set of competencies is universally taught within Canadian medical schools. While this may be suggestive of the worth associated with transgender health, it also represents an opportunity to create humanistic, patient-informed competencies that embrace the reality of intersectionality for this marginalized group of individuals.

3. *Avoid* teaching transgender health through the traditional PBL case approach that medicalizes or pathologizes the "other" and reinforces the binary perspective of *us* and *them*. If case studies are to be used, it is critical to avoid positioning the unique health needs of the transgender patient as problematic. While cases are normally written, narratives shared by transgender individuals in person allow the immediacy of discrimination to be experienced by the healthcare learner rather than safely read about from a distance. Supporting transgender individuals as authors or coauthors in curriculum content and materials not only lends authenticity to these works, but is also a way to recognize and honour the experiential voice.

4. *Never* assume that teaching faculty are all cisgender and recognize that educators who make their sexuality known need institutional support. Educators who are transgender may face unique challenges within the classroom and should be supported by their teaching institutions in ways that are collaboratively created. For example, the stress of decision-making concerning coming out to peers and students, combined with the lack of mentors to offer guidance about professional issues related to LGBTQ identity, has to be considered. Alternatively, when an educator is known to be transgender, the expectation that they will teach others about transgender issues can become onerous to them and removes the necessity of students and colleagues doing their own professional development and discovery.

5. *Every* approach should incorporate an interprofessional lens when teaching about sexualities. The complexity and range of care, due to the intersection of physical, emotional and cultural/social discourses, requires an approach that crosses professional or disciplinary boundaries to ensure a truly comprehensive teaching approach.

Such an approach reflects an appreciation of the different strengths and limitations each profession or discipline brings and capitalizes on building respect in the classroom, which can provide a practice template on graduation.

Conclusion

Healthcare and medical education systems hold vast potential to lead the delivery of compassionate, informed, and truly person-centred care, regarding transgender individuals. Positioning such care within the class-rooms of higher education for both educators and future healthcare providers alike normalizes the idea that ongoing education is important for all and must be reflective of professional humility. The offer of the above transgender-informed clinical and teaching pearls brings with it the intimation that teaching sexualities is neither static nor definitive, but rather an ongoing process of critical reflection, education, humility, as well as a stance that places oneself in a position of active learning that is intentional rather than accidental.

REFERENCES

American College of Obstetricians and Gynecologists. (2011). *Health care for transgender individuals.* No. 512. Committee on Health Care for Underserved Women. Retrieved from https://www.acog.org/Clinical-Guidance-and -Publications/Committee-Opinions/Committee-on-Health-Care-for-Underserved -Women/Health-Care-for-Transgender-Individuals?IsMobileSet=false

Anwer, L. A., & Ahmed Abu-Zaid. (2014). Transparency in medical error disclosure: The need for formal teaching in undergraduate medical education curriculum. *Medical Education Online, 19.* https://doi.org/10.3402/meo.v19.23542

Bauer, G. R., Scheim, A. I., Deutsch, M. B., & Massarella, C. (2014). Reported emergency department avoidance, use, and experiences of transgender persons in Ontario, Canada: Results from a respondent-driven sampling survey. *Annals of Emergency Medicine, 63*(6), 713–720.e1. https://doi.org /10.1016/j.annemergmed.2013.09.027

Bauer, G.R., Zong, X., Scheim, A.I., Hammond, R., & Thind, A. (2015). Factors impacting transgender patients' discomfort with their family physicians: A respondent-driven sampling survey. *PLoS ONE, 10*(12), e0145046. https:// doi.org/10.1371/journal.pone.0145046

Bell, J., & Purkey, E. (2019). Trans individuals' experiences in primary care. *Canadian Family Physician, 65*(4), e147–e154. Retrieved from https://www .cfp.ca/content/65/4/e147?rss=1

Bonvicini, K. A. (2017). LGBT healthcare disparities: What progress have we made? *Patient Education and Counselling, 100*(12), 2357–2361. https://doi.org/10.1016/j.pec.2017.06.003

Brotman, S., Ryan, B., Jalbert, Y., & Rowe, B. (2002). Reclaiming space-regaining health: The health care experiences of two spirit people in Canada. *Journal of Gay & Lesbian Social Services, 14*(1), 67–87. https://doi.org/10.1300/j041v14n01_04

Brown, J. F., & Fu, J. (2013). Emergency department avoidance by transgender persons: Another broken thread in the "safety net" of emergency medicine care. *Annuals of Emergency Medicine, 63*(6), 721–722. https://doi.org/10.1016/j.annemergmed.2013.11.020

Cahill, S., & Makadon, H. (2014). Sexual orientation and gender identity data collection in clinical settings and in electronic health records: A key to ending LGBT health disparities. *LGBT Health, 1*(1), 34–41. https://doi.org/10.1089/lgbt.2013.0001

Dubin, S. N., Nolan, I. T., Streed, C. J., Greene, R. E., Radix, A. E., & Morrison, S. D. (2018). Transgender health care: Improving medical students' and residents' training and awareness. *Advances in Medical Education and Practice, 9,* 377–391. Retrieved from https://www.ncbi.nlm.nih.gov/pmc/articles/PMC5967378/pdf/amep-9-377.pdf. https://doi.org/10.2147/amep.s147183

Henkel, G. (2014). Transgender patients in the ED. *American College of Emergency Physicians, 33*(3), 1–13

Kaldjian, L.C., Jones, E. W., Wu, B. J., Forman-Hoffman, V. L., Levi, B. H., & Rosenthal, G. E. (2007). Disclosing medical errors to patients: Attitudes and practices of physicians and trainees. *Journal of General Internal Medicine, 22*(7), 988–996. https://doi.org/10.1007/s11606-007-0227-z

Kattari, S. K., Walls, E., Speer, S. R., & Kattari, L. (2016). Exploring the relationship between transgender-inclusive providers and mental health outcomes among transgender/gender variant people. *Social Work in Health Care, 55*(8), 635–650. https://doi.org/10.1080/00981389.2016.1193099

Kosenko, K., Rintamaki, L., Raney, S., & Maness, K. (2013). Transgender patient perceptions of stigma in health care contexts. *Medical Care Issue, 51*(9), 819–822. https://doi.org/10.1097/mlr.0b013e31829fa90d

Lorin, M. I., Palazzi, D. L., Turner, T. L., & Ward, M.A. (2008). What is a clinical pearl and what is its role in medical education? *Medical Teacher, 30*(9–10), 870–874, https://doi.org/10.1080/01421590802144286

Mayer, K. H., Bradford, J. B., Makadon, H. J., Stall, R., Goldhammer, H., & Landers, S. (2008). Sexual and gender minority health: What we know and what needs to be done. *American Journal of Public Health, 98*(6), 989–995. https://doi.org/10.2105/ajph.2007.127811

Medina, J. (2013). The epistemology of resistance: Gender and racial oppression, epistemic injustice and the social imagination. Oxford Scholarship Online. https://doi.org/10.1093/acprof:oso/9780199929023.001.0001

Metastasio, A., Negri, A., Martinotti, G., & Corazza, O. (2018). Transitioning bodies: The case of self-prescribing sexual hormones in gender affirmation in individuals attending psychiatric services. *Brain Sciences*, *8*(5), 88. https://doi.org/10.3390/brainsci8050088 https://www.ncbi.nlm.nih.gov/pmc/articles/PMC5977079/

Morrison, S. D., Wilson, S. C., & Smith, J. R. (2017). Are we adequately preparing our trainees to care for transgender patients? *Journal of Graduate Medical Education*, *9*(2), 258. https://doi.org/10.4300/jgme-d-16-00712.1

National Center for Transgender Equality (2016). *National Transgender Discrimination Survey: Executive summary*. Retrieved from https://transequality.org/sites/default/files/docs/resources/NTDS_Exec_Summary.pdf

Obedin-Maliver, J., Goldsmith, E. S., Stewart, L., White, W., Tran, E., Brenman, S., Wells, M., Feterrman, D. M., Garcia, G., & Lunn, M. R. (2011). Lesbian, gay, bisexual, and transgender-related content in undergraduate medical education. *JAMA Internal Medicine*, *306*(9), 971–977. https://doi.org/10.1001/jama.2011.1255

Ontario Human Rights Commission. Appendix 1: Glossary of human rights terms. Retrieved from http://www.ohrc.on.ca/en/teaching-human-rights-ontario-guide-ontario-schools/appendix-1-glossary-human-rights-terms

Proctor, R. N., & Schiebinger, L. (Eds.). (2008). *Agnotology: The making and unmaking of ignorance*. Standford, CA: Standford University Press.

Rosen, D. H., & Hoang, U. (2017). *Patient centered medicine: A human experience*. New York, NY: Oxford University Press.

Roter, D. L., & Hall, J. A. (2006). *Doctors talking with patients/patients talking with doctors: Improving communication in medical visits*. Westport, CT: Praeger Publishers.

Rotondi, N. K., Bauer, G. R., Scanlon, K., Kaay, M., Travers, R., & Travers, A. (2013). Nonprescribed hormone use and self-performed surgeries: "Do-it-yourself" transitions in transgender communities in Ontario, Canada. *American Journal of Public Health*, *103*(10), 1830–1836. https://doi.org/10.2105/ajph.2013.301348

Rotzinger, K. (2018). Experiences of transgender people in the healthcare system: A complex analysis. *University of Ottawa Journal of Medicine*, *8*(1), 56–61. https://doi.org/10.18192/uojm.v8i1.2390

Rubertson, P. M., Huynh, H. P., Miller, T. A., Kruse, E., Chancellor, J., & Lyubormirsky, S. (2016). The relationship between physician humility, physician-patient communication, and patient health. *Patient Education and Counseling*, *99*(7), 1138–1145. https://doi.org/10.1016/j.pec.2016.01.012

Safer, J. D., Coleman, E., Feldman, J., Garofalo, R., Hembree, W., Radix, A., & Sevelius, J. (2016). Barriers to healthcare for transgender individuals: Current opinion in endocrinology. *Diabetes, and Obesity*, *23*(2), 168–171. https://doi.org/10.1097/med.0000000000000227. Retrieved from https://www.ncbi.nlm.nih.gov/pmc/articles/PMC4802845/

Scheim, A. I., Bauer G. R., & Coleman, T. A. (2016). Socio-demographic differences by survey mode in a respondent-driven sampling study of transgender people in Ontario, Canada. *LGBT Health, 3*(5), 391–395. https://doi.org/10.1089/lgbt.2015.0046

Shires, D. A., Stroumsa, D., Jaffee, K. D., & Woodford, M.R. (2018). Primary care clinicians' willingness to care for transgender patients. *The Annals of Family Medicine, 16*(6), 555–558. https://doi.org/10.1370/afm.2298

Simmenroth-Nayda, A., Weiss, C., Fischer, T., & Himmel, W. (2012). Do communication training programs improve students' communication skills? A follow-up study. *BMC Research Notes, 5*,1–9. https://doi.org/10.1186/1756-0500-5-486

Sukhera, J., & Chahine, S. (2016). Reducing mental illness: Stigma through unconscious bias-informed education. *MedEdPublis*. Retrieved from https://doi.org/10.15694/mep.2016.000044

Witman, A. B., Park, D. M., & Hardin, S. B. (1996). How do patients want physicians to handle mistakes? A survey of internal medicine patients in an academic setting. *Archives of Internal Medicine, 156*(22), 2565–2569. https://doi:10.1001/archinte.1996.00440210083008

Wittlin, N. M., Fovidio, J. F., Burke, S. E., Przedworski, J. M., Herrin, J., Onyeador, I. N., Phelan, S. M., & Tyn, M. (2019). Contact and role modeling predict bias against lesbian and gay individuals among early-career physicians: A longitudinal study. *Social Science & Medicine, 238*. https://doi.org/10.1016/j.socscimed.2019.112422

PART TWO

At the Margins: Diverse Voices and Perspectives

SUSAN HILLOCK

Part 2, "At the Margins: Diverse Voices and Perspectives," further develops intersectional analysis and examines how current heteronormative, risk-focused, white, straight-centric, and cisgender attitudes and sex-denying practices harm vulnerable groups. Celebrating diversity while interrogating discriminatory attitudes, a variety of important subjects are presented. This part begins with a critical analysis of the intersections of art, representation, and media images in Chapter 7, "Porn and Pedagogies: Reflections on Queer and Feminist Porn Studies in Academia." In this chapter, sexual diversity studies expert Laine Zisman Newman and her students Sarah Lima, Stuart MacLeod, Oreoluwa Adara, and Imogen Tam examine what it means to bring the topic of sex (and porn) into the classroom, where they reflect upon and imagine the possible formats of future porn courses, and consider how to break away from straight white-male settler perceptions and beyond canonical content in porn studies to consider the contemporary issues and concerns relevant to young queer adults. The authors recommend approaching porn as a genre, rather than focusing solely on censorship or stigmatization. They believe that this helps create important opportunities to analyse equitable practices in the development, production, and reception of porn and sexual representation. Given how widely such media texts are produced and consumed, the authors argue that despite these obstacles, developing critical media literacy in relation to porn is essential scholarship to the fields of popular culture, sexual diversity, and broader academic landscapes.

Next, Chapter 8, "Past Practices: How to Think about Sex Historically," features historian El Chenier's work, in which they caution us to think about the relationship between present understandings of sexual identity(ies) and evidence of past behaviours, as well as the role of Christianity and colonialism in shaping contemporary notions of sexuality at the intersection of gender, race, and class. Chenier makes the case that without a foundation in what it means to think critically about the past, we miss out on the deep work that archival materials allow us to do. They then offer an introduction to historical consciousness, focusing on pertinent questions that the history of sexuality invites us to consider. By expanding our understanding of the critical framework and historical thinking, they suggest that we can get much more mileage out of the images and texts we use to enliven our sex education lectures and readings. Further developing that notion, Chenier postulates that the value of historical consciousness is in the questions it generates, not the answers it provides. As well, it offers the ideal space for deep critical reflection on just what we think sexuality is and how we might imagine it, ourselves, and our world differently.

A timely chapter follows next, with early childhood studies educator Adam Davies discussing queer masculinities in Chapter 9, "Queering Masculinity in Early Childhood and Higher Education Classrooms: Gendered Regulation and the Double Blind of Queer Masculinities." Through an autobiographical queer life-narrative approach, Davies explores his own lived experiences as a queer male-identified early childhood educator and the regulation of queer masculinities within the profession, especially the "double bind" of queer men failing to embody tenets of hegemonic masculinity, while simultaneously constituting themselves as overly feminized subjects of care. Davies explains that there is still a dearth of literature exploring the lived experiences of queer men who are early childhood educators and the regulation of queer masculinity within the fields of ECE and preservice teacher education. Furthermore, he argues that through practices of policing and regulation, the gendered expressions of queer men who are educators – specifically expressions of effeminacies – are pathologized and subjugated in work with young children.

Indeed, Davies states that queer men within early childhood settings are caught in a double bind of failing to embody tenets of hegemonic masculinity due to their queerness, while simultaneously being recruited into the field through discourses that seek out men as masculinizing influences in early learning settings. He explains that for many queer men, the fears and cultural anxieties surrounding the presence of men in the classroom might limit their career trajectories or place them in a double bind, by which their masculinity is both required and reviled. Thus, he recommends having deeper conversations about supporting gender diversity for *both* children and educators. His hope is that his reflections and recommendations might inspire further conversations about the importance of embracing the vulnerability and openness of being visibly queer in the classroom, particularly within the fields of preservice teacher education and ECE, while crafting more space for open conversations with young children about gender and sexual diversity.

Then, grounded in an intersectional-theory model developed to understand the unique social, cultural, and political positioning of LGBTQ Muslims' lived experiences and identities in Western and European contexts, social work professor Maryam Khan brings a critical intersectional feminist approach to her contribution, Chapter 10, "Working with Muslim LGBTQ Service Users: Assessing and Locating Supportive Care and Teaching Practices." This chapter illuminates how to move beyond essentialized culturally competent ways of working with sexual and gender Muslim minorities to support LBTQ Muslim women and their families and provides lessons about sexuality(ies) that mainstream service providers and agencies need to learn to more effectively work with Muslim LGBTQs and allies. Khan illustrates a gap in current social work practice, in relation to service provision and programming, concerning how to best support LGBTQ Muslim sexuality(ies), queer individuals, and their families. She draws on her lived and professional experiences, in practice and as an educator, with Salaam (a LGBTQ Muslim support group) to advocate for an integration of minority stress, intersectional, and narrative perspectives in teaching and practice. She also argues for social work practitioners and educators to decolonize sexuality and gender by rejecting essentialist-based understandings of Islam and LGBTQ Muslim sexualities. Moreover, Khan suggests that drawing on homocolonialism, implementing critically reflexive social work practices, and incorporating the lived experiences of LGBTQ Muslims can be helpful in dismantling Islamophobic discourses.

Following this, in Chapter 11, "Sexuality and Aging," social work professors Lorna Guse and Hai Luo suggest a life-course perspective, with dual emphasis on the impact of societal events on aging persons and the notion that people shape their own lives through making choices. They provide specific teaching exercises to help readers reflect on growing old and aging as a sexual being. Guse and Luo define sexuality as the way that we see ourselves as sexual beings, the way we feel about ourselves, and how we choose to identify ourselves. The authors explain that as human beings our sexual self-perceptions and behaviours are shaped over the entire life course, and that sexuality remains crucial into later life for life satisfaction and physical and psychological well-being. It is also true that age-related changes in health and functional ability, loss of partners, and ageist attitudes have an impact on the continuity of sexual interest and activities. However, even though sex is generally beneficial to one's physical health, may reduce loneliness, and increase one's sense of self, Guse and Luo state that healthcare and social service practitioners and students often report discomfort and lack of competence in providing support to better older adults' sexuality. Thus, the authors maintain that acknowledging and learning more about sexuality and aging is important, complicated, and currently lacking breadth and depth. To help with this, they share specific teaching materials and resources that they have found to be useful. The authors also recommend that as sex educators we need to expand the research and knowledge base; should introduce future healthcare and helping professionals to theoretical perspectives, concepts, and discussions that equip them to link classroom learning to their life experiences and go beyond individual interpretation to broader understandings of diversity, choice, and sexual expression among older adults; and that in terms of sexuality, both teachers and students should reflect on their own values and attitudes to acknowledge the elderly as sexual beings.

Then, in Chapter 12, "Uncertain Subjects: (Un)Teaching Pain(ful) Sexualities, Power, and Pedagogy," doctoral candidate and clinical social worker Renee Dumaresque challenges narratives that focus solely on pleasure and invites us to think about, and teach about, painful sexualities. They use an auto-ethnographic approach to grapple with the murky distinction between pain and pleasure, argue chronic vulvar pain as a site of erotic protest and potentiality, demonstrate the intersection of medicalization, disablism, sanism, hetero-/cis-normativity, colonization, and racism in the making of harmful gender and sexed subjectivities, and rearticulate disabled and sick sexuality(ies) by enlisting queer and utopian performativity to expose the social construction of normative sexuality. Dumaresque resources personal knowledge acquired through their encounters with vulvar pain, and from their previous inquiries of vulvar pain, to engage with literature related to teaching and interrogate the approaches most often taken, across disciplines, in teaching sexualities in higher education.

Accordingly, they aim to disrupt totalizing knowledge of normative sexuality, to contribute to the intelligibility of crip and pain(ful) sexualities, and to grapple with mechanisms of power within education with respect to content and pedagogy that inform the subjectivities of teachers, learners, and sexual subjects. They explain that multiple and diffuse relations of power shape and show up in higher education, generating explicit knowledge that is circulated in the classroom, through, for example, the influence of dominant discourse in crafting content, as well as the affects, norms, modes of surveillance, and conformability that constitute teacher/student subjects through the normalizing impulse of schooling. By engaging a queer critical approach to auto-ethnography, an ethic of wonder, and a reading practice informed by Foucauldian ethics, Dumaresque contributes to knowledge of painful sexualities, disrupts totalizing discourse, offers an accounting of sexuality education, and proposes a transdisciplinary intervention for teaching sexuality that fosters an analysis of subjectivity as mediated and fluid.

7 Porn and Pedagogies: Reflections on Queer and Feminist Porn Studies in Academia

LAINE ZISMAN NEWMAN, SARAH LIMA, STUART MACLEOD, OREOLUWA ADARA, AND IMOGEN TAM

In the fall of 2018, the University of Toronto's Centre for Sexual Diversity Studies offered a fourth-year elective seminar course entitled "Sexual Aesthetics/Sexual Representation." Throughout the course, queer theories were used to explore the fetishization of gender variance and race, the absence of disability in sexual representation, the criminalization of sex work in Canada, and porn and sex as alternative technologies of resistance and healing. Approaching porn as a genre, rather than focusing solely on censorship or stigmatization, created important opportunities to analyse equitable practices in development, production, and reception of porn and sexual representation.

In the chapter that follows, we (four students and the lecturer for the course) examine learning about sex and porn studies in a university setting. Reflecting on our own experiences teaching and learning about sex, and thinking more broadly about sex education, we enter this discussion with the following questions in mind: what is essential to developing and producing a course focused on porn; how might we engage porn in relation to labour practices, race and marginalization, and crip and disability studies; what is the role of porn in informal sex education; and, how might we reframe a discussion on porn and sex work to position it as a component of wellness practices?

Course Title and Structure

While none of us were involved in naming the course, we discussed the course title at length throughout the semester and in our subsequent conversations. On one level, the title "Sexual Aesthetics/Sexual Representation" is advantageous as it opens up conversation to include broader themes than a course titled "Porn Studies" might; on another, its vagueness buries one of the key genres discussed in the course. Indeed, without the word "porn" in the title of the course, students entering the classroom on the first day confessed that they had not known exactly what the course was about.

Our active consideration of the course title makes evident the course's explicit focus on reflexive learning. Using Linda Williams's article "Pornography, Porno, Porn: Thoughts on a Weedy Field" (2014) as an entry point into a discussion on the influence and process of naming this field of study, we discussed practical implications and concerns pertaining to the course name. Recognizing that, for students, "Porn Studies" on a transcript could negatively influence opportunities, we were compelled to ask what the consequences were in explicitly naming porn on a syllabus in our current political climate. This concern seemed particularly relevant in the Canadian context, in which academics and influencers such as Jordan Peterson continue to make it difficult to speak openly about many fields deemed "progressive" in the humanities.[1]

The structure of the course further aimed to emphasize student participation and collective lateral learning. Recognizing that everyone has different experiences with porn and comes to the course with subjective perspectives, the seminar, by and large, refused a top-down approach. We tried to centralize students' standpoints alongside the voices of workers in the industry, an objective which was reflected in our textbook, *The Feminist Porn Book* (Taormino, Shimizu, Penley, & Miller-Young, 2013), an edited volume which presents perspectives from artists and sex workers in the industry rather than academics offering a peripheral analysis. The text was particularly beneficial, given that many of us have had limited interaction with literature on sex work, especially texts authored by industry professionals themselves.

Course Format

Our course ran once a week, in the fall of 2018. Taking advantage of our small class size (10 students), each class began with a brief check-in. Students were asked to reflect on their week, respond to readings and viewings, and share any questions or concerns. The lecturer would then provide a brief introduction to the weekly topic. For the remainder of the class, two students took on the role of discussion facilitators – a

---

1 In 2017, Peterson released a plan to create a website to "help students and parents identify postmodern content in courses so that they can avoid them" (Canadian Broadcaster CTV). The plan to create the website was later abandoned, but the threat of it had some professors concerned about harassment, anxious about an increasing climate of fear and intimidation in the academy.

major course assignment, which accounted for the majority of their final grades. Student facilitators were encouraged to incorporate activities to vary the format of discussion and analysis. For example, contributing to our ongoing discussion of what constitutes pornography, one student showed a series of images and asked the class to assess if they were pornographic or not. This discussion revealed that what is considered pornographic often relies heavily on context and personal bias. By calling into question what porn was to each of us as individuals, we were able to critically unpack *how* we came to hold these values and definitions, and relatedly, consider ways we could interrogate our positions on porn moving forward. We addressed topics ranging from censorship, self-care, and mainstream sexual representation to discussions of live performance and "nerdlesque."[2] Using a student-led approach, our conversations prioritized topics most relevant to those in the classroom.

Recurring Themes

Throughout the course, several themes persistently surfaced, based in part on the planned course syllabus and in part on the topics to which students gravitated. Below, we consider some of the most pertinent themes and discussion topics that emerged.

Trigger Warnings and Safer Spaces

It is not always obvious what is "triggering" to someone, and that was a learning experience for me as well this year. Part of the learning process is learning how to talk about this stuff in a way that is safe for everyone.

Imogen

In a course focusing on sexual representation and porn, there are many discussions that broach difficult and at times triggering topics. Therefore, one recurring theme in the course was the purpose and implementation of "trigger warnings" in the classroom. The word "trigger" here is not used to demarcate topics that elicit discomfort; instead, "trigger" is used, as Eli Clare notes, to "reflect the abrupt, visceral tailspin some of us experience when encountering or being caught off-guard by particular images or stories, smells or sounds, memories or emotions" (Clare, 2017, p. xx). In a class dealing with sex and sexuality, where we

---

2 Nerdlesque is a subset a burlesque, which combines traditional burlesque routines with geek culture.

explicitly analysed the concept of consent, we situated trigger warnings as a consent-based practice. Trigger warnings played an important role in this course, as they provided time for everyone to prepare themselves for the content about to be addressed, and gave everyone an opportunity to consent to being in that environment. Instead of framing warnings within the context of censorship or discomfort, we utilized them as necessary descriptions of subject matter to provide students time to explore healthy boundaries related to learning. Through this approach, we remain accountable by asking for consent for everything we do.

Admittedly, there has been a backlash against the use of trigger warnings in the classroom (Rae, 2016), with some faculty and professors feeling that the necessity to provide trigger warnings actually works to censor content and poorly prepares students for navigating the world (in which, indeed, there will be unanticipated triggering content). However, creating a safer space that encourages participation begins by recognizing that experiences and positionality impact the individual and collective learning experience. In the context of our classroom, trigger warnings served as a prompt to describe *all* content, prior to it being discussed or screened, because privileging only explicitly pornographic or violent content as worthy of trigger warnings flattens the nuance of one's relationship to trauma. Indeed, we never know what may be triggering to those in the classroom, nor should we assume to know.

Agency, Equity, and Stigmatization

What interested me the most about these conversations was a kind of "a-ha!" moment that happened early on in the course. Realizing that we could talk about the porn industry as just another industry, the genre as just another genre.

Stuart

There is indeed exploitation, abuse, and objectification in the porn and sex-work industry. However, it is certainly not the only profession facing these kinds of challenges. Factory workers, clothing manufacturers, even university faculty and staff all experience exploitation, sexual assault, sexism, and racism to varying degrees. We should *always* be talking about labour laws, sexism, racism, and classism when we talk about any employment. These conversations are important as they highlight the criminal dependencies of capitalist industries. But as theorists and as consumers we rarely define industries based on their illegal or exploitative elements. For example, when we talk about fashion, we might discuss a desire to develop more equitable labour practices (Connell, 2019; Joy et al., 2012; Park, 2016), but we do not define the field by sweatshops or argue for its inherent relation to exploitation. When individuals conversely define pornography and sex work solely through mistreatment and abuse, they strip the workers of rights and agency – they take away their voices and obstruct their pursuits of safe work environments.

When we talk about (and teach about) pornography as a genre of film and sex work as an industry or profession, we centralize and validate the *choice* to work in these industries. This enables us to talk about important conversations pertaining to labour laws, equity, and safety – conversations we have regarding all professions, in order to protect worker rights and welfare. We already have labour laws that work to structure a safe and equal workspace – hours, pay, breaks, and protections against sexual harassment already exist.[3] By talking about sex work *as work*, we encourage conversations around safety that refute stigmatization while emphasizing rights.

Important to our course discussions of equity was the distinction between optics and agency – analysing the difference between the empty appearance of the inclusion of marginalized people within a potentially oppressive normative framework and the productive power of porn produced *outside* this hegemony – namely porn created by and for marginalized groups. The presence of marginalized peoples in porn does not make it inclusive and progressive. However, that does not preclude the possibility for porn to move beyond presence toward meaningful visibility. For example, in our course, a student facilitated a discussion on trans representation in feminist porn through the work of Shine Louise Houston, creator of the award-winning *Crash Pad* series (Houston, 2005). *Crash Pad* presents gender-diverse, performer-directed scenes emphasizing authenticity, fluidity, and performer pleasure over mainstream pornographic tropes that primarily serve a cis male consumer base.

Sticky Porn/Straight Porn/White Porn

Desirability is something people learn in part from porn, and unfortunately in mainstream porn dangerous dynamics are shaped and replicated. Some bodies are desired, objectified, or fetishized, and we learn from watching that. As much as we don't want to just criticize porn, we do need to understand power dynamics that are learnt through porn.

Oreoluwa

One difficult part of planning and facilitating this course was finding ways to talk about "straight porn." While we did not want to fall into a trap

---

3 In Ontario, see, for example, the Employment Standards Act (ESA), and the Occupational Health and Safety Act (OHSA).

of centralizing straight-white-male porn – a topic that is often tirelessly critiqued – we recognized the need to address concerns with straight porn to outline what queer and feminist porn subverts. Unpacking straight porn (and all media representation for that matter) means critically analysing its relationship to all that bolsters the nation state: capitalism, classism, settler colonialism, ableism, racism, sexism; homophobia/transphobia, and heterosexism and cissexism (among other systems of inequity and oppression). The porn industry is inherently connected to capitalism and profit: it is shaped by settler colonialism; it propagates normalized forms of racism; and it often perpetuates sexist, homophobic, and transphobic tropes. So, even while we might opt to focus on the positive potential of queer and feminist porn, conversations around equity and oppression are necessary starting points. It is important to initiate a discussion that identifies why and how straight porn can be problematic, but also to emphasize that porn itself is not inherently problematic.

In discussing straight porn – and feminist and queer acts to subvert it – we thought critically about what attributes "stick" to certain bodies. Sara Ahmed (2015) uses the term "sticky" to describe how emotions and responses are not detached from bodies or inside of bodies: they shape bodies and relationships between them. Stickiness is the way in which repetition of emotion and response becomes impression. It is *"an effect of the histories of contact between bodies, objects, and signs"* (p. 90, emphasis in original). Porn is a "sticky" subject. It is "sticky" in that certain emotions pertaining to participation, creation, and viewership stick to certain things or certain bodies. As ideas are repeated, they accumulate value. So fetishizing racialized bodies, fat bodies, or disabled bodies has an ongoing (sticky) impact. Notions of desirability and experiences of fetishization – based on inequitable systemic oppression – *stick*: they cling to our bodies and influence the way we move through space. Mainstream porn could even be perceived as sticky glue, holding in place the associations between particular signs and bodies, through which stereotypes are promoted. While teaching porn might not make such sticky emotions unstick, the act of acknowledging and decoding such stickiness, changes the conversation.

One way, in which we attempted to unstick normalized perceptions of desirability, was to move away from conversations of cis-het (cisgender-heterosexual) porn and viewership and turn the conversation to one about queer and feminist bodies and experiences. When we are talking about queer porn and feminist porn, we are not necessarily just talking about who is fucking. We are talking about subversive and radical form and content, about approach and aesthetic (e.g., queering a typical work environment, prioritizing labour equity, and consent from both crew and performers). In our course, a student referred to "queer" as a superpower: one that is not necessarily bound by the limitations and labels of heteronormativity. You do not have to get married, have children, or be in a monogamous relationship. None of this necessarily applies to you.

When we talked about studying queer porn, we observed the same kind of superpower. It does not have to be bound by the expectations or norms of other fields. While all porn can engage in fantasy, "queer porn" is targeting a different audience and is not just a reproduction or amplification of power dynamics that already exist in the "real world." For Tristan Taormino (2013), feminist and queer porn (though she does not explicitly use the term "queer") represents a counteraction toward the formulaic male-centred scenes of mainstream studios. Taormino extends the conversation beyond audience fantasy, explaining,

> I want to empower the performers to show us what they want to do, to share a part of their sexuality with the camera. So much of porn asks performers to act out someone else's fantasy or do what someone else thinks looks sexy: what if they were given the opportunity to do their own thing. (p. 258)

These antithetical approaches use porn as an avenue to more readily explore spectrums of sexual encounters and organic connections.

Entry Points to Sex Education through Porn, Pop Culture, and Fandom

I didn't learn about queer culture in school. The first time I ever saw two women embrace was in Buffy the Vampire Slayer. *These kinds of shows don't just increase visibility for queer intimacies, they also provide an alternative accessible perspective that diverges from the conservative heteronormative logics we have access to in the classroom.*

Sarah

Despite popular focus on formal sex education curriculum, much of what we learn about sex comes through intersecting and overlapping lived experiences of community, popular culture, social media, and porn. Indeed, scholars have theorized on the use of porn and pop culture in sex education (see for example: Albury, 2014; Dawson, 2017; Goldstein, 2019; Spieldenner, 2018) and have noted the ways youth interact with and learn from porn.[4] For many students in our

---

4 An intersectional analysis could be brought to bear related to differences in youth's porn interest, access, and use, as well as its impact. Every standpoint and positionality we inhabit will influence our interactions with porn, whether that be gender, race, geography, religion, class, ability, or sexual orientation. Taking an intersectional approach to our classroom and readings of porn, we continually attempt to debunk essentialist assumptions that one isolated social location (for example, young cis men) will determine frequency of engagement and consumption of porn.

class, mainstream curriculums not only failed to accurately reflect the diversity of sexual identities, but also actively suppressed opportunities to see our sexualities presented as normal and healthy.[5]

Students in the course noted that much of their sexual knowledge came from informal sexual education, such as pop culture and fan fiction, because of censorship in their youth. By discussing fan fiction and pop culture as informal sex ed curriculums throughout our course, we allowed for analysis of not only content, but also authorship and consumption. Discussing fan fiction and other news media validated experiences of creating, sharing, and consuming as processes of personal sexual pedagogy. This means that rather than dismissing or trivializing these mediums, we acknowledged the ways in which we learn from each other and explore our identities.

Care Work and Collective Care

Learning about porn in class was a different experience from what I had imagined. A lot of the porn we examined was not mainstream porn. In a few courses I took, porn was about care work and consent and spatial recognition and intimacy. It was focused on queer-crip porn and counterpublic porn. While we talked about porn and intimacy, it was the way we used porn as a touchstone in the course that was so engaging and different.

Sarah

Porn studies and sexual representation need not only be about pleasure; they are also about care work, consent, spatial recognition, and intimacy. Additionally, they are about how porn and sex work create alternative futurities and imaginations, particularly for bodies that are typically desexualized or objectified. Self-described "poly queer femmegimp porn star academic" Loree Erickson (2013) creates porn to heal from a lack of representation (p. 320). She reflected on her 2013 film *want*, saying,

> I wanted to see bodies that looked and moved and felt like mine represented in the exciting, but clearly still problematic, queer sexual culture. I wanted to see something that reflected my desires! I wanted to know that

---

5 For example, Doug Ford government's regressive proposal to reintroduce Ontario's 1998 sexual education curriculum failed to include gender or sexual diversity, cyber safety, or consent. While Ford's proposal inevitably did not come to fruition, it nonetheless is evidence to the precarity of sexual education curriculum and the ways in which students' access to formal sexual education in the classroom is subject to the political policies of that moment.

desiring people like me was possible. I resolved then and there to become a porn star. (Erickson, 2013, p. 324)

In creating counterpublic porn, Erickson creates space to transform norms through resistance, grapple with harmful logics, and rewrite old narratives.

In counterpublic porn, people reimagine ways of wanting and sharing bodies as well as minds, rejecting ascribed and standardized expectations of desirability. In this way, counterpublic porn dovetails resistance work in exchanging new modes of desire across the practice of retelling stories that detach shame from "cultures of undesirability" (Erickson, 2016, p. 18). Cultures of undesirability refocus our collective attention, validating not only queercrip[6] passions, but also underpredicted and underproduced sites of arousal, and political possibilities for what it means to feel cared for (even if this means how we organize our lives around people's care needs). Alongside Erickson, we can think about sexual representation through the lens of crip theory and examine porn in the context of transformational justice and worldmaking across pleasure and desirability, using Erickson's inspirational work around "sites of shame as sites of resistance" (Erickson, 2007).

Although porn and sex work have the capacity to create collective networks of care, these practices can also be coopted and subsumed within individualistic neoliberal systems. In *Care Work: Dreaming Disability Justice*, Leah Lakshmi Piepzna-Samarasinha (2018) considers how care-work and the healing justice movement reproduce organizational cultures that are founded on individualism and resiliency. In their work, they quote Yashna Maya Padamsee's work on "Communities of Care":

> If we let ourselves be caught up in the discussion of self-care we are missing the whole point of Healing Justice (HJ) work … Too often self-care in our organizational cultures gets translated to our individual responsibility to leave work early, go home – alone – and go take a bath, go to the gym, eat some good food and go to sleep. So, we do all that "self-care" to return to organizational cultures where we reproduce the systems we are trying to break. (p. 109)

The complexities of porn as care work must therefore be considered in relation to neoliberal notions of wellness and productivity. To combat tropes of resilience through individualism, we might instead think about porn, care, and resistance through collective potentiality.

---

6 For more on the intersections of crip theory and queer theory, see Kafer, 2013; McRuer, 2006; Sandahl, 2003; Trace, 2014; Wood, 2014.

Conclusion: Course Recommendations

Thinking with and through our experiences in the classroom, we conclude here by providing five practical recommendations for developing and running a porn course. This is by no means an effort to construct an essentialized or universal framework but is instead an offering of perspectives based on our reflections and experiences:

1. Trigger warnings: Although trigger warnings were regularly provided in our course, we believe that including them within a syllabus *and* during lectures would give students the opportunity to better prepare and negotiate their own engagement prior to entering the physical space.
2. Guest lecturers: To ensure that conversations around porn and sex work prioritize first-hand experiences and experiential knowledge, it is necessary to integrate voices from those who are working in sex work and the porn industry. Lecturers should intentionally consider compensation and respectful student–speaker interaction in planning and inviting professionals into the classroom.
3. Collective viewing: In our course, we did not engage in collective viewing of porn in the classroom. Decentralizing film as the primary subject for pornographic analysis broadened our conversations to include multifaceted definitions of porn and the general economy of desirability as industry. However, this also created a pedagogical degree of separation from explicit material itself. With specific content warnings and descriptions, the collective viewing of porn could provide unique opportunities to not only decode content but also to specifically consider the impact of collective versus individual viewership.
4. Indigenous voices and settler colonialism: In a settler colonial context, it is essential to explore how power operates to construct Western understandings of gender identity, expression, and pleasure. There is a need to not only explore how settler colonialism shapes perceptions of desirability in the West, but also to recentralize Indigenous perspectives and experiences in relation to gender representation, sex work, and porn.
5. Student engagement: Recognizing the value in experiential knowledge and diverse readings of media text, it is imperative to develop a student-led learning experience through an open, communicative, and trauma-informed approach (Fava and Bay-Cheng, 2013). A commitment to student engagement makes room for diverse standpoints and centralizes the needs of the individuals present in the room.

There are undeniable challenges in bringing porn courses into academic institutions, ranging from a university's response, to student experiences, and discomfort. However, given how widely such media texts are produced and consumed, we argue that despite these obstacles, developing critical media literacy in relation to porn is essential scholarship in the fields of popular culture and sexual diversity, and in broader academic landscapes.

REFERENCES

Ahmed, S. (2015). *The cultural politics of emotion.* New York: Routledge, Taylor & Francis Group.

Albury, K. (2014). Porn *and* sex education, porn *as* sex education. *Porn Studies, 1*(1–2), 172–181. https://doi.org/10.1080/23268743.2013.863654

Clare, E. (2017). *Brilliant imperfection: Grappling with cure.* Durham: Duke University Press.

Connell, K. Y. H. (2019). Utilizing political consumerism to challenge the 21st century fast fashion industry. In M. Boström, M. Micheletti, & P. Oosterveer (Eds.), *The Oxford handbook of political consumerism* (pp. 293–312). New York: Oxford University Press.

Dawson, K. (2017). Porn as sex education: Findings from a public screening of queer porn. *The Journal of Sexual Medicine, 14*(5), 291. https://doi.org/10.1016/j.jsxm.2017.04.402

Employment Standards Act, 2000, SO 2000, c 41. http://canlii.ca/t/53kh1, retrieved on 2019–09–25.

Erickson, L. (2007). Revealing femmegimp: A sex-positive reflection on sites of shame as sites of resistance for people with disabilities. *Atlantis, 31*(2), 42–52.

Erickson, L. (2013). Out of line: The sexy femmegimp politics of flaunting it. In T. Taormino (Ed.), *The feminist porn book: the politics of producing pleasure* (pp. 320–328). New York: Feminist Press at the City University of New York.

Erickson, L. (2016). Transforming cultures of (un)desirability: Creating cultures of resistance. *Graduate Journal of Social Science, 12*(1), 11–22.

Fava, N. M., & Bay-Cheng, L. Y. (2013). Trauma-informed sexuality education: Recognising the rights and resilience of youth. *Sex Education, 13*(4), 383–394. https://doi.org/10.1080/14681811.2012.745808

Goldstein, A. (2019). Beyond porn literacy: Drawing on young people's pornography narratives to expand sex education pedagogies. *Sex Education, 20*(1), 1–16.

Houston, S. L. The *Crash Pad* series (2005–). Available at: http://crashpadseries.com/.

Joy, A., Sherry, J. F., Venkatesh, A., Wang, J., & Chan, R. (2012). Fast fashion, sustainability, and the ethical appeal of luxury brand. *Fashion Theory, 16*(3), 273–296. https://doi.org/10.2752/175174112x13340749707123

Kafer, A. (2013). *Feminist, queer, crip*. Bloomington, IN: Indiana University Press.

McRuer, R. (2006). *Crip theory: Cultural signs of queerness and disability*. New York: New York University Press.

Occupational Health and Safety Act, RSO 1990, c O.1, http://canlii.ca/t /53nnv, retrieved on 2019–09–25.

Park, H., & Kim, Y. K. (2016). An empirical test of the triple bottom line of customer-centric sustainability: The case of fast fashion. *Fashion and Textiles, 3*(1). https://doi.org/10.1186/s40691-016-0077-6

Piepzna-Samarasinha, L. L. (2018). *Care work: Dreaming disability justice*. Vancouver: Arsenal Pulp Press.

Rae, L. (2016). Re-focusing the debate on trigger warnings: Privilege, trauma, and disability in the classroom. *First Amendment Studies, 50*(2), 95–102. https://doi.org/10.1080/21689725.2016.1224677

Sandahl, C. (2003). Queering the crip or cripping the queer? Intersections of queer and crip identities in solo autobiographical performance. *GLQ: A Journal of Lesbian and Gay Studies, 9*(1–2), 25–56. https://doi.org/10.1215 /10642684-9-1-2-25

Spieldenner, A. R. (2018). Object lessons: Using trans porn in class to explore gender fluidity. *Communication Teacher, 33*(3), 215–220. https://doi.org/10 .1080/17404622.2018.1467569

Taormino, T. (2013). Calling the shots: Feminist porn in theory and practice. In Taormino, T., Parreñas-Shimuzu, C., Penley, C., Miller-Young, M. (Eds.), *The feminist porn book: The politics of producing pleasure* (pp. 253–264). New York, NY: Feminist Press.

Taormino, T., Shimizu, C. P., Penley, C., & Miller-Young, M. (2013). *The feminist porn book: The politics of producing pleasure*. New York, NY: The Feminist Press at the City University of New York.

Trace, K. (2014). *Hot, wet, and shaking: How I learned to talk about sex*. Halifax, Nova Scotia: Invisible Publishing.

Williams, L. (2014). Pornography, porno, porn: Thoughts on a weedy field. In T. Dean, S. Ruszczycky, D. Squires (Eds), *Porn archives* (29–43). Duke University Press.

Wood, C. (2014). *Criptiques*. United States: May Day Publishing.

8 Past Practices: How to Think about Sex Historically

EL CHENIER

There are few things more fun to spice up a lecture than an eye-catching historical image, and when it comes to sexuality, there are an endless number to choose from. This is especially true now that more and more materials are available online. We need never set foot in an archive: many of us will encounter captivating material on our social media feeds. Without a foundation in what it means to think critically about the past, however, we miss out on the deep work archival materials allow us to do. In this chapter, I offer an introduction to historical consciousness, focusing on questions that the history of sexuality invites us to consider. With a deeper understanding of the critical framework historical thinking offers, we can get much more mileage out of the historical images and texts that we use to enliven our lectures and readings on human sexuality, regardless of the discipline in which we may teach.

During the first class of a 100-level Introduction to the History of Sexuality course that I teach, I project onto the screen a page from Andreas Vesalius's 1593 medical text *De Humani corporis fabrica Libri septem* (see Figure 8.1). Based on Vesalius's meticulous dissections of human cadavers, *De Humani corporis fabrica Libri septem* greatly advanced the science of anatomy and earned him an appointment as imperial physician to the court of Charles V, Holy Roman Emperor. "What," I ask the room full of students, "is this a drawing *of*? Half of the students look up, down, around, everywhere except at me. The other half look directly at me, wondering if it is a trick question. Eventually, one brave student will finally say what everyone is thinking: "It's a penis." Students shift in their seats. Nervous laughter ripples through the room.

"No," I explain, "it is a vagina."[1]

---

1 Even this is not right, as this part of the female body had not yet been given that name (see Laqueur, 1990, pp. 159–161).

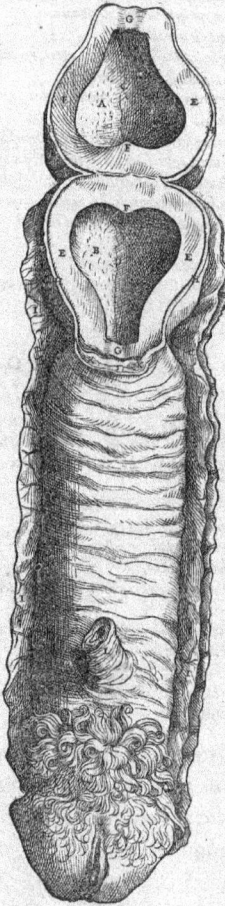

Figure 8.1. Image of reproductive organs in Andreas Vesalius's *De Humani corporis fabrica Libri septem* (1543).

Source: From Andreas Vesalius, *De Humani corporis fabrica Libri septem* (p. 381). Lugduni: Apud Joan. Tornaesium. (1552). Andreae Vesalii Bruxellensis, scholae medicorum Patauinae professoris De humani corporis fabrica libri septem. Wellcome Collection. Attribution 4.0 International (CC BY 4.0).

Until the eighteenth century, many Europeans conceived of men and women as one sex; women were simply men turned inside out.[2] As the widely distributed seventeenth-century text *Aristotle's Masterpiece* put it,

> ... tho' they of different sexes be,
> Yet in the whole they are the same as we:
> For those that have the strictest Searchers been,
> Find Women are but Men turn'd Out side in.   (Harvey, 2005, p. 83)

Thus, the vagina was thought to be an inverted penis; the labia, foreskin; the uterus, a scrotum; and the ovaries, testicles. Because it had no equivalent in the male body, the clitoris was largely ignored until the 1850s, when the study of embryos showed the clitoris, not the vagina, shared a common origin with the penis.[3]

The idea that women and men were copies of each other did not mean that they were social or political equals. Medical theories held that females and males existed on a continuum of heat and perfection, with men being more hot, active, and perfect; women cooler, sluggish, and less perfect (Harvey, 2005). The sexism of the one-sex model is plain for even the most distracted undergraduate to see.

Vesalius's vagina illuminates change and continuity, key foci of historical study. It shows how Western European ideas about the human body have changed over time, yet we see continuity in theories about the biological basis of male superiority; many continue to believe men to be physically and mentally superior to women. For most people, this is where the lesson ends: people in the past thought differently from us because they were more sexist and because scientific knowledge was still rudimentary. Yes, they reason, sexism still exists, but as science advances, residual beliefs in fundamental differences between women and men will gradually fade away. Indeed, Western education is based on this very premise: knowledge, especially scientific knowledge, will liberate us from our limiting beliefs and bring equality, justice, and freedom to all.

What the history of sexuality teaches us, however, is that this is simply not true. Facts, even biological ones, never speak for themselves. They must be interpreted, and as they are, they are given meaning. Knowledge, therefore, is inextricably linked to culture and ideology and embedded

---

2 The one-sex model was originally proposed by historian Thomas Laqueur (1990). European medievalist and Renaissance historians have argued that the one-sex model coexisted with a two-sex model.
3 Laqueur, 1990, p. 10, but see Park, who shows that sixteenth-century French doctors discussed the clitoris (1997, p. 173).

in relations of power. Biology has never been *and can never be* a science based on value-free, objective facts.

Not convinced? Consider abortion. Safe abortion is now easy and inexpensive to provide, but its availability depends on the prevailing meaning given to biological tissue growing in a uterus. Here is where values and ideology enter. Moreover, because the management of bodies is in the interest of the state, women's reproductive functions are one of the few areas of healthcare subject to government oversight via criminal regulation. There are no bodies, no biological sciences, and no abortion services that exist outside politics.

Indeed, we can use the past to develop our own and students' capacity for complex thinking (and hopefully, feeling and experiencing), not by showing how far we have come as a society, but by opening ourselves up to critical reflection on the truisms of our own age. Critical historical approaches to sexuality offer teachers and students across disciplines an opportunity to see how our beliefs about sex and sexuality are no less subjective than those of seventeenth century Europeans.

Now that we know that the image is of a vagina, I ask, "Is this image accurate"? More confident about where this is all going, they call out, "No"! Unfortunately, they have once again missed history's mark. When thinking historically, the image is absolutely accurate. It accurately represents the beliefs, views, and values of the time in which it was produced. Although this may seem pedantic, my objective is to orient us away from reading scientific renderings of the body as evidence of an objective truth, toward seeing how representations of the body – *including* those in contemporary biology texts – are filtered through culture and ideology, both of which are rooted in relations of power. As historian Joan Scott points out,

> The shaping of the categories "male" and "female" and the process of defining a female body – how it should look, move, and function – takes place in a specific context, and that context will be reflected in or reinforced by these ideas about bodies. What is defined as "the female body" ... is a political act. (Scott, 1988, p. 2)

While it is easy to see how struggles for lesbian, gay, women's, intersex, and trans rights are political acts, seeing the definition of male and female bodies as political is a new and, for some, a profoundly uncomfortable proposition. It is essential, however, to grasp the critical insights offered by the history of sexuality. Only by denaturalizing that which we think is natural – male and female, for example – can we begin to grasp the profound opportunity queer, intersex, and trans experience offers us to unpack our limited ways of thinking, seeing, and feeling.

By now, it should be clear that the history of sexuality is not the study of the truth about sex. It is the study of truth claims about sex. To begin to unpack truth claims about sex, and in terms of teaching about sexuality(ies), we must let go of the idea that there *is* a truth about sex at all. To do this, we must make strange not only the past, but also the present. To this end, I share a brief quote from a 1970s interview with American essayist, novelist, and intellectual Gore Vidal. Vidal defies history: in 1948, when fear and hostility toward homosexuals dominated the American zeitgeist (Johnson, 2006), he published a novel featuring a neutral gay male character (Vidal, 1948). Although the novel did enormous damage to his literary career, he remained a favoured guest of liberal elites, among them the Kennedys. All the while, he was openly bisexual (Barnes, 1973). When talking about same-sex sex became more acceptable in the 1970s, a journalist asked him if his first sexual experience was heterosexual or homosexual. Gore replied, "I was too polite to ask" (Vidal & Stanton, 1980, p. 23). Gore's response throws into sharp relief our culture's reliance on the sexed body to give meaning to sexual desire and sexual acts, and to determine a sexual identity. It opens up the possibility of experiencing and thinking about sexual desire and activity untethered from gender and the sexed body. It makes present ways of knowing strange.

If untethered from the sex or gender of the other (or others), what shape would pleasure and desire take? How would we relate to the person or persons we desire? How would we relate to ourselves? How might others relate to us? Vidal is an important bisexual author to be celebrated for his willingness to resist the restrictive sexual culture of his time, but historical analysis provides us with an opportunity to do much more than honour brave souls who dared to live a queer life under oppressive conditions. When used as a pathway to expand our conceptual thinking beyond the familiar, attention to this brief exchange with a journalist in the 1970s reveals how our own understanding of sex and sexuality relies on the biological body for its meaning. Rather than affirming what we already think we know about sexuality (that bisexuals were oppressed and it was brave to be open about it), Gore's passing comment provides an alternative way to imagine ourselves, our relationship to others, and to the world around us. In this way, historical thinking hones our ability to queer the present.

Most of us, however, use the past merely to validate and affirm what we already believe to be true. Educators present evidence of same-sex desire in the past to show that same-sex attracted people have always existed. Evidence suggests that simply being represented in a positive light validates LGBTQ2+ people's right to exist today.[4] Images, personal accounts, and other records of strong, accomplished, successful communities like our own and individuals like ourselves is a powerful antidote to the barrage of negative representations we encounter (Hillock, 2016). They affirm our essential human dignity and empower us in our present-day lives.

A common example of the use of history to advance minority rights is the mobilization of evidence of sex between men in ancient Greece, a strategy used since at least the nineteenth century, to call for either a softening of attitudes or even decriminalization (Colligan, 2003; Ross, 2013). Classic texts like Plato's *Symposium* and plays by Aristophanes, as well as Greek artwork, drinking vessels, and vases show that sex between male citizens was celebrated as an honourable and pleasurable practice (Dover, 1978). (See Figure 8.2.) Given that ancient Greece is the foundation of Western civilization, argued men like sex reformer John Addington Symonds and writer Oscar Wilde, surely homosexual practices should not be treated as criminal (Heacox, 2004).

While this strategy enjoyed some success in the political realm, its logic is ahistorical. If we reduce the significance of same-sex sex to the physical act itself – a male-bodied person stroking the penis of another male-bodied person, for example – then what two men did in ancient Greece and what two men might do today are virtually the same. The *act* is transhistorical. But is it gay or even homosexual?

Sexuality, as historians see it, is the "product of distinct and change-able social circumstances, especially discourses around sexuality, which determined the 'nature' of all sexual experience" (Buffington, Luibhéid, & Guy, 2014, p. 3). Thus, sexual acts cannot be divorced from the social and political context in which they occur. Throughout the global north, same-sex attraction is currently considered the expression of an identity or orientation essential to one's nature. Today, one does not just *have* same-sex sex but *is* homosexual or gay (or lesbian, or bisexual, or heterosexual, and so on). The notion that each individual has what we now call a sexual orientation was invented in the mid-1800s by same-sex attracted European men who challenged the criminalization of sodomy. It was subsequently developed by sexologists Richard von Krafft-Ebing (1840–1902) and Havelock Ellis (1859–1939) (Terry, 1995).

---

4 It needs to be pointed out that white historians and anthropologists of the Two-spirit past have long used queer Indigenous histories in ways that prop up colonialism. See Morgensen (2011).

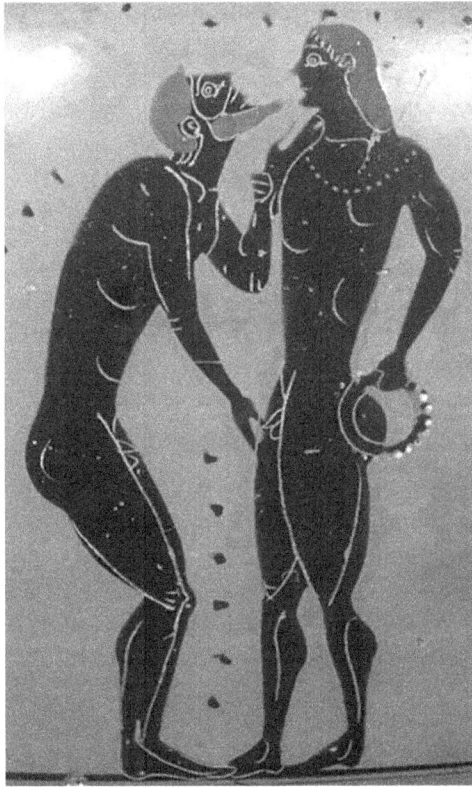

Figure 8.2. Athenian amphora, c. 540 BCE.

Source: Painter of Cambridge, Staatliche Antikensammlungen 1468, Munich. GNU Free Documentation License (CC-BY-SA 3.0).

In ancient Greece, however, homosexuality and heterosexuality simply did not exist. A distinction was made between sex between people of the same sex and sex between opposite sexes. It was even understood that some people, such as Alexander the Great (Johansson, 2016), preferred their own sex. However, the sexual culture between men that flourished in ancient Greece was not separate from the sexual culture between women and men in the way that homosexuality is distinct from hetero-sexuality today. Men who engaged in sex with other men were not con-sidered "gay" or "homosexual" or anything remotely similar.

Sex between men was structured according to a very particular set of social rules (Halperin, 1990). Whereas in our present-day culture, the central distinction in a sex act is the biological sex of the participants, in ancient Greek culture, it evolved around who took an insertive role versus who took a penetrated role. The penetrated role was acceptable only for women, slaves, or male youths who were not yet citizens, all of whom were considered inferior to male citizens. Adult men pursued younger adolescents. They wooed them as one would a female, and they played the insertive role in sexual relations. Attraction to young men was regarded as a sign of masculinity, not effeminacy. Indeed, in the *Symposium*, Plato argued that the ideal army would be comprised of same-sex male lovers (Benardete, 2001, p. 83). Love and sexual attraction were not male or female directed; they were inspired by character and beauty (Pickett, 2018). As a character in Plutarch's Erotikos explains, "The noble lover of beauty engages in love wherever he sees excellence and splendid natural endowment without regard for any difference in physiological detail" (Greenberg, 1988, p. 146).

The context, not just the physical act itself, plays a key role in giving sex acts meaning and shaping the experience and identity of the actors themselves. How ancient Greeks understood same-sex sexual relationships was so fundamentally different from the way gay- and bisexual-identified male Westerners today understand themselves (and the way our culture makes meaning of same-sex attraction) that it simply cannot be said that homosexuality has existed throughout time. Homosexual and bisexual are modern concepts, cultural – not scientific – "truths." To be a gay or bisexual male today is to be a minority, socially marginalized, and in some places, a social pariah and criminal. In ancient Greece, to have sex with a younger man was manly. It was wholly compatible with social respectability and conventional family life (i.e., marriage and fatherhood) (Greenberg, 1988, pp. 141–151).

What about historical examples from the more recent past? Radclyffe Hall was out and proud half a century before gay pride was even a thing. Born Marguerite Radclyffe Hall in 1880, near Bournemouth, England, Hall pursued sexually and emotionally intimate relationships exclusively with women (Vanita, 2007). With two novels – the second earning two major literary prizes – behind them, Hall took the enormous risk of writing a novel whose main protagonist is an invert, a term that some would later argue was equivalent to lesbian. Hall was determined to present "the life of a woman who is a born invert" with "sincerity and truth" in the hope that this would encourage others to come out publicly and engender "a more tolerant understanding" of inverts among "normal" people (Baker, 1985, p. 202). Hall crafted the narrative around protagonist Stephen Gordon (whose parents had hoped for a boy and decided to give their female child the male name they had selected), a fictional character

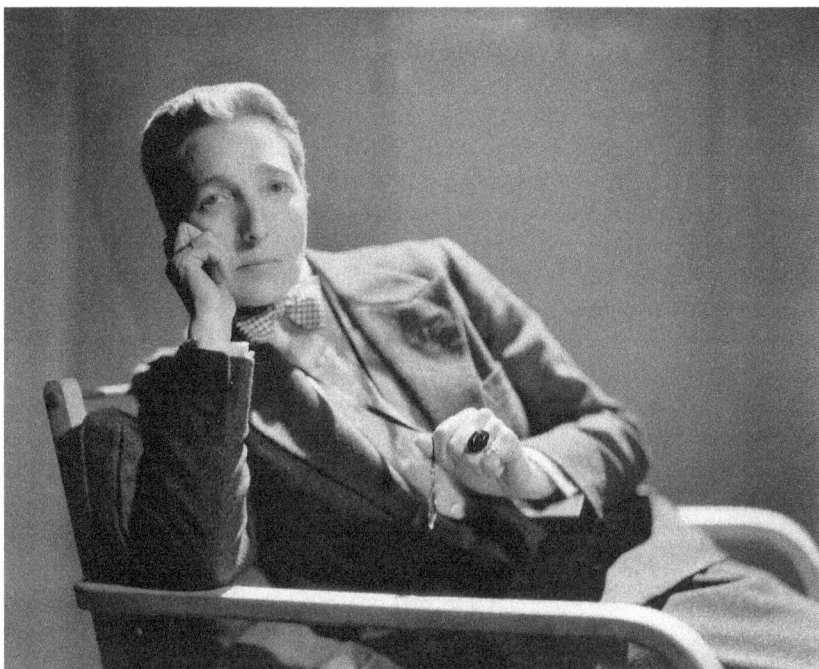

Figure 8.3. Radclyffe Hall.

Source: Photo by Howard Coster. © National Portrait Gallery, London.

who shared Hall's sexual attraction to women and affinity to masculine dress and deportment. Gordon discovers her desire for women at an early age, and, after perusing her father's library, learns she is an invert, a term used by sexologists to describe women and men who are attracted to the same sex and show traits in appearance, affect, or behaviour of the opposite sex. Gordon later becomes lovers with Mary, but because their relationship condemns Mary to a life of misery, she pushes Mary into the arms of a male character, thus ensuring Mary will have a chance at happiness. The novel closes with Gordon pleading with God for "the right to our existence" (Hall, 1928, p. 403).

It surprised no one, least of all Hall, when the Crown laid obscenity charges against the publisher. The trial was a media sensation that generated both sympathy and condemnation. Hall considered herself a martyr, an image many upheld long after her death in 1943. Hall was a genuine historical hero.

But a hero for whom? Neither Hall nor protagonist Stephen Gordon used the word lesbian to describe themself even though it was in use at the time. Instead, Hall identified and depicted Gordon as a congenital invert. The term, invented by sexologists, built upon a theory first proposed by Karl Ulrichs (1825–1895), a former civil servant with a background in law. In a series of booklets titled *Researches on the Riddle of Male-Male Love*, he proposed that same-sex attracted men had a female psyche confined in a male body. Drawing on Plato, Ulrichs named such people Urnings (the term homosexual was not coined until 1869). Although his booklets were published under a pen name, he eventually presented arguments in public in favour of repealing sodomy laws (Kennedy, 1997).

Sexologists Krafft-Ebing and Ellis subsequently theorized that same-sex attracted people were gender inverts, meaning that, as Ulrichs suggested, they were born in the body of one sex, but their disposition was that of the other. Thus, they represented a third sex, a unique combination of male and female traits and attributes (Hovey, 2007). While neither Krafft-Ebing nor Ellis was as reformist as Ulrichs, many same-sex attracted people, including Hall, saw sexological theories as providing compelling arguments against the stigmatization and criminalization of "their kind."[5]

Although many of Hall's lesbian contemporaries criticized *The Well of Loneliness* as "a ridiculous book, trite, superficial," and "loathsome," it was for decades considered a lesbian bible. It was the only novel written about a lesbian by an out lesbian, and many readers related to the suffering Stephen Gordon endured. That changed in the 1970s, when a new generation of same-sex attracted women embraced lesbianism as love for and attraction to sameness, not difference. For them, lesbianism was synonymous with the celebration of female autonomy from traditional gender categories and roles. They rejected conventional femininity, and masculinity was condemned as oppressive and patriarchal. Hall was again a pariah, but for new reasons. In 1984, cultural

---

5 Ellis was hardly a champion of homosexual rights, but his arguments were nevertheless embraced by same-sex attracted people who insisted that their sexuality was not criminal, depraved, or perverse, but merely a benign variation. In a bitter irony, however, these same theories were used to further isolate and penalize homosexuals. By the middle of the twentieth century, homosexuality was treated as a mental illness, and people who were same-sex attracted were incarcerated in mental health institutions and subject to a diverse range of treatments, usually against their will. What Hall and others once saw as a pathway to liberation became a new source of even more cruel oppression.

anthropologist Esther Newton (Newton, 1984) argued that Hall's version of lesbianism must be understood in historical context. At a time when sexual passion was normal for men but deemed deviant in women, and when female intimacy was desexualized, congenital inversion and masculinity were languages that allowed Hall to give shape and meaning to female same-sex desire. In other words, Hall tapped into discourses available to her.

But *was* Hall a lesbian? Is *The Well of Loneliness* a lesbian novel? Post-Newton, Hall became a lesbian history exemplar, despite Hall never themself using the word lesbian. Was that purely strategic on their part, or was it because congenital inversion, which explained same-sex desire through a paradigm of gender inversion, resonated more strongly for Hall than did the term lesbian, which did not necessarily imply a relationship to either masculinity or femininity?

Hall dropped their first name – Marguerite – when they began publishing fiction, and in their personal life went by John, a name given by their first lover, Mabel Batten. Like Stephen Gordon, the female protagonist in *The Well of Loneliness*, Hall dressed in a decidedly masculine style, wearing tailored suits, although with skirts, not pants, and hairstyles popular among cisgender males. Hall characterized Gordon as having a body more male than female. Is Hall better understood as trans?

In 1993, queer theorist Judith Halberstam took up this question directly and concluded that the meaning of the term lesbian is particular to the post-1950s era and cannot be used to describe women who lived even as recently as Hall (Halberstam, 2001). Halberstam argues that rather than fit Hall into our categories, we recognize female masculinity as a category particular to Hall's era and experience. Humanities scholar Jay Prosser disagrees. His interpretation of *The Well of Loneliness* indicates that Gordon (and perhaps, by extension, Hall) is transgender, not lesbian (Prosser, 2001).

Literary scholar Katherine A. Costello (2018) points out that both interpretations rely on a fixed and secure notion of male and female bodies – Gordon either is female and masculine (Halberstam) or trans (Prosser) – and miss a more interesting interpretation. Costello argues that *The Well of Loneliness* embraces sexual indeterminacy. Gordon's sense of self "unmoors identity from [biological] sex"; the novel proposes "a deliberate suspension of knowledge about a body's sex, and especially genitalia" and "open[s] up the possibility of a new taxonomy of identity," an identity based on sexual indeterminacy, defined as "a mobility between maleness and femaleness that turns ambivalence into its own place" (p.3). This is what Gordon meant when referring to the "no-man's-land of sex" (Costello, 2018, p. 3). It is not lesbianism or trans but rather "the recognition of the tragic difficulty of living out such indeterminacy in the face of a hegemonic heterosexuality that is grounded in sexual determinacy and claims love as its exclusive privilege" (p. 6). Like Gore Vidal, who made biological sex irrelevant to his sexual experience, *The Well of Loneliness* asks us to "sustain the discomfort of unknowingness" so that we might build "new forms of embodiment and thus new forms of identity" (Costello, 2018, p. 180).

The desire to claim ancient Greeks and even Hall as forebears to the lesbian, gay, bisexual, and trans present is an approach Laura Doan (2013) calls "ancestral genealogy," whereby historians search the archives for antecedents of contemporary identities to produce a narrative of origins. Even though the vast majority of historians of sexuality reject the notion that lesbian or gay identity is a transhistorical phenomenon, their scholarship nevertheless leans toward origin stories, demonstrating "the tremendous power of identity itself ... [which] like an undertow [,] drag[s] the researcher back to the familiar" (Doan, 2013, p. 92). Even the most sophisticated historians have an "impulse to relate the lesbian, gay, or queer present to the past" (p. 60). They struggle to develop, "a critical history practice that is profoundly skeptical of identities and concepts" to "regard the past as 'radically unknowable'" (p. 60). She argues that what we need to develop and teach is a queer critical history that "constructs the historical meanings of sex and sexuality ... not by tracing back modern sexual identities with a knowingness of what these identities mean to us now but by acknowledging at the outset the unknowability and indeterminacy of the sexual past" (p. 61).

Such an approach is not unique to the history of sexuality. As Sam Wineburg (2001) argues in *Historical Thinking and Other Unnatural Acts,*

> We discard or just ignore vast regions of the past that either contradict our current needs or fail to align tidily with them ... Because we more or less know what we are looking for before we enter this past, our encounter is unlikely to change us or cause us to rethink who we are. (p. 21)

But it is the "strangeness of the past [that] heightens our awareness of how we conceptualize ourselves as human beings" (p. 21). A historian, he argues, is an expert in "cultivat[ing] puzzlement" (p. 21). By developing a critical stance toward "the handful of labels ascribed to us at birth" (Wineburg, 2001, p. 7), historical consciousness – which is the practice of developing understanding beyond our own experience so that we come to know people through a deep and nuanced understanding of their, not our, conditions and circumstances – has the potential to humanize us. Whereas liberal tolerance for difference encourages us to find that which is similar among us, history teaches us that we can never fully – perhaps not even partially – grasp the experience of another. Costello suggests that we may not even be able to grasp our own experience. Our perceptions and judgments will always be partial and imperfect; sometimes, there are no words or no names to capture our complex feelings and emotions. As historian Richard White (Wineburg, 2001) put it, good history begins in strangeness. The past should not be comfortable; it should not be "a familiar echo of the present" (p. 11). Indeed, the most common misperception about the discipline of history is that it is about facts and certainties. Nothing could be further from the truth. The value of historical consciousness is in the questions it generates, not the answers it provides. It offers the ideal space for deep critical reflection on just what we think sexuality is and how we might imagine it, ourselves, and, our world, differently.

Conclusion: Teaching Implications

Using evidence of past beliefs, values, and practices is a wonderful way to engage students in lecture and course material, especially when those practices and beliefs appear radically different from our own. But we must not make the mistake of reinforcing the false notion that we moderns are more knowledgeable, more progressive, or more liberated than our ancestors. For instance, although there is no doubt that women in the West have more social, political, economic, and sexual autonomy than they did just 50 years ago, if we make this the sole point of our engagement with the past, we reinforce a false sense of certainty about the rightness of the historical present.

Western European ideas about the human body have changed over time, yet there are important continuities in theories about the biological basis of male superiority, for example. But facts – even biological ones – never speak for themselves. They must be subjected to the same rigorous scrutiny that we bring to an analysis of pop culture, for example. The jewel in the history of sexuality's crown is its capacity to denaturalize that which we think is natural, to "queer" what appears as just common sense, and to see facts as ideologies in motion. By bringing not just history, but historical consciousness, into our teaching and the classroom, we can deepen students' capacity for critical analysis of sexuality, build exciting pathways across multiple disciplines, and entertain our students with images of penises. Or was it a vagina?

REFERENCES

Baker, M. (1985). *Our three selves: The life of Radclyffe Hall.* London: Hamish Hamilton.

Barnes, S. (1973, September 16). Behind the face of the gifted bitch. *The Sunday Times Magazine. Sunday Times*, p. 44[S]+.

Benardete, S., & Bloom, A. (2001). *Plato's symposium.* Chicago: University of Chicago Press.

Buffington, R. M., Luibhéid, E., & Guy, Donna J. (Eds.). (2014). *A global history of sexuality: The modern era.* Hoboken, NJ: John Wiley & Sons.

Colligan, C. (2003). "A race of born pederasts": Sir Richard Burton, homosexuality, and the Arabs. *Nineteenth-Century Contexts, 25*(1), 1–20. https://doi.org/10.1080/0890549032000069131

Costello, K. A. (2018). A no-man's-land of sex: Reading Stephen Gordon and "her" critics. *Journal of Lesbian Studies, 22*(2), 165–184. https://doi.org/10.1080/10894160.2017.1342457

Doan, L. (2013). *Disturbing practices: History, sexuality, and women's experience of modern war.* Chicago: University of Chicago Press.

Dover, K. (1978). *Greek homosexuality.* Cambridge, Mass.: Harvard University Press.

Greenberg, D. (1988). *The construction of homosexuality.* Chicago: University of Chicago Press.

Halberstam, J. (2001). "A writer of misfits": "John" Radclyffe Hall and the discourse of inversion. In L. Doan & J. Prosser (Eds), *Palatable poison: Critical perspectives on* The well of loneliness (pp. 145–161). New York: Columbia University Press.

Hall, R. (1928). *The well of loneliness.* Garden City, N.Y.: Sun Dial Press.

Halperin, D. (1990). *One hundred years of homosexuality: And other essays on Greek love.* New York: Routledge.

Harvey, K. (2005). Sexuality and the body. In H. Barker & E. Chalus (Eds.), *Women's history: Britain, 1700–1850: An introduction* (pp. 79–99). London: Routledge.

Heacox, T. (2004). "Idealized through Greece": Hellenism and homoeroticism in works by Wilde, Symonds, Mann, and Forster." *Sexuality and Culture, 8*(2), 52–79. https://doi.org/10.1007/s12119-004-1012-3

Hillock, S. (2016). Social work, the academy, and queer communities: Heteronormativity and exclusion. In S. Hillock & N. J. Mulé. (Eds.). *Queering social work education* (pp. 73–92). Vancouver: UBC Press.

Hovey, J. (2007). Third sex. In F. Malti-Douglas (Ed.), *Encyclopedia of sex and gender* (Vol. 4, pp. 1461–1462). Detroit, MI: Macmillan Reference USA. Retrieved from https://link-gale com.proxy.lib.sfu.ca/apps/doc/CX2896200637/GVRL?u=sfu_z39&sid=GVRL&xid=3c42f5af.

Johansson, W. (2016). Alexander the Great. In *Encyclopedia of homosexuality* (Vol. I, pp. 39–40). New York: Routledge.

Johnson, D. (2006). *The lavender scare: The Cold War persecution of gays and lesbians in the federal government.* Chicago: University of Chicago Press.

Kennedy, H. (1997). Karl Heinrich Ulrichs: First theorist of homosexuality. In V. Rosario (Ed.), *Science and homosexualities* (pp. 26–45). New York, NY: Routledge.

Laqueur, T. (1990) *Making sex: Body and gender from the Greeks to Freud.* Cambridge: Harvard University Press.

Morgensen, S. L. (2011). *Spaces between us: Queer settler colonialism and Indigenous decolonization.* Minneapolis: University of Minnesota Press.

Newton, E. (1984). The mythic mannish lesbian: Radclyffe Hall and the New Woman. *Signs, 9*(4), 557–575. https://doi.org/10.1086/494087

Park, K. (1997). The rediscovery of the clitoris: French medicine and the tribade, 1570–1620. In C. Mazzio & D. Hillman (Eds.), *The body in parts: Fantasies of corporeality in Early Modern Europe* (pp. 171–193). New York: Routledge.

Pickett, B. (2018). Homosexuality. In E. N. Zalta (Ed.), *The Stanford encyclopedia of philosophy* (Spring 2018 ed.). Retrieved from https://plato.stanford.edu /archives/spr2018/entries/homosexuality/.

Prosser, J. (2001). "Some primitive thing conceived in a turbulent age of transition": The transsexual emerging from *The well.* In L. Doan & J. Prosser (Eds.), *Palatable poison: Critical perspectives on* The well of loneliness (pp. 129–144). New York: Columbia University Press.

Ross, I. (2013). *Oscar Wilde and Ancient Greece.* Cambridge: Cambridge University Press.

Scott, J. W. (1988). *Gender and the politics of history.* New York: Columbia University Press.

Terry, J. (1995). Anxious slippages between "us" and "them": A brief history of the scientific search for homosexual bodies. In J. Terry & J. L. Urla (Eds.), *Deviant bodies: Critical perspectives on difference in science and popular culture* (pp. 129–69). Indiana University Press.

Vanita, R. (2007). Hall, Radclyffe 1880–1943. In F. Malti-Douglas (Ed.), *Encyclopedia of sex and gender* (Vol. 2, pp. 669–670). Macmillan Reference, USA. Gale eBooks, https://link-gale-com.proxy.lib.sfu.ca/apps/doc/CX2896200284/GVRL?u=sfu _z39&sid=GVRL&xid=905256b2. Accessed 13 Oct. 2019.

Vidal, G. (1948). *The city and the pillar.* New York: New American Library.

Vidal, G., & Stanton, R. (1980). *Views from a window: Conversations with Gore Vidal* (1st ed.). Secaucus, N.J.: L. Stuart.

Wineburg, S. (2001). *Historical thinking and other unnatural acts: Charting the future of teaching the past.* Philadelphia: Temple University Press.

9 Queering Masculinity in Early Childhood and Higher Education Classrooms: Gendered Regulation and the Double Bind of Queer Masculinities

ADAM W.J. DAVIES

While much work has begun to address the regulation of genders and sexualities in early learning settings and early childhood education (ECE) (Davies, 2003; Robinson, 2005), there is still a dearth of literature exploring the lived experiences of queer men who are early childhood educators and the regulation of queer masculinity within the fields of ECE and preservice teacher education. Through practices of gender policing and regulation, the gendered expressions of queer men who are educators – specifically expressions of queer masculinities – are pathologized and subjugated in work with young children (Moosa & Bhana, 2019). The field of ECE is often feminized and structurally underappreciated due to societal femmephobia – the regulation and policing of femininity (Davies, 2020; Davies & Hoskin, 2021; Hoskin, 2017) – and the devaluation of care work (Davies & Hoskin, 2021). Queer men within early childhood settings are caught in a double bind of failing to embody tenets of hegemonic masculinity due to their queerness, while simultaneously being recruited into the field through discourses that seek out men as "masculinizing" influences in early learning settings (Davies & Hoskin, 2021; Warin, 2018).

In this chapter, I explore my lived experiences working and teaching, and use them as a framing device to discuss how gender and sexuality norms operate to gender police both educators and children in ECE settings. Teaching is inherently both a personal and political endeavour that weaves through the autobiographical self (Pinar, 1975). Reflecting on my experiences provides me with a starting point for understanding how crucial it is to cultivate safer educational spaces for both gender-diverse children *and* educators. Grace (2006) states that writing the queer self as a form of narrative praxis can "create a space to confront homophobia; to transgress heteronormativity as the normative perspective on sex, sexuality and gender; and to explore an illimitable array of queer positionalities" (p. 828). With this, I begin.

My Social Location

To start this chapter, I should locate myself as a white, queer, openly disabled,[1] cisgender male academic. I am currently an assistant professor at the University of Guelph, teaching in the Family Relations and Human Development program, where many of my undergraduate students are entering the field of ECE or planning to undertake bachelor of education preservice elementary teaching programs. Previously, I taught courses at Ryerson University in Early Childhood Studies. I focus much of my scholarly work on issues of gender and sexuality and inclusion in early years and school-age education. After receiving my official certification with the College of Early Childhood Educators through my master's degree, which was a teacher education preservice program with a specialization in elementary education and ECE, I worked in the field of ECE as I continued my graduate education. A great deal of my work experience comes from working within childcare and after-school programming. Before entering my preservice teacher education degree program, I completed an undergraduate degree in music education, with a focus on elementary music education. Throughout my postsecondary education, I was fairly frequently one of the only men in my classes; this was also true of my workplace experiences. Moreover, I was commonly the only queer individual in my work and educational settings, where little discussion of gender or sexual diversity occurred. This often left me feeling as though I was the sole representative of all gender and sexual diversity, which felt partial and flawed. For many in the field of education, whether to come out or disclose one's sexual identity is a difficult issue. Because my effeminate[2] gender expression often meant I was read as queer instantaneously, I often did not have the option of whether or not to declare my sexuality to others.

---

1 Here I use "identity first language" to openly identify with my disabilities and the disability community by not neatly separating or distinguishing disability from my personhood (Titchkosky, 2001). The politics of various disabilities and diagnostic categorizations are beyond the scope of this chapter, but I openly note my experiences with/in diagnostic categorization to challenge ableism in the academy.

2 There are many complexities surrounding the usage of the word "effeminate." I use this term to denote male femininity, the open visibility of queerness in men, and being outside the bounds of heteronormative constructs for masculinity (Davies, 2020). However, I note important work that has critiqued this term, its pathological history, and how it has been used to place constructions of masculinities as higher than femininities (Hoskin, 2017, as cited in Davies, 2020).

ECE and Men as Educators

Within the field of ECE, few men work as educators. Accordingly, the research literature describes how men are "missing" in the field of ECE (Wernersson, 2015). In 2013, the Ontario College of Early Childhood Educators reported that about there are approximately 599 male registered early childhood educators (RECEs) in Ontario, or 1.4% of a total of 41,700 certifications (Irish, 2013). This gap highlights several issues that relate to the gendering of ECE as a "feminized" field (Scurfield, 2017). Moreover, focusing on the numbers gap between men and women employed as ECEs, as Peeters, Rohrmann, and Emilsen (2015) state, "can lead to the idealization of male workers even when they lack experience and training. At the same time, it raises suspicions when a man 'lowers' himself to work with young children" (p. 308). In short, while there is a low percentage of male educators in the field of ECE, the research literature constructs this "gender gap" based on several problematic presumptions (Davies & Hoskin, 2021; Warin, 2018).

Studying ECE as a Queer Man

While I was studying ECE and elementary education in my preservice teacher education program and undergraduate degree, I observed that explicit conversations about gender and sexual diversity were missing from course curricula; no individual courses on gender and sexual diversity from critical theory or psychosocial perspectives were offered in the early years or elementary education. Taking a predominantly developmental and psychological standpoint (Ainsworth, 1973; Bowlby, 1969; Erikson, 1968; Piaget, 1936, 1945, 1957; Volpe, 2010; Vygotsky, 1978), classes importantly focused on children's mental health, developmental psychology, literacy instruction and professional ethics. Still, classes infrequently mentioned LGBTQ+ identities. For me as one of very few queer students, it was often challenging to find others who could relate to my lived experiences. The respectability politics of preservice teaching and early childhood education, as with many professions, including social work and the social services fields, heterosexualize and pathologize open conversations about sexuality, particularly queer sexualities (DePalma & Jennett, 2010; Mizzi, 2016). Personally experiencing many feelings of isolation and displacement, I struggled at times in postsecondary education at both the undergraduate, preservice, and graduate levels, to find a sense of belonging. Feeling fractured, I had to compartmentalize my various selves and conform to the dominant norms within the professionalized environment of the field of education. My own lived experiences as a young queer man and my life within queer circles – particularly gay men's cultures and communities – were very different than the hetero-sexualized environment of my educational trajectory.

During my field placements and practicums, I would often try to incorporate conversations of gender and sexual diversity into the pre-existing curriculum. For example, teaching in a grade one classroom, I taught students the LGBTQ+ (lesbian, gay, bisexual, transgender, queer) acronym and the various identities each letter represents. Following this, I read a different storybook each day depicting a specific identity under the LGBTQ+ umbrella and discussed different family and relationship structures with my students. I was fortunate enough to be in a placement setting near Toronto's Church and Wellesley Gay Village, where these conversations of gender and sexual diversity were normalized for children. As well, the associate teacher with whom I worked was supportive of these conversations taking place in his classroom and was aware that the Grades 1–8 2015 Health & Physical Education Curriculum (OME, 2015), recently updated, now included content regarding diverse family structures and gender and sexual identities. It is critical for early childhood educators to have administrative and educator support when discussing gender and sexuality in the classroom (Kroeger & Regula, 2017), as well as curricular backing, such as embedded curricular expectations for addressing LGBTQ+ content (Balter, van Rhijn, & Davies, 2016, 2018).

In my differing placements, I was continually informed of the paucity of male educators in the fields of ECE and elementary education. The low number of male ECEs in Ontario has inspired recruitment efforts. These efforts, although important, often result in reinforcing the notion that men have essentially different traits than women, and that it is, therefore, important to recruit "male role models" who can embody tenets of maleness and impart traditional notions of masculinity (Davies & Hoskin, 2021; Martino, 2008; Warin, 2019; Warin & Adriany, 2017). In a Swedish context, Wernersson (2015) discusses how conversations about the low numbers of men in the field of ECE can rely on biologically essentialist notions that promote binarized ideas of essential sex differences in characteristics between men and women. Within my practicum placements, as much as I was commonly praised for being a man in the field of ECE and elementary education, I was still seen as failing to meet the markers of hegemonic masculinity (Connell, 1995) by not being sporty or athletic enough.

Within units in my placements, I discussed diverse family structures with students and attempted to incorporate a plurality of families and family dynamics into our conversations. Taking an approach in which I discussed different kinds of families without specifically emphasizing one structure, I incorporated photos of polyamorous families and families with more than one or two adult or parental figures into the class display board and conversations. I again feared that my visible queerness would position me in a tokenistic fashion, whereby I would be identified as the primary reason why LGBTQ+ content was being incorporated into classroom discussions. I primarily feared that I would receive pushback for incorporating LGBTQ+ content – specifically, open discussion of polyamorous relationships and families – and that because of my queerness, parents and community members would see me as solely responsible for these conversations. In truth, my mentor teacher with whom I worked strongly supported me in beginning LGBTQ+ conversations within this placement. My fear carried over into many other placements and practicum experiences. In education, as in other disciplines and fields, including social work, there are still many normative assumptions about family structures (Williams & Prior, 2015). These normative assumptions stigmatize polyamorous families and prevent open conversations about queer families and how to ensure greater comfortability and access to services for queer families (Boyd, 2017; Pallotta-Chiarolli, Haydon, & Hunter, 2013). Further research is necessary, particularly in a Canadian context, on polyamorous families' experiences navigating social services and childcare settings (Boyd, 2017; Pallotta-Chiarolli, Sheff, & Mountford, 2020; Williams & Prior, 2015).

During placements, I considered whether or not to come out about my sexuality, and what the ramifications might be. This is a dilemma for many queer educators, as coming out is a personal journey that can be filled with questions and struggles. When children asked me if had a wife, girlfriend, or female partner, I answered that I did have a partner at the time, but that he was a boy; or I would state that I had a boyfriend and then inform the children that "princes sometimes love princes instead of princesses" – an approach that is rather simplistic, binarized, and imperfect but does open the door slightly for further conversations regarding queer sexualities and relationships. As well, I often introduced the children's books: *The Princes and the Treasure* by Jeffrey A. Miles (2014) or *King & King* by Linda de Haan and Stern Nijland (2002). These stories are picture books for young children that explain male same-sex relationships through colourful photos and whimsical fairytales. These texts proved key to opening conversations in my various placements and were useful guides whenever students asked about my relationship status. (See Box 9.1 later in this chapter for a list of LGBTQ+ children's books.)

While these texts are important, using books that depict same-sex relationships in a fairy tale style comes with limitations. Structures of whiteness and class privilege in such books can constitute what Taylor (2012), drawing on Duggan (2003), deems the "homonormative subject" in LGBTQ+ children's literature. Many producers are actively working to create LGBTQ+ children's literature that is diverse and intersectional (such as the Toronto LGBTQ+ independent press Flamingo Rampant – also see Davies & skelton, 2017).

Queer Masculinities in Childcare Settings

As I worked in the field of ECE, I quickly discovered how deeply entrenched gendered norms and the heterosexualization of young children are in the field (Davies, 2003; Robinson, 2005). Robinson (2005) describes the interconnections between heterosexuality and gender normativity as desirable outcomes for young children by explaining how, through "processes of gendering, children are constructed as heterosexual beings" (p. 19). It is common for educators to regulate toy and sticker choices for boys and girls (through binary notions), identify items using gendered colours (i.e., blue for boys and pink for girls), celebrate pretend marriages for children, or state that children of the opposite sex are "dating." My presence as someone visibly queer within these heterosexualized settings often disrupted the notion that children will naturally develop into heterosexual adults or that binarized gendered norms and heterosexuality are compulsory (Rich, 1980).

Regulating the Queer Male Body

Children are not the only ones policed in educational settings. Throughout my years working in childcare settings, pursuing undergraduate and graduate studies, and eventually teaching in ECE at the higher education level, I have always been positioned as having a visibly queer body. All bodies are regulated under what Foucault (1977) theorizes as "panoptic surveillance," a concept based on English philosopher Jeremy Bentham's panoptic prison design. Bentham designed the panoptic prison to position the prison guard in a tall central tower and to hold inmates in prison cells with open walls facing the tower. Thus, inmates would not be aware of exactly when the prison guard was watching and would constantly regulate their own behaviours and actions as if they were always being watched. Expanding on the idea of the panopticon, Foucault (1977) theorized that modern society operates under dispersed yet omnipresent forms of social control. Within the panopticon, the body's movements are policed and regulated continuously through societal norms and the gaze of others. Because of this social control, individuals willingly change their behaviours, actions, and appearances to conform to societal norms for fear of being noticed as out of place or abnormal. Foucault (1977) describes how panopticism operates through the visibility of the body, saying, "she [sic] who is subjected to a field of visibility, and who knows it, assumes responsibility for the constraints of power" (p. 202). Within my own professional practices, I felt the continual gaze of others, particularly as I interacted with children (see Davies, Vipond, & King, 2019, for another application of panopticism; or Ingrey, 2012).

In one childcare setting within a community centre, the entire front wall of the room I worked in was a glass window. People who were exercising or using the centre for recreational purposes could look into the room to see how I and the other care workers were interacting with their children. While individuals often stopped and glanced into the room, there were many quiet times where the hallway was empty. Still, I never knew when individuals would be stopping to look, so I regulated my interactions with children as though I were always being watched. For many male early childhood educators, cultural panics about men having physical contact with young children are common barriers to men being hired. In Alison Jones's (2003) qualitative research regarding the place of pleasure, desire, and sensuality in ECE, a participant states, "with the rooms the way they are I would not hire a male in this centre probably. I'd be getting questions from the parents. It's not open enough" (p. 241). Correspondingly, Jones (2003) explains how the field of ECE fears the "spectral pervert" (p. 241) in the space of the washroom. Without an open environment where the male educator can be surveilled, panics emerge about potential pedophilia.

Paranoia about men, particularly queer men, in classrooms with young children works in contrast to discourses that construct men as "missing" from the field of ECE. In the Swedish context, Eidevald, Bergström and Broström (2018) discuss how male early childhood educators manoeuvre and position themselves in relationship to discourses of male pedophilia. Eidevald et al. (2018) state there is

> a risk for men who provide care to children in ECEC that includes physical contact, as the pedophile discourse points them out as potential perpetrators. Care is at the same time seen as important for children's well-being, and physical contact in a diaper change, nap-time, comforting and dressing is seen as necessary to professional work in ECEC. (p. 409)

Within this double bind, men are constructed as potentially predatory, while simultaneously being enjoined to use physical touch to support the well-being and positive development of children. The specific double bind of queer masculinity positions queer men as simultaneously included and excluded in ECE spaces. That is, as men, they are sought after to provide masculinizing influences in the field of ECE. At the same time, they are excluded should they fail to meet heteronormative standards of masculinity (Davies, 2020; Davies & Hoskin, 2021). In addition, as men, they are seen as potentially predatory, especially if they are visibly queer. Eidevald et al. (2018) suggest that cultural anxieties and surveillance emerge related to the bodies of both male educators and children in ECE settings. This cultural anxiety positions male educators in general as a potential threat to children; and, as Moosa and Bhana (2019) state, this "terror of sexual abuse is further entrenched within the construction of the gay man as the ultimate sexual predator" (p. 4).

Gender and Sexuality in ECE Higher Education

After completing my teacher education program, I moved into graduate studies and decided to focus on gender and sexuality in ECE as one of my research areas, with my doctoral thesis being on gay masculinities and the politics of emotional intimacies and connections between gay men (Davies, 2021). During my doctoral studies, I began teaching in early childhood studies programs. In my teaching, I addressed topics related to gender and sexuality, even though my courses were not described as being about these topics. While gender and sexuality are increasingly being discussed in elementary and secondary education classrooms (Davies & skelton, 2017; Greensmith & Davies, 2018; Simons, Grant, & Rodas, 2021), the field of ECE still addresses gender and sexual diversity in a limited and binarized fashion, particularly in terms of training preservice educators (Kroeger & Regula, 2017) and cultivating space for educators to deconstruct gendered assumptions (Kroeger, Recker, & Gunn, 2019). In a research study I was involved with (Balter, van Rhijn, & Davies, 2016, 2018), our informal examination of postsecondary ECE programs in Ontario discovered that no courses on gender and sexuality, specifically, were being offered to preservice ECE students in Ontario. When I began to teach in the higher education system, I found opportunities to incorporate gender and sexuality into my early childhood education courses through a "topic of the week" approach. While this approach to addressing gender and sexuality can be seen as tokenistic or additive, I purposely included my week on gender and sexual diversity in ECE at the beginning of the course. This way, I was able to reference material discussed during this week throughout the remainder of the course.

Indeed, discussions of gender and sexuality are often absent from higher education ECE programs (Balter et al., 2016) but are still ingrained in the "hidden curriculum," or the embedded and underlying values and beliefs of educational institutions (Balter et al., 2018; Giroux, 1981; Giroux & Purpel, 1983; Jackson, 1968; Robinson & Davies, 2017). These values can be communicated through preservice educators' pre-conceived notions of children as innocent, asexual, or "cute" (Balter et al., 2018; Robinson & Davies, 2017). As mentioned previously, many educators see children within a gender binary, limited to stereotypical ideas about boys and girls (Balter et al., 2016, 2018; Davies, Vipond, & King, 2019; Ingrey, 2012) To help counter these tendencies, I strive to incorporate gender and sexuality into my teachings as much as possible. In doing so, here are some of the challenges I have encountered.

Challenges

Allen and Rasmussen (2015) discuss how teaching queer theory in higher education programs is limited because education programs often consider queer theory as only being about gender and sexuality – not about teaching practices (i.e., limiting the idea of *queering* pedagogical practices). Therefore, discussions of gender and sexuality are seen as outside the bounds of the required curricula. As the only queer educator and theorist in many early learning settings, I was often asked, "Do all gay men look and act like you?" These comments provide one example of the systemic denigration and regulation of femininity – i.e., femmephobia (see Davies, 2020; Davies & Hoskin, 2021; Hoskin, 2017) – in men in ECE and society at large (Davies & Hoskin, 2021).

Kroeger and Regula's (2017) research suggests ways that postsecondary ECE educators who teach preservice candidates can openly address gender diversity with young children and families through an antibias approach. An antibias approach to teaching and early childhood curricula seeks to counteract forms of bias and discrimination that arise in the form of preconceived notions, hidden ideologies, and taken-for-granted norms in the classroom by encouraging critical self-reflection, collective community, and dialogue (Kroeger & Regula, 2017). Such an approach addresses the diverse ways that gender diversity presents itself in young children. Kroeger, Recker, and Gunn (2019) describe how an LGBTQ-affirming antibias approach to teaching cultivates spaces for young children to ask questions about gender openly and freely with educators and each other, holds space for LGBTQ children's literature that features diverse characters, and incorporates materials and content that do not reinforce or reify any gender norms or centre heterosexual narratives.

I argue that an antibias approach can be equally useful in preservice ECE classrooms for dismantling gender biases regarding both children and educators (Kroeger & Regula, 2017; Kroeger, Recker, & Gunn, 2019).

In my own experience as an educator, my queer self-presentation and flexible masculinity disrupts the expectation of heteronormativity within these classrooms; therefore, I effectively employ my own visibility as part of my teaching approach, given that my visibility is not a choice (see also hicks, 2016). This is true for many gender-nonconforming educators as well (not that visibility should *always* be equated with queerness or gender nonconformity – see Hoskin, 2017). Trans educator and activist benjamin lee hicks (2016) writes in the context of elementary education,

> I needed to learn what sort of access I would allow others to assume when it came to the visibility/vulnerability of my own queerness. I now see that learning to articulate how I feel about my right to privacy co-existing with the hyper-visibility that I can't always control is analogous to creating safe(r), queer(er) classroom spaces with my students. (hicks, 2016, p. 131)

This explanation conveys the inherent vulnerability that arises when an educator is unable to control how their queerness (and others' readings of their queerness) positions them within the classroom. As a queer man in early childhood postsecondary classrooms, my embodied presence means that I am either hyper-visible or unrecognizable as a properly male subject (Davies, 2020; Davies & Hoskin, 2021; Hoskin, 2017); I am continually positioned as an "other" in contrast to the heterosexual norm. The vulnerability of this position provides me with both opportunities and challenges. Ultimately, by embracing the visibility and vulnerability of my queerness, I am able to move toward new conversations with my students (hicks, 2016).

Teaching Resources and Exercises

Based on my experiences teaching and learning within higher education ECE settings, as well as early learning and childcare locations, I would like to propose a few lessons and next steps to consider. By bringing our queer selves into our professional praxis as educators in various forms – for instance, by speaking openly about our partners, lovers, and queer friends – we can shift discourses that cast queerness and gender nonconformity as failures, disturbances, or dangers, particularly as it pertains to the highly professionalized fields of preservice teacher education and ECE (Grace, 2006; hicks, 2016). Bringing diverse stories into the classroom to provide narratives beyond and outside heteronormativity is important for moving beyond merely including gender and sexual diversity.

With my preservice ECEs, I used the story *I Am Jazz*, written by Jazz Jennings (Herthel & Jennings, 2014), a transgender teenager and advocate who has been open about her journey transitioning throughout her

---

Box 9.1: Recommended LGBTQ Children's Books

Bergman, S. B., & Dougherty, R. (2015). *Is that for a boy or a girl?* Toronto, ON: Flamingo Rampant.

De Haan, L., & Nijland, S. (2002). *King & king.* San Francisco, CA: Tricycle Press.

Herthel, J., & Jennings, J. (2014). *I am Jazz.* New York, NY: Penguin.

Hoffman, S., & Hoffman, I. (2014). *Jacob's new dress.* Chicago, IL: Albert Whitman and Company.

Kilodavis, C. (2011). *My princess boy.* New York, NY: Simon and Schuster.

Miles, J. (2014). *The princes and the treasure.* Handsome Prince Publishing.

Newman, L., & Thompson, C. (2009). *Daddy, Papa, and me.* Berkeley, CA: Tricycle Publishing.

Newman, L., & Thompson, C. (2009). *Mommy, Mama, and me.* Berkeley, CA: Tricycle Publishing.

Parker, G. & Orchard, S. (2017). *Bell's knock birthday!* Toronto, ON: Flamingo Rampant.

---

childhood and adolescence. Instead of reading the story myself, I showed a video of Jazz herself reading the story. This allowed my students to see her facial expressions and emotions as she narrated her gender transition. Following this reading, I asked my students to reflect on how adult figures in Jazz's life listened to her words, validated her feelings, and supported her through her transition. I asked my students to picture themselves in the role of an adult figure in Jazz's life and to imagine how they would support Jazz and what they would say to her to ensure she felt safe in their care. I asked them to take note of the ways in which she advocates for herself. I then asked students how they would respond to Jazz if she was one of their siblings, their best friend, or a child in their care. Moving through this progression, students began to reflect upon how they could translate the care they would provide for a loved one to their everyday practices with children. I also recommend the books listed Box 9.1.

Conclusion

My experiences as a queer man in the field of ECE leads me to recommend having deeper conversations about supporting gender diversity for *both* educators' and children's well-being. For many queer men, the fears and cultural anxieties surrounding the presence of men in the classroom might limit their career trajectories or place them in a double bind by which their masculinity is both required and reviled. My hope is that these self-reflections and recommendations might inspire further conversations about the importance of embracing the vulnerability and openness of being visibly queer in the classroom (hicks, 2016), particularly within the fields of pre-service teacher education and ECE, while crafting more space for open conversations with young children about gender and sexual diversity.

REFERENCES

Ainsworth, M. D. S. (1973). The development of infant-mother attachment. In B. Cardwell & H. Ricciuti (Eds.), *Review of child development research, Vol. 3* (pp. 1–94). Chicago: University of Chicago Press.

Allen, L., & Rasmussen, M. L. (2015). Queer conversation in straight spaces: An interview with Mary Lou Rasmussen about queer theory in higher education. *Higher Education Research & Development, 34*(4), 685–694. https://doi.org /10.1080/07294360.2015.1062072

Balter, A. S., van Rhijn, T. M., & Davies, A. W. (2016). The development of sexuality in childhood in early learning settings: An exploration of early childhood educators' perceptions. *The Canadian Journal of Human Sexuality, 25*(1), 30–40. https://doi.org/10.3138/cjhs.251-a3

Balter, A. S., van Rhijn, T., & Davies, A. W. (2018). Equipping early childhood educators to support the development of sexuality in childhood: Identification of pre-and post-service training needs. *The Canadian Journal of Human Sexuality, 27*(1), 33–42. https://doi.org/10.3138/cjhs.2017-0036

Bowlby J. (1969). *Attachment. Attachment and loss: Vol. 1. Loss.* New York: Basic Books.

Boyd, J. P. (2017). *Polyamory in Canada: Research on an emerging family structure.* Alberta, Canada: Canadian Research Institute for Law and the Family. Retrieved from https://prism.ucalgary.ca/bitstream/handle/1880/107495 /Boyd%20Polyamorous%20Families%201.pdf?sequence=1

Brownhill, S. (2015). Male role models in education-based settings (0–8): An English perspective. In S. Brownhill, J. Warin, & I. Wernersson (Eds.), *Men, masculinities and teaching in ECE* (pp. 44–53). London, UK: Routledge.

Connell, R. W. (1995). *Masculinities.* Berkeley, CA: University of California Press.

Davies, A. W. (2020). "Authentically" effeminate? Bialystok's theorization of authenticity, gay male femmephobia, and personal identity. *Canadian Journal of Family and Youth/Le Journal Canadien de Famille et de la Jeunesse, 12*(1), 104–123. https://doi.org/10.29173/cjfy29493

Davies, A. W. (2021). Queering app-propriate behaviours: The affective politics of gay socio-sexual applications. [Unpublished doctoral dissertation]. University of Toronto, Toronto, Canada.

Davies, A. W., & Hoskin, R. A. (2021). Using femme theory to foster a feminine-inclusive early childhood education practice. In Z. Abawi, R. Berman, & A. Eizadirad (Eds.), *Equity as praxis in early childhood education and care*. Toronto: Canadian Scholars.

Davies, A. W., Vipond, E., & King, A. (2019). Gender binary washrooms as a means of gender policing in schools: A Canadian perspective. *Gender and Education, 31*(7), 866–885. https://doi.org/10.1080/09540253.2017.1354124

Davies, A. W., & wallace skelton, j. (2017). Queer and trans at school. *Education Canada, 57*(2), 42–44. Retrieved from: https://www.edcan.ca/articles/queer-trans-school/

Davies, B. (2003). *Frogs and snails and feminist tales: Preschool children and gender*. New York: Hampton Press.

DePalma, R., & Jennett, M. (2010). Homophobia, transphobia and culture: Deconstructing heteronormativity in English primary schools. *Intercultural Education, 21*(1), 15–26. https://doi.org/10.1080/14675980903491858

Duggan, L. (2003). *The twilight of equality? Neoliberalism, cultural politics, and the attack on democracy*. Boston, MA: Beacon Press.

Eidevald, C., Bergström, H., & Broström, A. W. (2018). Maneuvering suspicions of being a potential pedophile: Experiences of male ECEC-workers in Sweden. *European Early Childhood Education Research Journal, 26*(3), 407–417. https://doi.org/10.1080/1350293x.2018.1463907

Erikson, E. H. (1968). *Identity: Youth and crisis*. New York, NY: Norton.

Flamingo Rampant Press. [Home page]. (n.d.). *Flamingo Rampant*. Retrieved October 19, 2019, from https://www.flamingorampant.com

Foucault, M. (1977/2012). *Discipline and punish: The birth of the prison*. New York, NY: Vintage.

Giroux, H. A. (1981). Schooling and the myth of objectivity: Stalking the politics of the hidden curriculum. *McGill Journal of Education, 16*(3), 282–304.

Giroux, H., & Purpel, D. (1983). *The hidden curriculum and moral education*. Berkeley, CA: McCuthchan Publishing Corporation.

Grace, A. P. (2006). Writing the queer self: Using autobiography to mediate inclusive teacher education in Canada. *Teaching and Teacher Education, 22*(7), 826–834. https://doi.org/10.1016/j.tate.2006.04.026

Greensmith, C., & Davies, A. W. J. (2017). Queer and trans at school: Gay-straight alliances and the politics of inclusion. In X. Chen, R. Raby, & P. Albanese (Eds.), *The sociology of childhood and youth in Canada* (pp. 314–334). Toronto: Canadian Scholars.

Herthel, J., & Jennings, J. (2014). *I am Jazz*. New York, NY: Penguin.

hicks, b. l. (2016). Gracefully unexpected, deeply present, and positively disruptive: Love and queerness in community classroom. In D. Linville (Ed.), *Queering education: Pedagogy, curriculum, policy* (pp. 130–145). Retrieved from https://files.eric.ed.gov/fulltext/ED573409.pdf

Hoskin, R. A. (2017). Femme theory: Refocusing the intersectional lens. *Atlantis: Critical Studies in Gender, Culture & Social Justice, 38*(1), 95–109.

Ingrey, J. C. (2012). The public school washroom as analytic space for troubling gender: Investigating the spatiality of gender through students' self-knowledge. *Gender and Education, 24*(7), 799–817. https://doi.org/10.1080/09540253.2012.721537

Irish, P. (2013, February 7). Men stand out as daycare workers. *The Toronto Star.* Retrieved from https://www.thestar.com/life/parent/2013/02/07/men_stand_out_as_daycare_workers.html

Jackson, P. (1968). *Life in classrooms.* New York, NY: Holt, Rinehart and Winston, Inc.

Jones, A. (2003). The monster in the room: Safety, pleasure and early childhood education. *Contemporary Issues in Early Childhood, 4*(3), 235–250. https://doi.org/10.2304/ciec.2003.4.3.2

Kroeger, J., Recker, A. E., & Gunn, A. C. (2019). Tate and the pink coat: Exploring gender and enacting anti-bias principles. *YC Young Children, 74*(1), 83–92.

Kroeger, J., & Regula, L. (2017). Queer decisions in early childhood teacher education: Teachers as advocates for gender non-conforming and sexual minority young children and families. *International Critical Childhood Policy Studies Journal, 6*(1), 106–121.

Martino, W. (2008). The lure of hegemonic masculinity: Investigating the dynamics of gender relations in two male elementary school teachers' lives. *International Journal of Qualitative Studies in Education, 21*(6), 575–603. https://doi.org/10.1080/09518390701546732

Mizzi, R. C. (2016). Heteroprofessionalism. In N. M. Rodriguez, W. Martino, & J. Ingrey (Eds.), *Critical concepts in queer studies and education* (pp. 137–147). Palgrave Macmillan, New York.

Moosa, S., & Bhana, D. (2019). Masculinity as care: Men can teach young children in the early years. *Early Years, 40*(1), 1–15.

OME. (2015). The Ontario curriculum, grades 1–8: Health & physical education. Retrieved from https://www.oaith.ca/assets/files/2015%20Health%20and%20Physical%20Education%20Curriculum.pdf

Pallotta-Chiarolli, M., Haydon, P., & Hunter, A. (2013). "These are our children": Polyamorous parenting. In A. E. Goldberg & K. R. Allen (Eds.), *LGBT-parent families: Innovations in research and implications for practice* (pp. 117–131). Springer: New York, NY.

Pallotta-Chiarolli, M., Sheff, E., & Mountford, R. (2020). Polyamorous parenting in contemporary research: Developments and future directions. In A. E. Goldberg (Ed.), *LGBTQ-parent families: Innovations in research and implications for practice* (pp. 171–184). Springer: New York, NY.

Peeters, J., Rohrmann, T., & Emilsen, K. (2015). Gender balance in ECEC: Why is there so little progress? *European ECE Research Journal, 23*(3), 302–314. https://doi.org/10.1080/1350293x.2015.1043805

Piaget, J. (1936). *Origins of intelligence in the child.* London, UK: Routledge & Kegan Paul.

Piaget, J. (1945). *Play, dreams and imitation in childhood.* London, UK: Heinemann.

Piaget, J. (1957). *Construction of reality in the child.* London, UK: Routledge & Kegan Paul.

Pinar, W. F. (1975). Currere: Toward reconceptualization. In W. F. Pinar (Ed.), *Curriculum theorizing: The reconceptualists.* Berkeley, CA: McCutchan Publishing Corporation.

Rich, A. (1980). Compulsory heterosexuality and lesbian existence. *Signs: Journal of Women in Culture and Society, 5*(4), 631–660. https://doi.org/10.1086/493756

Robinson, K. H. (2005). "Queerying" gender: Heteronormativity in early childhood education. *Australasian Journal of Early Childhood, 30*(2), 19–28. https://doi.org/10.1177/183693910503000206

Robinson, K. H., & Davies, C. (2017). Sexuality education in early childhood. In L. Allen & M. L. Rasmussen (Eds.), *The Palgrave handbook of sexuality education* (pp. 217–242). London: Palgrave Macmillan.

Scurfield, I. (2017). Walking gendered lines: The contradictory expectations of men who work in ECE. *Inquiries Journal, 9*(11). Retrieved from http://www.inquiriesjournal.com/articles/1708/walking-gendered-lines-the-contradictory-expectations-of-men-who-work-in-early-childhood-education

Simons, J. D., Grant, L., & Rodas, J. M. (2021). Transgender people of color: Experiences and coping during the school-age years. *Journal of LGBTQ Issues in Counseling, 15*(1), 16–37. https://doi.org/10.1080/15538605.2021.1868380

Taylor, N. (2012). US children's picture books and the homonormative subject. *Journal of LGBT Youth, 9*(2), 136–152. https://doi.org/10.1080/19361653.2011.649646

Titchkosky, T. (2001). Disability: A rose by any other name? "People-first" language in Canadian society. *Canadian Review of Sociology/Revue canadienne de sociologie, 38*(2), 125–140. https://doi.org/10.1111/j.1755-618x.2001.tb00967.x

Volpe, R. (Ed.). (2010). *The secure child: Timeless lessons in parenting.* Charlotte, NC: IAP.

Vygotsky, L. S. (1978). *Mind in society: The development of higher psychological processes.* Cambridge, MA: Harvard University Press.

Warin, J. (2018). *Men in ECE and care: Gender balance and flexibility.* Switzerland Springer.

Warin, J. (2019). Conceptualising the value of male practitioners in early childhood education and care: Gender balance or gender flexibility. *Gender and Education, 31*(3), 293–308. https://doi.org/10.1080/09540253.2017.1380172

Warin, J., & Adriany, V. (2017). Gender flexible pedagogy in early childhood education. *Journal of Gender Studies, 26*(4), 375–386. https://doi.org/10.1080/09589236.2015.1105738

Wernersson, I. (2015). More men? Swedish arguments over four decades about "missing men" in ECE and care. In S. Brownhill, J. Warin, & I. Wernersson (Eds.), *Men, masculinities and teaching in ECE* (pp. 31–43). Switzerland: Routledge.

Williams, D. J., & Prior, E. E. (2015). Contemporary polyamory: A call for awareness and sensitivity in social work. *Social Work, 60*(3), 268–270. https://doi.org/10.1093/sw/swv012

10 Working with Muslim LGBTQ Service Users: Assessing and Locating Supportive Care and Teaching Practices

MARYAM KHAN

An LGBTQ[1] Muslim intersectionality has gained some visibility in social science research (Rahman & Valliani, 2016) yet remains largely ignored within normative LGBTQ communities in higher education and the arenas of program and service provision in the global north.[2] There especially exists a gap concerning how to best support LGBTQ Muslims and their families within the scope of social work and other helping professions in regard to service provision and programming (Khan, 2016a, 2016b). In this chapter, Islam is used as a tradition in a broad sense that informs the social, political, cultural, spiritual, and diasporic experiences (i.e., lives and identities) of LGBTQ Muslims, irrespective of religious practice. In this way, LGBTQ Muslims' varying experiences and relationships within the tradition can be framed inside the inherent pluralism that exists locally and globally in practices and approaches to Islam. The literature exploring the nexus of helping professions (such as social work, nursing, psychotherapy, psychology, and psychiatry) and supporting Muslims can be classified under mental health and cultural competency models and approaches (Crabtree, Husain, & Spalek, 2008). For example, this scholarship informs service providers and educators in higher learning about "how to" support Muslims through knowledge mobilization related to (normative) Islam and its practices; how to navigate traditional gender roles and etiquette in Muslim families; Muslim

---

1 This acronym is used predominantly in the global north (in scholarship and as an identity) to discuss Muslim nonnormative sexualities, gender identities, and expressions. Many Muslims may use the LGBTQ identity label to access services but may not identify personally under this term. I am using "sexually and gender diverse" and "LGBTQ" interchangeably to honour the myriad lived experiences.
2 I am referring to nation states that are situated in the northern hemisphere such as Canada, the United States, and Europe.

dietary restrictions; understanding of hijab; emphasis on collectivism versus individualist cultures; Muslim responses to "help" from service providers; and an overall focus on culture and ethnicities (Crabtree, Husain, & Spalek, 2008; Hodge, 2005; Hodge, Baughman, & Cummings 2006; Humeidan, 2012; Mohiuddin & Maroof, 2012; Nadir & El-Amin, 2012). These works focus on normative understandings of Islam as they relate to heterosexuality, gender roles, and sexuality.

In this chapter, I draw on my lived, teaching, and professional social work experiences as a former peer group facilitator with Salaam Canada,[3] a LGBTQ Muslim support group, to offer reflexive reflections – beyond essentialized culturally competent ways – on teaching in higher education and supporting LGBTQ Muslims and their families in frontline interdisciplinary practice, taking into consideration modernity, secularism, Islamo-racism,[4] and colonialism. I then conclude with a discussion on what lessons about sexuality(ies) mainstream service-provider agencies and educators in higher learning institutions need to be more cognizant of to more effectively support Muslim LGBTQs.

Understanding LGBTQ Muslim Intersectionality

The exact number of LGBTQ Muslims is unknown in Canada. This gap in research knowledge makes it challenging to apply for funding to support the development of programs and services. According to Salaam Canada's (conservative) estimates using 2011 Statistics Canada data, there are approximately 50,000 LGBTQ Muslims residing in Canada as of 2019 (Salaam Regional Convening, 2019). Notably, Muslims comprise approximately 3.2% of the Canadian national population, making Islam the second largest religious group, after Christianity (Environics, 2016). The Environics (2016) survey also reported that Muslim Canadians aged 45 to 59 (which is 55%) abhorred notions of same-sex marriage and did not agree with homosexuality, and "Muslims 18–34 (47%) and those born in Canada (52%)" were identified as accepting of same-sex marriage and homosexuality (p. 33). These statistics suggest that older Canadian Muslims harbour negative attitudes toward same-sex marriage and homosexuality, whereas the younger cohort is seen as more accepting.

---

3 https://www.salaamcanada.info/
4 This term coined by Singh (2016) and taken up by Beck, Charania, Al-Issa, and Wahab (2017) refers to the nexus of Islamophobia and racism operating in nuanced ways (micro, meso and macro levels) in social work education and practice that engage colonial and racist tropes about Muslims, Islam, and racialized communities that are orientalist in nature.

There are many hegemonic discourses that construct and influence the lives and identities of LGBTQ Muslims. The most common hegemonic discourse asserts that Islam is antithetical to diverse gender identities and sexualities. This powerful hegemonic discourse is fuelled and maintained by many macro-level factors, perspectives, and intentional practices that operate within social, historical, cultural, and political realms (El-Tayeb, 2011, 2012).

Further, there is the discrimination and marginalization encountered by LGBTQ Muslims, orchestrated through heterosexism, transphobia, biphobia, and homophobia found in mainstream Muslim communities (Environics Institute, 2016; Pew Research Centre, 2015) and Muslim majority regions across the globe (Mulé, Khan, & McKenzie, 2017). There are many Islamic nation states where prohibitions against holding same-sex assemblies exist and where "homosexuality" is illegal and punishable (Carroll & Itaborahy, 2015). As well, there are some nation states, such as Jordan and Turkey, where punishments for "homosexuality" are not state mandated, yet violence, negative attitudes, and marginalization still persist against sexual and gender minorities (Kıraç, 2016). Historically, colonization and imperialism have been identified as cornerstone shifts in the changing attitudes and legal sanctions against sexual and gender diversity in Muslim societies. For example, El-Rouayheb's (2005) work on Arab societies documents the influence and adoption of Victorian morals, values, and beliefs about sexuality by the Arab elites, which resulted in the removal of pedastric references in poetry. Further, many local Indigenous[5] expressions of same-sex homoeroticism and categories used in popular discourse and literature were disbanded by the Victorian colonial powers and made to fit under a singular overarching identity category, which over time was rendered as sexually perverse and abnormal (i.e., "shudhudh jinsi") (El-Rouayheb, 2005, p. 158). In the South Asian context, colonization and imperialism led to the suppression of sexual and gender diversity in public and private spheres to appease colonial appetites (Gopinath, 2005; Kugle, 2002). Other examples are Singapore, India, Malaysia, and Bangladesh: all former British colonies that introduced legislation to criminalize same-sex relationships and supported conservative interpretations of Islamic jurisprudence (Ibrahim, 2016).

Scholars have critiqued at length the practice of some LGBTQ organizations travelling to the southern hemisphere to propagate Western

---

5 This term refers to land, people, culture, customs, and traditions that are local and native to a given geographic region and exists in relation to colonial occupation.

understandings of sexuality, and gender (Grewal, 2005; Massad, 2007). In a similar vein, Christian-based missionary and civilizing mission organizations forge alliances with anti-LGBTQ Indigenous groups (e.g., conservative religious) in these nation states to support bi-, trans-, and homophobic efforts. For example, there is a history of missionary-based (anti-LGBTQ and anti-abortion) organizations that undermine political, cultural, and social-consciousness-raising organizing by minority-based NGOs (women and equity-seeking groups) working toward gender and sexual parity in former colonial nation states. Globally, there exist human rights defenders who are working against imperial and colonial legacies through LGBTQ community mobilizing to decolonize discourses related to gender and sexuality (Lennox & Waites, 2013; Vance, Mulé, Khan, & McKenzie, 2018).

In this geopolitical identity rights-based landscape, it is common practice to situate nation states in the global north (compared to the rest of the globe) as progressive champions of LGBTQ rights, as these nation states provide legal and human-rights-based protections for LGBTQ persons. Notably, these rights and freedoms are relatively recent developments in these nation states, with support for trans persons still lacking (Hildebrandt, 2014; Lennox & Waites, 2013). Further, sexual and gender minorities continue to experience discrimination, prejudice, and violence, especially racialized newcomer, immigrant, and refugee Muslims in these nation states (Canada Research Team of Envisioning Global LGBT Human Rights, 2015; Kahn, 2015).

Homocolonialism and LGBTQ Muslim Sexualities

Rahman's (2014, 2018) approach to understanding Muslim LGBTQ sexuality(ies) is one that accounts for the roles played by modernity, colonialism, orientalism, Islamophobia, and conservative Muslim intolerance for LGBTQ rights – all as triangulated processes referred to as "homocolonialism." Modernity is a social, political, and cultural force that equates nation states' modernization with progress and is measured by legal rights afforded to sexual minorities. In making this leap, nation states in which identity-based sexual-minority rights are absent are constructed in orientalist ways as nonprogressive, primitive, and uncivilized. Islamo-racism has a history in the establishment of Euro-Western nationhood and national identity that heavily relies on colonial tropes (e.g., occident versus orient) to distinguish itself (occident) as separate from the traditional and nonassimilable Muslims (El-Tayeb, 2011, 2012)

This blanketing casts Islamic regions and Muslims as nonaccepting of sexual and gender diversity, erases colonial and imperial occupation histories (alongside the vast histories of sexual and gender diversity in Islamic societies), and obscures alternative (non-Western) ways of understanding sexuality and gender (Khan & Mulé, 2021). For example, in contemporary Iran, "homosexuality" (as understood in the global north) is considered illegal and is an offence punishable by the state. This case example is often cited to assert that Islam is antithetical to LGBTQ Muslim intersectionality. Often elided are the intermediate spaces for sexual and gender fluidity and experiences carved out by gender confirmation surgeries that are funded by the state (Najmabadi, 2014). The point here is that painting Islam as inherently homophobic based on specific Euro-Western manifestations and understandings of sexuality and gender is highly problematic and further fuels Islamo-racism by evoking civilizational and orientalist discourses (Najmabadi, 2014).

Secularism can also be added to this triangulation, since it assumes that sexual and gender parity can be achieved through secularization of the nation state (Asad, 2003). The connection made between modernity, secularism, gender, and sexual parity can be problematic as it assumes that secular states (such as Canada) have transcended religious dogma and conservatism but ignores the bi-, trans-, and homophobia present in mainstream society and its institutions. Rahman's (2018) homocolonialism extends Puar's (2007) analysis of homo-nationalism (i.e., LGBTQ identity and performance as normalizing imperial force) to further account for international relations in a geopolitical context surrounding gender and sexual minorities and their construction. Homocolonialism has three main aspects that triangulate and feed into each other. The first two aspects address how gender and sexual-minority rights are perceived as solely developed by and belonging to the nation states in the global north. LGBTQ rights are constructed as signs of civilizational progress; that is, as a natural step in modernity and enlightenment. These are then used as "pinktesting" yardsticks to measure Islamic nation states as being neither progressive nor enlightened enough, because they do not follow suit with notions of identity rights as advanced by LGBTQ agencies and nongovernmental bodies in the global north. Homocolonialism involves fostering essentialist, universalizing, and ahistorical hegemonic discourses that confer specific ways of being LGBTQ that are grounded in Euro-Western histories and are seen as the only legitimate models for identity development, progress, and living a LGBTQ life. This configuration allows such nation states to maintain their civilizational and exalted superiority over the Islamic nation states.

The third aspect involves positioning Islam and Muslims as alien to and as existing external to Euro-Western modernity; and anti-LGBTQ

Muslim sentiment and attitudes are seen as resisting progress and modernity (Rahman, 2018). This positioning is evidenced in the discourses and debates in Québec regarding immigration and the hijab controversy and its banning – as if Muslims and Islam have no place in the secular modernist nation state of Canada (Bilge, 2012). Muslim nation states that oppose sexual and gender-based imperialism from the global north assert claims to their sovereign right to govern, and on this basis, reject identity-based sexual and gender minority claims. It must be noted that claiming nation state sovereignty does not eradicate or excuse Muslim bi-, trans-, and homophobia, which is often grounded in conservative Islamic theological and culture-based arguments (Ibrahim, 2016; Mulé, Khan, & McKenzie, 2017).

The triangulation of the aspects of homocolonialism described above can render invisible the sexualities of LGBTQ Muslims, as their identities and lived experiences transcend hegemonic norms found in both LGBTQ and Muslim communities. The impact of homocolonialism is evident in the scholarship on LGBTQ Muslims. For example, social science research asserts that most LGBTQ Muslims experience prejudice, violence, and discrimination in normative Muslim communities, and may stay closeted as a result and may compartmentalize their identities by withholding some intersectional identity facet in normative Muslim and LGBTQ communities. For example, they may abandon and/or minimize same-sex desire within their families of origin (Abdi, 2014; Abdi & Gilder, 2016; Jaspal, 2012; Jaspal & Cinnirella, 2010). Some research argues that shame, upholding family honour, and reputation play a role in the lives of LGBTQ Muslims (Fattah & Fierke, 2009; Siraj, 2011). Further, sexual and gender diversity is perceived as a result of Euro-Western influence (Al-Sayyad, 2010; Mahomed, 2016), and racialized LGBTQ Muslims are seen as too Westernized and as inauthentic ethnic and cultural diasporic subjects (Habib, 2019; Jaspal, 2012).

Within LGBTQ communities, sexual- and gender-diverse Muslims also experience Islamophobia, racism, and are marginalized for not adhering to normative ideals around coming out and the performance of LGBTQ identities (Esack & Mahomed, 2011). Nonetheless, there is a growing body of studies that locate an LGBTQ Muslim intersectionality as reconcilable with Islam by drawing on nonnormative, feminist, liberatory, and affirmative approaches to the Islamic tradition. For example, such approaches include unpacking patriarchal and misogynist influences on Islam and the Quran (Kugle, 2014, 2016). Another example is engaging in re-interpretations of Quranic exegesis that are mindful of diversity, pluralism, and are gender and sexuality sensitive (Shah, 2016; Siraj, 2016a, 2016b).

Practice Recommendations for the Helping Professions

In the section below, I outline specific interdisciplinary recommendations that will support the engagement of LGBTQ Muslims, both in practice and in higher education.

Learnings from Support Groups

Many LGBTQ Muslims seek services from LGBTQ Muslim support groups such as Salaam Canada, El-Tawhid Juma Circle (ETJC)[6] as part of the Unity Mosque, and Muslims for Progressive Values (MPV)[7] to develop strategies to ameliorate familial, cultural, religious, spiritual, and ethnic matters related to positionality. These nonprofit groups are dedicated to fostering supportive and affirmative practices, and offer resources to support LGBTQ Muslims. Based upon my experiences with LGBTQ Muslim support groups (as recipient and provider), especially my involvement with Salaam Toronto[8] (a chapter of Salaam Canada) as a peer facilitator, LGBTQ Muslims access such groups to counter social, cultural, and political isolation and to meet and build alliances with other sexually and gender diverse Muslims and allies where a sharing of lived experiences (of resistance, agency, and marginality) can happen in an inclusive setting.

I have found that most LGBTQ Muslims express a desire to connect with resources (e.g., find theological/spiritual support, meet racialized LGBTQs, and access role models) to be more content with their identity. In service provision, programming, and teaching, it is important to discuss matters related to spirituality and faith from affirmative perspectives, as these arise for LGBTQ Muslims. Also, the inclusion of diverse critical content, such as abortion, fertility planning, STI/HIV, and AIDS testing, is highly recommended. These issues can be challenging to introduce and discuss due to educator and service-provider discomfort, so another recommendation is to bring in expert guest speakers and facilitators who self-identify as part of the Muslim community and/or work as sex therapists to help foster discussion related to difficult topics. In programming, service providers can also support LGBTQ Muslims by going beyond the individualized and self-based models to include community and critical perspectives (Kumsa, 2011).

Research on sexually and gender diverse Muslims states that integrating religious and/or spiritual facets into therapeutic relationships from

---

6 http://www.jumacircle.com/who-we-are

7 http://www.mpvusa.org/

8 https://www.salaamcanada.info

an intersectional approach can often be beneficial (Langroudi & Skinta, 2019; McMichael, 2002). LGBTQ Muslims may access services to counter the Islamo-racism found in mainstream LGBTQ service agencies where LGBTQ Muslims may feel pressured and forced to hide aspects of who they are due to hostile political climates for Muslims (Khan & Mulé, 2021). Alternatively, religion and spirituality may be connected with experiences of trauma, marginalization, and persecution, so such aspects may not be welcomed (Furness & Gilligan, 2010; Kahn, 2015). In light of these complexities, it remains important to not make assumptions and to ask service users about their needs.

Helpful Approaches in Teaching and Practice

To address the diverse intersectional needs of LGBTQ Muslims, social work educators and practitioners can engage with critical self-reflexivity and decolonization, and work toward incorporating socially just practices that are mindful of minority stress theory (MST), are narrative based as well as intersectionality focused, and maintain an analysis of resilience and trauma (Chapman, Hoque, & Utting, 2013; Langroudi & Skinta, 2019; Meyer, 2015; Rahman & Valliani, 2016). The deployment of such approaches can allow practitioners and educators to challenge commonly held assumptions about LGBTQ Muslims based on their experiences, values, beliefs, and positionality, lack of knowledge, and/or exposure to Islam or Muslims (Graham, Bradshaw, & Trew, 2009).

MST

MST argues that racial and sexual minorities are exposed to prejudice and stigma, which results in a greater risk for mental and physical health problems, depression, suicide, substance use, and addictions (Ghabrial, 2017; Meyer, 2015). MST takes into account barriers, stressors, oppressions, and challenges (on micro, miso, and macro levels) that can result from identification with a minority identity. Additionally, MST takes into account any social supports and systems (at individual and community levels) that allow for the emergence of agency, resistance, and resilience. In this case, resistance and resilience refer to the strategies and tools used by racial and sexual minorities to navigate stressors and overcome individual and/or community-based barriers. Consideration of how a minority identity impacts individuals and their communities provides a more complete picture of LGBTQ Muslims' needs for their physical, psychological, and social well-being (Meyer, 2015).

Narrative

Narrative approaches used in individual and group therapies can be helpful in supporting LGBTQ Muslim intersectional approaches (Buchanan, Dzelme, Harris, & Hecker, 2001; Hammoud-Beckett, 2007). For example, narrative approaches can enable the creation of counter-stories and discourses (White, 1995) that are grounded in the lived realities and experiences of LGBTQ Muslims (Etengoff & Rodriguez, 2021). In higher learning and practice, narrative approaches are recommended since they do not advocate for a removal of Muslim identity, sexuality, or gender identity, but instead undertake an "and" approach, as in "LGBTQ and Muslim," versus an "or" approach, as in "LGBTQ or Muslim" (Advocates for Youth, 2018a, 2018b).

Intersectionality

Moreover, centring the intersectional identities and lived experiences in higher learning has been documented as beneficial (Ghabrial, 2017). This practice challenges homocolonialism by bringing together resistance and agency against pervasive hegemonic discourses in identifying and living LGBTQ *and* Muslim lives. This intersectional space is legitimate and cannot be reduced to a "minority within a minority" framing, but instead is an actual way of being and is an identity that is equal to, and different from, dominant hegemonic expectations (Rahman, 2018).

In higher learning and teaching, instructors can assign readings, documentaries, films, and invite guest speakers with lived experiences (LGBTQ and Muslim) to the classroom. Notably, instructors must ensure that the content of the material and presentation undertakes perspectives on Islam, gender, and sexuality that are critical and not orientalist. For example, instructors could get in touch with LGBTQ Muslim support groups via email or websites to discuss appropriate resources (e.g., materials, guest speakers, experiential exercises) that are affirmative and do not further marginalize LGBTQ Muslim sexualities (i.e., lived experiences of nonbinary, trans-identified, gender-bending, and fluid Muslims).

Critique of Cultural Competence Models

Another important consideration related to practice and education is to remain wary and cautious of culturally competent models and approaches. These models can set up service users, educators, and practitioners in colonial and rigid stances, which can lead to essentialized and orientalist constructions of the race, gender, and sexuality of Muslims and their families. Further, the colonial idea that knowledge(s) about the *other* can somehow be quantified into strategies, practices, and approaches requires critique (Said, 1978). Notably, LGBTQ Muslims service users are the *experts* in their own lives. Ritualistically adhering to competency models can provide false practice knowledge(s) based on *otherness* that are situated through an object/subject approach. This can undermine the expertise of the service user and place it (expertise) in the hands of the practitioner. Instead of endorsing culturally competent models that are mainly geared toward "teaching" normative social workers about LGBTQ Muslim sexualities, instructors can encourage students to undertake critical approaches that are nonessentialist and ask students to examine reflexively (through their many selves, experiences, and knowings) their Islamophobia, trans-, bi-, and homophobia (Khan, 2016a; Kumsa, 2011).

Decolonization

Decolonizing contemporary understandings of gender and sexuality begins with a broadening of such terms to be more responsive to varying community, cultural, social, and political contexts (Lennox & Waites, 2013; Rahman, 2018). For example, in Pakistan and India, a gay identity may not fit neatly: some men engage in sexual acts with other men, but this has no bearing on their social, cultural, and political identities, as these acts are not used as criteria for identity-based claims (Khan, 2001). This is an important distinction to be made, as sexual acts may not be primary markers of social, political, and cultural identities; and knowing the context(s) is imperative. Therefore, if a sexually or gender diverse diasporic Muslim denies identification as gay, this does not automatically equate to internalized homophobia. In practice, it would be imperative to explore the individual and community contexts (including psychosocial, historical, religious, ethnic, and political) and understandings of sexuality and gender that inform the individual, and her/zer/his experiences. With respect to teaching, attention can be placed on the (historical and contemporary) expressions of sexualities and genders found in Islamic and Muslim societies (i.e., conceptualizations of gender identity and experiences in Islam not limited to two genders; historic and contemporary examples of nonbinary, trans and cross-dressing experiences), alongside the impact of colonial and imperial legacies on contemporary constructions of these, viewed from transnational and queer feminist perspectives (see Gopinath, 2005; Grewal, 2005).

Families and Communities of Origin

As mentioned previously, it is important that service providers not make assumptions; rather, they should ask service users what their relationship is with Islam to get to know their specific contexts. For example, there are many types of Muslims (e.g., cultural, political, religious, spiritual, nonpractising, practising, atheist, converts, and re-verts), with varying sects, approaches (Ahmadiyya, Shia, Ismaili, Sufi, and Sunni), and experiences with Islam. LGBTQ Muslims whose families and communities of origin may or may not be religious can still partake in cultural and social aspects of Islam, connected to an ethno-racial diasporic community that celebrates and observes high holidays such as Eid and Ramadan alongside births, funerals, and marriages within their respective traditions, all within the cultural context of Islam (with or without the religious rituals) (Khan & Mulé, 2021).

Normative understandings and practices of Islam do not represent all Muslim-identified individuals and communities. For example, sexual and gender diversity in normative Muslim understandings is identified as sinful and *haram* (prohibited) (Alvi & Zaidi, 2019; Killawi, 2012), based on conservative approaches to the Quran and Islam (Kugle, 2010). In contrast, the Quran, which is the main scriptural source for Muslims, is sex positive. Sex, sexuality, and intimate relations are seen as important facets of the human experience and are addressed in positive ways. For example, Muslims who maintain ethical sexual relations with spouses and/or partners are seen to be engaging in acts of worship (Kugle, 2010). A Muslim individual's or families' approaches to sex, sexuality, and relationships is contingent on values and beliefs shaped by socioeconomic statuses, upbringing and background, and experiences of religiosity to name a few. There is no set formula used to determine how any given Muslim will respond to conversations about sex, sexuality, LGBTQ sexuality, abortion, STI's, HIV/AIDS, contraception, fertility, and so on. Given this, normative understandings of such topics in Islam are constructed mainly in heteronormative ways and can be considered taboo subjects. As a result, LGBTQ Muslims may not feel comfortable discussing sex and sexuality among other topics with peers and family members, as well as (normative) Muslim social services, due to fears related to social isolation and safety.

In a similar vein, LGBTQ Muslims may feel sensitive about discussing their families' responses and attitudes with service providers. This may be because LGBTQ Muslims do not want their families painted in orientalist fashion (as homophobic); also, they do not want to face pressure to come out in normative ways. Countless Salaam attendees have asserted that they have experienced pressure from normative LGBTQ organizations and Gay and Straight Alliances to abandon their family, leave Islam, and come out. There are many ways to live and perform a LGBTQ Muslim life, and these do not need to mirror normative ways of being. A rejection of the aforementioned identity label does not equate to internalized trans-, bi-, and homophobia. In other words, coming out is not synonymous with identity legitimization (Esack & Mahomed, 2011).

Moreover, breaking ties with family members may or may not be a feasible option due to financial instability for diasporic Muslim LGBTQ individuals. Families serve an important function as social and cultural support buffers against Islamo-racism and provide a sense of belonging and community. Service provision in normative LGBTQ organizations tends to focus on the identities and rights of the individual, and may not consider families of LGBTQ Muslims in a positive light due to the pervasive belief that Islam equals gender and sexual intolerance. LGBTQ Muslims' families cannot be constructed as solely against sexual and gender diversity and taboo topics (such as sexuality, abortion, fertility issues, HIV-AIDS, and STI testing); as every family can vary in its response and acceptance, and may have experience with such issues in varying degrees. In terms of intervention, service providers could explore how to establish clear boundaries with families and help service users enhance coping skills and be content with their intersectional identity.

Conclusion

In this chapter, I drew on my lived and professional (practice and educator) experiences with Salaam, a LGBTQ Muslim support group that advocates an integration of minority stress, intersectional, and narrative perspectives in teaching and practice. I also argued for social work practitioners and educators to decolonize sexuality and gender by rejecting essentialist understandings of Islam and LGBTQ Muslim sexualities. Drawing on homocolonialism, implementing critically reflexive social work practices, and incorporating the lived experiences of LGBTQ Muslims can be helpful in dismantling Islamophobic discourses in social work education and practice.

REFERENCES

Abdi, S. (2014). Staying I(ra)n: Narrating queer identity from within the Persian closet. *Liminalities: A Journal of Performance Studies, 10*(2), 1–20.
Abdi, S., & Gilder, B. V. (2016). Cultural (in)visibility and identity dissonance: Queer Iranian-American women and their negotiation of existence. *Journal of*

International and Intercultural Communication, 9(1), 69–86. https://doi.org/10.1080/17513057.2016.1120850

Advocates for Youth. (2018a). *I'm Muslim and I might not be straight.* Retrieved from: https://advocatesforyouth.org/resources/health-information/im-muslim-and-i-might-not-be-straight

Advocates for Youth. (2018b). *#MuslimAnd Toolkit.* Retrieved from: https://www.advocatesforyouth.org/wp-content/uploads/2020/03/MuslimAnd-Toolkit-1.pdf

Al-Sayyad, A. A. (2010). "You're what?": Engaging narratives from diasporic Muslim women on identity and gay liberation. In S. Habib (Ed.), *Islam and homosexuality* (pp. 373–394). Santa Barbara, California: Greenwood Publishing.

Alvi, S., & Zaidi, A. (2019). "My existence is not haram": Intersectional lives in LGBTQ Muslims living in Canada. *Journal of Homosexuality, 68*(6), 993–1014. https://doi.org/10.1080/00918369.2019.1695422

Asad, T. (2003). *Formations of the secular: Christianity, Islam, modernity.* Stanford, CA: Stanford University Press.

Beck, E., Charania, M., Al-Issa, A. F., & Wahab, S. (2017). Undoing Islamophobia: Awareness of orientalism in social work. *Journal of Progressive Human Services, 28*(2), 58–72. https://doi.org/10.1080/10428232.2017.1310542

Bilge, S. (2012). Mapping Québécois sexual nationalism in times of "crisis of reasonable accommodations." *Journal of Intercultural Studies, 33*(3), 303–318. https://doi.org/10.1080/07256868.2012.673473

Buchanan, M., Dzelme, K., Harris, D., & Hecker, L. (2001). Challenges of being simultaneously gay or lesbian and spiritual and/or religious: A narrative perspective. *American Journal of Family Therapy, 29*(5), 435–449. https://doi.org/10.1080/01926180127629

Canada Research Team of Envisioning Global LGBT Human Rights. (2015). *Envisioning LGBT refugee rights in Canada: Is Canada a safe haven?* Retrieved from: http://envisioninglgbt.blogspot.ca/p/publicationsresources.html

Carroll, A., & Itaborahy, L. (2015). *State sponsored homophobia 2015: A world survey of laws: Criminalisation, protection and recognition of same-sex love.* Retrieved from: https://ilga.org/downloads/ILGA_State_Sponsored_Homophobia_2015.pdf

Chapman, C., Hoque, N., Utting, L. (2013). Fostering a personal-is-political ethics: Reflexive conversations in social work education. *Intersectionalities: A Global Journal of Social Work Analysis, Research, Polity, and Practice, 2*, 24–50.

Crabtree, S. A., Husain, F., & Spalek, B. (2008). *Islam and social work: Debating values, transforming practice.* Bristol, UK: The Policy Press University of Bristol.

El-Tayeb, F. (2011). *European others: Queering ethnicity in postnational Europe.* Minneapolis: University of Minnesota Press.

El-Tayeb, F. (2012). "Gays who cannot properly be gay": Queer Muslims in the neoliberal European city. *European Journal of Women's Studies, 19*(1), 79–95. https://doi.org/10.1177/1350506811426388

El-Rouayheb, K. (2005). *Before homosexuality in the Arab-Islamic world, 1500–1800.* Chicago: The University of Chicago Press.

Environics Institute. *Survey of Muslims in Canada 2016.* Retrieved from: https://www.environicsinstitute.org/projects/project-details/survey-of-muslims-in-canada-2016

Esack, F., & Mahomed, N. (2011). Sexual diversity, Islamic jurisprudence and sociality. *Journal of Gender and Religion in Africa, 17*(2), 41–57.

Etengoff, C. M., & Rodriguez, E. M. (2021). *"I feel as if I'm lying to them"*: Exploring lesbian Muslims' experiences of rejection, support, and depression. *Journal of Homosexuality,* 68(7), 1169–1195. https://doi.org/10.1080/00918369.2021.1888586

Fattah, K., & Fierke, K. M. (2009). A clash of emotions: The politics of humiliation and political violence in the Middle East. *European Journal of International Relations, 15*(1), 67–93. https://doi.org/10.1177/1354066108100053

Furness, S., & Gilligan, P. (2010). *Religion, belief, and social work: Making a difference.* Bristol, UK: The Policy Press.

Ghabrial, M. A. (2017). "Trying to figure out where we belong": Narratives of racialized sexual minorities on community, identity, discrimination, and health. *Sexuality Research & Social Policy, 14,* 42–55. https://doi.org/10.1007/s13178-016-0229-x

Gopinath, G. (2005). *Impossible desires: Queer diasporas and South Asian public cultures.* Durham, NC: Duke University Press.

Graham, J. R., Bradshaw, C., & Trew, J. L. (2009). Adapting social work in working with Muslim clients. *Social Work Education, 28*(5), 544–561. https://doi.org/10.1080/02615470802400729

Grewal, I. (2005). *Transnational America: Feminisms, diasporas, neoliberalisms.* Durham, NC: Duke University Press.

Habib, S. (2019). *We have always been here: A queer Muslim memoir.* Toronto: Penguin Random House.

Hammoud-Beckett, S. (2007). Azima ila Hayati – An invitation in to my life: Narrative conversations about sexual identity. *The International Journal of Narrative Therapy and Community Work, 39*(1), 29–39. www.dulwichcentre.com.au

Hildebrandt, A. (2014). Routes to decriminalization: A comparative analysis of the legalization of same-sex sexual acts. *Sexualities, 17*(1–2), 230–253. https://doi.org/10.1177/1363460713511105

Hodge, D. R. (2005). Social work and the house of Islam: Orienting practitioners to the beliefs and values of Muslims in the United States. *Social Work, 50*(2), 162–173. https://doi.org/10.1093/sw/50.2.162

Hodge, D. R., Baughman, L. M., & Cummings, J. A. (2006). Moving toward spiritual competency. *Journal of Social Service Research, 32*(4), 211–231. https://doi.org/10.1300/j079v32n04_12

Humeidan, M. (2012). University counselling centres. In S. Ahmed & M. M. Amer (Eds.), *Counseling Muslims: Handbook of mental health issues and interventions* (pp. 213–226). New York, NY: Routledge.

Ibrahim, N. A. (2016). Homophobic Muslims: Emerging trends in multireligious Singapore. *Comparative Studies in Society and History, 58*(4), 955–981. https://doi.org/10.1017/s0010417516000499

Jaspal, R. (2012). "I never faced up to being gay": Sexual, religious and ethnic identities among British Indian and British Pakistani gay men. *Culture, Health & Sexuality, 14*(7), 767–780. https://doi.org/10.1080/13691058.2012.693626

Jaspal, R., & Cinnirella, M. (2010). Coping with potentially incompatible identities: Accounts of religious, ethnic, and sexual identities from British Pakistani men who identify as Muslim and gay. *British Journal of Social Psychology, 49*, 849–870. https://doi.org/10.1348/014466609x485025

Kahn, S. (2015). Experiences of faith for gender role non-conforming Muslims in resettlement: Preliminary considerations for social work practitioners. *British Journal of Social Work, 4*(7), 2038–2055 https://doi.org/10.1093/bjsw/bcu060

Khan, M. (2016a). Coming out with God in social work? Narrative of a queer religious woman in the academe. In S. Hillock & N. J. Mulé (Eds.), *Queering Social Work Education* (pp. 186–212). Toronto: UBC Press.

Khan, M. (2016b). Queering Islam through ijtihad. In S. Hussain (Ed.), *The Muslimah who fell to Earth: Personal stories by Canadian Muslim women* (pp. 23–32). Toronto, ON: Mawenzi House Publishers.

Khan, M., & Mulé, N. J. (2021). Voices of resistance and agency: LBTQ Muslim women living out intersectional lives in North America. *Journal of Homosexuality.* https://doi.org/10.1080/00918369.2021.1888583

Khan, S. (2001). Culture, sexualities, and identities: Men who have sex with men in India. In G. Sullivan & P. A. Jackson (Eds), *Gay & lesbian Asia: Culture, identity, and community* (pp. 99–115). New York: Haworth Press.

Killawi, M. (2012). Sexuality and sexual dysfunctions. In S. Ahmed & M. M. Amer (Eds), *Counseling Muslims: Handbook of mental health issues and interventions* (pp. 329–354). New York, NY: Routledge.

Kıraç, F. (2016). The role of religiosity in satisfaction with life: A sample of Turkish gay men. *Journal of Homosexuality, 63*(12), 1594–1607. doi: https://doi.org/10.1080/00918369.2016.1158002

Kugle, S. S. (2002). Sultan Mahmud's makeover: Colonial homophobia and the Persian-Urdu literary tradition. In R. Vanita (Ed.), *Queering India: Same-sex love and eroticism in Indian culture and society* (pp. 30–46). New York: Routledge.

Kugle, S. S. (2010). *Homosexuality in Islam: Critical reflection on gay, lesbian, and transgender Muslims.* Oxford: Oneworld.

Kugle, S. S. (2014). *Living out Islam: Voices of gay, lesbian, and transgender Muslims.* New York: New York University Press.

Kugle, S. S. (2016). Strange bedfellows: Qur'an interpretation regarding same-sex female intercourse. *Theology & Sexuality, 22*(1–2), 9–24. https://doi.org/10.1080/13558358.2017.1296685

Kumsa, M. K. (2011). A resettlement story of unsettlement: Transformative practices of taking it personally. In D. Baines (Ed.), *Doing anti-oppressive practice: Social justice social work,* 2nd ed. (pp. 229–248). Halifax & Winnipeg: Fernwood Publishing.

Langroudi, K. F., & Skinta, M. D. (2019). Working with gender and sexual minorities in the context of Islamic culture: A queer Muslim behavioural approach. *The Cognitive Behaviour Therapist, 12,* 1–12. https://doi.org/10.1017/s1754470x19000096

Lennox, C., & Waites, M. (Eds.). (2013). *Human rights, sexual orientation and gender identity in the Commonwealth: Struggles for decriminalisation and change.* London: School of Advanced Study, University of London.

Mahomed, N. (2016). Queer Muslims: Between orthodoxy, secularism and the struggle for acceptance. *Theology & Sexuality, 22*(1–2), 57–72. https://doi.org/10.1080/13558358.2017.1296688

Massad, J. A. (2007). *Desiring Arabs.* Chicago: The University of Chicago Press.

McMichael, C. (2002) "Everywhere is Allah's place": Islam and the everyday life of Somali women in Melbourne, Australia. *Journal of Refugee Studies, 15*(2), 171–188. https://doi.org/10.1093/jrs/15.2.171

Meyer, I. H. (2015). Resilience in the study of minority stress and health of sexual and gender minorities. *Psychology of Sexual Orientation and Gender Diversity, 2*(3), 209–213. https://doi.org/10.1037/sgd0000132

Mohiuddin, S., & Maroof, S. (2012). Inpatient psychiatric units. In S. Ahmed & M. M. Amer (Eds.), *Counseling Muslims: Handbook of mental health issues and interventions* (pp. 183–196). New York, NY: Routledge.

Mulé, N. J., Khan, M., & McKenzie, C. (2017). The growing presence of LGBTQIs at the UN: Arguments and counter-arguments. *International Social Work, 61*(6), 1126–1138. https://doi.org/10.1177/0020872817702706

Nadir, A., & El-Amin, C. (2012). Home-based social services. In S. Ahmed & M. M. Amer (Eds.), *Counseling Muslims: Handbook of mental health issues and interventions* (pp. 197–212). New York, NY: Routledge.

Najmabadi, A. (2014). *Professing selves: Transsexuality and same-sex desire in contemporary Iran.* North Carolina: Duke University Press.

Pew Research Centre. (2015, November 3). *U.S. public becoming less religious: modest drop in overall rates of belief and practice, but religiously affiliated*

Americans are as observant as before. Retrieved from: https://www.pewforum
.org/2015/11/03/u-s-public-becoming-less-religious/

Puar, J. (2007). *Terrorist assemblages: Homonationalism in queer times.* Durham,
N.C.: Duke University Press.

Rahman, M. (2014). *Homosexualities, Muslim cultures and modernity.* Basingstoke:
Palgrave Macmillan.

Rahman, M. (2018). Postcolonialism and international relations: Intersections
of sexuality, religion and race. In R. Persaud & S. A. Sajed (Eds.), *Race, gender
and culture in international relations* (pp. 99–115). New York: Routledge.

Rahman, M., & Valliani, A. (2016). Challenging the opposition of LGBT
identities and Muslim cultures: Initial research on the experiences of LGBT
Muslims in Canada. *Theology & Sexuality, 22*(1–2), 73–88. https://doi.org
/10.1080/13558358.2017.1296689

Said, E. W. (1978). *Orientalism.* New York, NY: Vintage Books Edition.

Salaam Regional (Ontario and Québec) Convening held February 23 and 24,
2019 at the 519 Church St. Community Centre. Toronto, Ontario.

Salaam Toronto. (2019). https://www.salaamcanada.info.

Shah, S. (2016). Constructing an alternative pedagogy of Islam: The experiences
of lesbian, gay, bisexual and transgender Muslims. *Journal of Beliefs & Values,
37*(3), 308–319. https://doi.org/10.1080/13617672.2016.1212179

Shoeb, M., Weinstein, H., & Halpern, J. (2007). Living in religious time and
space: Iraqi refugees in Dearborn, Michigan. *Journal of Refugee Studies, 20,*
441–460. https://doi.org/10.1093/jrs/fem003

Singh, J. (2016). The death of Islamophobia and the rise of Islamo-racism.
Retrieved from: http://www.racefiles.com/2016/02/23/the-death-of
-islamophobia-the-rise-of-islamo-racism

Siraj, A. (2011). Isolated, invisible, and in the closet: The life story of a Scottish
Muslim lesbian. *Journal of Lesbian Studies, 15*(1), 99–121. https://doi.org
/10.1080/10894160.2010.490503

Siraj, A. (2016a). British Muslim lesbians: Reclaiming Islam and reconfiguring
religious identity. *Journal of Contemporary Islam, 10*(2), 185–200. https://doi
.org/10.1007/s11562-015-0348-9

Siraj, A. (2016b). Alternative realities: Queer Muslims and the Qur'an. *Theology &
Sexuality, 22*(1–2), 89–101. https://doi.org/10.1080/13558358.2017.1296690

Thobani, S. (2007). *Exalted subjects: Studies in the making of race and nation in
Canada.* Toronto: University of Toronto.

Vance, K., Mulé, N. J., Khan, M., & McKenzie, C. (2018). The rise of SOGI:
Human rights for LGBT people at the United Nation. In N. Nicol, A. Jjuuko,
R. Lusimbo, N. J. Mulé, S. Ursell, A. Wahab, & P. Waugh (Eds.), *Envisioning
global LGBT human rights: (Neo)Colonialism, neoliberalism, resistance and hope*
(pp. 223–246). London: Institute of Commonwealth Studies/Human Rights
Consortium.

Wagaman, M. A. (2016). Self-definition as resistance: Understanding identities among LGBTQ emerging adults. *Journal of LGBT Youth, 13* (3). https://doi .org/10.1080/19361653.2016.1185760

White, M. (1995). *Re-authoring lives: Interviews and essays.* Adelaide: Dulwich Centre Publications.

11 Sexuality and Aging

HAI LUO AND LORNA GUSE

Sexuality is the way we see ourselves as sexual beings, the way we feel about ourselves, and how we choose to identify ourselves. As human beings, our sexual self-perceptions and behaviours are shaped over the entire life course (Kasif & Band-Winterstein, 2017). Sexuality remains crucial for life satisfaction and physical and psychological well-being into later life (Bentrott & Margrett, 2011; Haesler, Bauer, & Fetherston-haugh, 2016). Indeed, the importance of sexuality in older adults is demonstrated by more than 2,000 results from a search of books with the key words "sex and aging," including *Naked at Our Age: Talking Out Loud About Senior Sex* (Price, 2011) and *The Ultimate Guide to Sex After Fifty: How to Maintain – or Regain – a Spicy, Satisfying Sex Life* (Price, 2015). Older adults have also reported that they would like their or their partner's physician to discuss sexual needs (Roney & Wallace Kazar, 2015). Even though Casta-Kaufteil (2004) points out that regardless of age, sex is generally beneficial to one's physical health, and Archibald (2002) indicates that sexual intimacy may reduce loneliness and increase one's sense of self, healthcare and social service practitioners and students often report discomfort and lack of competence in providing support to the betterment of older adults' sexuality (Sadovesky, Alam, Enecilla, Cosiquien, Tipu, & Etheridge-Oteym, 2006; Skultety, 2007). In this chapter, we will first define sexuality in later life and examine common biases and stigmas related to this issue; we will then provide theoretical considerations followed by the discussion of the intersection of the diversity of older adults and sexuality and sexuality in long-term care homes. The second half of the chapter presents approaches to teaching sexuality and aging in higher education, including utilizing examples of literature, film and television, and birthday cards to evoke discussion and learning in class.

Sexuality and Aging

Definition of Sexuality

The World Health Organization (2010) defines sexuality as "the integration of the somatic, emotional, intellectual and social aspects of sexual being in ways that are positively enriching and that enhance personality, communication and love" (p. 1). Sexuality was first viewed by healthcare professionals from physiological and biological aspects (Eyler, 1997; Jen, 2018; Tiefer, 1996) but quickly expanded to be more inclusive of emotional aspects of love, affection, intimacy, and companionship (Araujo et al., 2004; Cort et al., 2001; Kasif & Band-Winterstein, 2017). Syme (2014) argued that a holistic concept of sexuality "incorporates an integration of emotional, social, intellectual, and somatic experiences, represents diverse sexual experiences, reflects relationship context, and focuses on pleasure as well as on sexual dysfunction" (p. 36).

Across studies, sexuality in older adults seems to have been categorized into three groups to include a broad range of expression: 1) physical sexual expression: sexual intercourse, solo and partnered masturbation, oral sex, and engaging with fantasy material such as pornography or erotica; 2) physical–affectionate expression: personal grooming, touch, hand holding, dancing, dressing up, and displays of affection; and 3) sociopsychological expression: companionship, romance, and intimacy (Bentrott & Margrett, 2011; DeLamater & Karraker, 2009; Hajjar & Kamel, 2003a, 2003b).

Biases about Sexuality and Aging

Older adults can adapt to normative age-related changes and create or maintain satisfactory sexual lives (Skultety, 2007). An early longitudinal study on aging and sexuality revealed that sexual interest and activities continued on a consistent basis from midlife into later life for healthy older adults (Brestschneider & McCoy, 1988). Among couples, no significant differences were found in affectionate sexual behaviours (e.g., kissing, caressing) for middle-aged and older individuals; though older couples conducted less sexual intercourse, self-stimulation, and oral sex (AARP, 2005). The absence of a sexual partner due to divorce or separation, death, or illness has been reported repeatedly as the major barrier to sexual activities (Roney & Kazar, 2015; Skultety, 2007). Older adults without a sexual partner also expressed less interest in sex (Gott & Hinchliff, 2003). Deterioration in general physical health, as well as psychological causes (e.g., depression) in one or both partners can lead to decreased sexual function (Gott & Hinchliff, 2003). Kwon and Schafer (2017) reported that severe obesity changed sexual activity for couples, particularly for obese women and less so for obese men.

Sexual dysfunctions present barriers for older adults; however, men and women experience different dysfunctions. For older men, the most common dysfunction is erectile dysfunction. For women, the cause is more psychological – a lack of sexual interest (Nicolosi, Laumann, Galsser, Moreira Jr., Paik, & Gingell, 2004). It is interesting that early ejaculation, instead of erectile dysfunction, was reported as the most common male dysfunction among Central and South American and Southeast Asian men, but age was not a significant predictor; and women's lack of sexual interest was found across all age groups. Women's lack of sexual interest was found to be correlated with their beliefs of cultural norms in which aging reduces sexual desires and behaviour (Nicolosi et al., 2004) or in terms of sexual scripts that they acquire through the life course, described by Watson, Stelle, and Bell (2017) as passive, receptive, and monogamous. Older women, however, in recent studies on their perceptions of sexuality, claimed that they did not see aging as having a negative impact on their sexuality in later life (Watson et al., 2017). "Sexual dysfunction is not a part of aging per se, but rather a complex set of diagnoses determined partially by cultural standards, expectation about, and the recognition and definition of sexual problems by healthcare and other service providers in each area" (Skultety, 2007, p. 34). Consequently, healthcare and service providers should examine their own perspectives on the relationship between aging and sexual dysfunction as a potential source of bias and ageism.

The most influential and complex factors in older adults' sexuality are sociocultural messages about sex, age, gender role, attractiveness, sexual appeal, and relationships in later life. A study by Wada, Clarke, and Rozanova (2015) analyzing articles on older adults' online dating concluded that "the ideal of remaining young-looking, physically attractive and sexually active is dominant and marginalizes older adults who choose not to conform to that ideal or are unable to do so" (p. 47). Watson, Stelle, and Bell (2017) point out that women are expected to be "sexually monogamous within one heterosexual, married relationship" (p. 35). As they grew older, women from the study did not see sex as being as important and urgent as they had at earlier points of life but still saw it as a prevalent component in romantic relationships (Watson et al., 2017). As mentioned in a previous section, sex for these women was seen more as a way to experience intimacy, closeness, and companionship. Indeed, most research about sexuality and older adults has revealed that sex remains a vital part of many people's later lives (Fisher, 2010; Gray & García, 2012; Hinchliff, Gott, & Ingelton, 2010; Morrissey Stahl, Gale, Lewis, & Kleiber, 2019). For example, the majority of older participants in Lindau and Gavrilova's (2010) study and Clarke and Korotchenko's (2011) study expressed that for them sex was an integral component of quality of life.

Theoretical Considerations

In sexuality research literature, sexual expression has usually been associated with monogamous marriage, reproduction, and physical attractiveness, suggesting that sexual behaviour, other than for the aforementioned purposes, is unacceptable (Reingold & Burros, 2004). Sexuality, although personal and private, is a public, cultural, and social matter in which morality is deemed as correlated with sexual expression. Ageism, sexism, racism, classism, and heterosexism interact to shape sexual interest and behaviour. Yet the research so far has not offered sufficient and convincing theoretical analysis to such phenomena. Sexuality research has largely focused on younger people (Jen, 2018). Indeed, many conventional theories fail to address aging and sexuality. The lack of theorizing about sexuality and aging "weakens the link between theoretical and applied gerontology, while also limiting the cumulative nature of inquiry" (Jen, 2018).

We believe that the story of sexual pleasure is vital for older adults' well-being. Until recently, especially for older women, this story has not often been present in personal and public narratives or in scholarly literature, even in feminist, structural, and critical analysis (Jen, 2018). For instance, "prominent feminist writers have not considered aging issues until reaching mid- or late life themselves (e.g., Friedan's *The Fountain of Age* [1993]; de Beauvoir's *The Coming of Age* [1972]; Steinem's *Doing Sixty & Seventy* [2006])" (Jen, 2018). In contrast, some recent research explored edgy sexual expression among older adults. For example, Morrissey Stahl et al. (2019) document how older women (aged 57 to 91) satisfy themselves with conventional and controversial means (e.g., masturbation and vibrators) and how their sexual practices had been affected by societal and cultural influences including denial, censure, and judgment.

Life-course perspective and continuity theory have been recommended as promising gerontological theoretical frameworks to better understand sexuality in later life (Jen, 2018; Kasif & Band-Winterstein, 2017; Novak, Northcott, & Campbell, 2018). The life-course perspective posits that people develop and age at every stage of life, and historical conditions and people's social networks influence their experiences and opportunities (Elder, Johnson, & Crosnoe, 2003). For example, older widows have described their transitions to couplehood and widowhood, constructing sexual self-perceptions across the life course, through continuity and change (Kasif & Band-Winterstein, 2017). Transitions theory similarly emphasizes changes throughout life, but delves more deeply into the patterns and properties of transitions and identifies conditions that facilitate and inhibit progression (Meleis, Sawyer, Im, Hilfinger Messias, & Schumacher, 2000). This theory can be applied to social work, psychology, and nursing clinical practice to assist clients with transitions; for example, the transition of becoming a family caregiver or experiencing menopause (Im & Meleis, 2000; Meleis et al., 2000). This theory may be useful in research and practice to learn more about the transitions related to sexuality and aging.

Diversity in Sexuality and Aging

Accordingly, it is also clear how little we know about within-group differences between older adults. Current empirical evidence is mainly based on cross-sectional studies with either poor definitions or sex within heterosexual healthy Caucasian older adults (Skultety, 2007). Knowledge about sexuality among older adults of diverse ethnic or social backgrounds, LGBTQ* community members, or older adults with varied health conditions remains scarce (Morrissey Stahl et al., 2019; Skultety, 2007). A national study in the United States found that more than 90% of adults age 70 or older across all ethnic groups disagree that "sex is only for younger people" (AARP, 2005, p. 1). In an international study, the Global Study of Sexual Attitudes and Behaviors, similar opinions were found among more than 80% of participants across nations (Nicolosi et al., 2004). However, some between-group differences were also evident. For example, Caucasian and Asian Americans were more likely to believe that "sex becomes less important to people as they age" than their African and Hispanic counterparts (AARP, 2005, p. 20); and more participants in developing countries would agree that "older people no longer want sex" (Nicolosi et al., 2004, p. 994). As pointed out by Marshall (2014, 2018), most of our assumptions of sexuality and aging and, indeed, successful aging are anchored in gendered, heterosexual relationships. Practitioners, educators, and students in the field of aging need to be aware of these knowledge gaps and keep an eye on the latest literature updates. When providing safe and equitable care to older adults, healthcare providers must be cognizant of societal-based ageism and its impact on perceptions of diversity and aging.

Sexuality in Long-Term Care Homes

Long-term care homes (also known as nursing homes) are institutional living for older adults who, because of physical or cognitive impairment, can no longer provide their own personal and health care. Residents are sexual beings, and some are sexually active (Simpson, Brown Wilson, Brown, Dickinson, & Horne, 2018). Elias and Ryan (2011) studied sexuality and sexual expression in long-term care homes, reporting that interest does not change on admission but opportunities for sexual expression are limited by lack of privacy and family and staff attitudes. Some institutions have private rooms for each resident, but many do not. An early study suggested that home visits for residents should be facilitated when the sexual partner was willing and lived in the community (Mulligan & Palguta, 1991). A study of Spanish female residents reported that these older women "limited their expression of their sexuality" (Pslacios-Cena et al., 2016, p. 473) by not showing cleavage or wearing bright clothes that would create gossip among staff and other residents and cause embarrassment to their families. Similarly, Simpson et al. (2018) describe residents as "censuring [their] displays of affection" (p. 1494).

Long-term care home staff members' attitudes toward residents' sexuality have been investigated in several studies. Drawing on their review of these studies, Benbow and Beeston (2012) conclude that "attitudes and beliefs toward sexuality and aging are often strongly influenced by stereotypes and myths" (p. 1029) such as the assumption that older adults are asexual. In contrast, Simpson et al. (2018) identify staff and family members who acknowledge residents' sexuality needs and, in particular, describe staff efforts "to meet a range of legal, institutional and professional demands and negotiate diverse relationships and various obstacles that can deny satisfaction of intimacy needs" (p. 1494). This fits with another study that suggested that "aged care staff knowledge of later life sexuality is inadequate, but attitudes toward later life sexuality and about intimacy and dementia were relatively permissive" (Chen, Jones, & Osborne, 2017, p. 35). It may depend on a resident's behaviour because staff members tend to be more tolerant of sexual expressions such as handholding, while more erotic behaviours such as "sexual excitement or desire" are treated with anger and disgust (Taylor & Gosney, 2011, p. 541). Clearly, this is an area for further discussion, research, and education because feelings such as anger and disgust are not helpful therapeutically and are likely detrimental to positive staff–resident caregiving relationships.

Staff attitudes toward sexuality and aging become complicated when residents are living with dementia (Di Napoli, Lauren Breland, & Allen,

2013). Benbow and Beeston (2012) point to staff use of the label "sexually inappropriate behaviours" without a clear definition of what this really entails (p. 1029). Does masturbation in the privacy of one's room and being interrupted by staff members who have broken privacy and entered without knocking constitute inappropriate behaviour? The distinction between what is private or public can be blurred in these institutions. Residents living with dementia who remove their clothing in public areas likely are not expressing their sexuality; this behaviour is more likely an outcome of the resident's cognitive state and diminished orientation (Benbow & Beeston, 2012). Sexual behaviours of residents living with dementia toward other residents (especially those who are also living with dementia), bring additional concerns for capacity to make decisions and consent to participate (Benbow & Beeston, 2012). When unwanted sexual advances are made toward vulnerable residents, protection is the major concern (Benbow & Beeston, 2012; Di Napoli et al., 2013). "Indeed, for staff providing long-term care for people with dementia, the main source of tension in respect to sexuality is often the conflict between the need to protect people who lack capacity and allowing autonomy to residents who do have capacity" (Benbow & Beeston, 2012, p. 1031).

Teaching Sexuality and Aging in Higher Education

As the numbers of older adults continue to rise, so will healthcare providers' opportunities to discuss sexual concerns (Brandon, 2016). A key question for healthcare and social service practitioners and students working with older adults is, How do we make sexuality a routine part of our services? "How can healthcare and social service providers encourage discussions of this vital aspect of older adults' relationships" (Skultety, 2007, p. 31)? Adapted from recommendations by various researchers, here is a list of crucial issues for which practitioners and students should be prepared to provide support to older adults (Skultety, 2007; Jen, 2018; McInnis-Dittrich, 2020; Morrissey Stahl et al., 2019; Novak, Northcott, & Campbell, 2018):

1. Ask permission to talk about sexuality.
2. Be open to the idea that older adults' sexual expression is on a spectrum in which various types of desires and practice exist, as opposed to the dated views of older adults being both asexual and hypersexual.
3. Acknowledge discomfort and examine one's own ideas about aging and sexuality, relationships, and values and beliefs around this topic.

4. Discuss less about the details of sexual activity and more about relationship beliefs and ideas and how practitioners can facilitate and support older adults in pursuing the relationships they desire.
5. Allow and encourage a broad definition of sex and an inclusive range of sexual behaviours.
6. Do not assume the lack of sexual behaviour is part of the normative aging process, but inform older couples that most older couples enjoy sexual relationships.
7. Do not let the idea that sexuality and aging is a topic better left to specialists stop you from sending positive messages to older adults through asking a few simple questions about sexual interests and relationships.
8. Open the topic of sexually transmitted disease (including HIV and AIDS), the risks and the preventive measures.
9. Advocate for older adults about the needs of sexual well-being in healthcare, social service, and community settings.

(Point 1 adapted from McInnis-Dittrich, 2020; point 2 adapted from Morrissey Stahl et al., 2019; points 3, 4, 5, 6, & 7 adapted from Skultety, 2007; point 8 adapted from Novak, Northcott, & Campbell, 2018.)

Teaching about Sexuality and Aging: Classroom Activities

These crucial issues must find a place in the classroom for open discussion and learning. In terms of sex education in higher education, adult learners bring varied life experiences to the classroom. They may or may not know much about aging and sexuality but their life experiences contribute to and shape how they respond to the ideas presented in classroom. Our teaching role is to equip them to make connections between what they know and what they are learning. Once these connections are made, adult learners can internalize and extend their learning. Two educators, Sue Fostaty Young and Robert J. Wilson, have developed this notion in their Ideas, Connections, and Extensions (ICE) approach (Fostaty Young & Wilson, 2000). According to them, a successful final stage of learning leads to students' raising questions such as "So, what does this mean? How does this shape my view of the world?" (p. 5).

Based upon the ICE approach, we have constructed some examples of classroom activities on sexuality and aging. One limitation of these examples is that they tend to focus on heterosexual relationships, Caucasian and middle-class people, and women. Although a manual for classroom activities related to sexuality and aging does not seem to exist, other sources, such as the book *A Hands-on Approach to Teaching about*

Aging by Baker, Kruger, and Karasik (2018), offer a hands-on approach to teaching about aging, and some of these activities could be modified to address sexuality and aging.

Literature Example

Fiction (novels) and nonfiction (biography) literature, poetry, and academic journals are all good sources of ideas on aging and sexuality. For example:

> *All of us preserve time. We preserve the old versions of the people who have left us. And under our skin, under the layer of wrinkles and experience and laughter, we too, are older versions of ourselves. Directly below the surface, we are our former selves: the former child, the former lover, the former daughter.* (George, 2015, p. 137)

For preclass preparation, students receive a copy of the above quotation and write answers to the following questions:

1. What is George telling us about aging? What are her ideas about sexuality and aging?
2. What is the connection between her ideas and theoretical approaches such as the life-course perspective or transitions theory?
3. How do her ideas relate or not relate to your life experiences?

In the classroom, for further discussion, other questions are asked, either with the students as a large group or once students are placed in small working groups (no more than six students per group):

4. *All of us preserve time.* Do you/your group agree with this statement?
5. The quotation refers to *the former lover* along with the normative roles of child and daughter. How does this reflect George's perspective?
6. How would the quotation have had a different meaning if George had omitted the words *under the layer of wrinkles?*

Film and Television Examples

Films that contain content on sexuality and aging are valuable in the classroom. Gatling, Mills, and Lindsay (2017) analysed four comedy films with content on older adults' sexuality, two of which dealt with homosexual relationships. Their article could be a required reading for students, with questions aimed at whether or not the influence of the film industry will normalize societal perceptions of older adults' sexuality and sexual expression. Gatling et al. (2017) suggest as much, saying that "once the taboo topic of senior sexuality is normalized, those who assess the needs of the elderly in order to provide care will be able to broach the subject and ensure that a client's sexual health is not ignored" (p. 28).

Another film, *Away from Her* (Polley, 2006), depicts the life of a couple experiencing changes related to the wife's diagnosis of dementia, relocation to a nursing home, and her subsequent sexual attraction to another resident in the nursing home. Classroom discussion of this film can be guided to explore what is known about the relationship between three factors – capacity, consent, and autonomy – and whether or not the way sexuality is expressed should be taken into account when considering these factors.

A recent documentary, *Age of Love* (Loring, 2014), explores the lives of older adults (70 to 90 years of age) who have registered for a speed-dating event. It follows them prior, during, and after the speed dating, and depicts the differences among these men and women, along with their common interest in meeting someone new. The documentary stimulates interest in the classroom, and common themes come forth that reflect the research literature. After watching the film, one student shouted out, "They're just like us!" Quotations taken from the film can be highlighted to explore ideas, connections, and extensions.

From the two examples below, extensions related to desire, loneliness, and intimacy; and aging, beauty and sexuality are relevant to learning about changes associated with sexuality and aging. Students can be asked to compare and discuss what Janice and Lou are saying about their hopes and expectations for love and companionship, and how this relates to the definitions of sexuality and to students' life experiences and perspectives:

> *I'm not necessarily looking to find the love of my life. But, if it happens, it happens …* (Janice)

> *At my age, it's the companionship, wanting to be with the person, worrying about them, sharing the hardship and the laughter.* (Lou)

Similarly, comparing and discussing Linda and Frank's comments on aging, body image, and sexuality can lead students to relate these comments to younger age groups and societal views on beauty and attractiveness:

> *My arms are wrinkled and flabby. Do I want them to be? No, but this is who I am, and I think it's better just to be me.* (Linda)

> *At this age, beauty is. It's not about wrinkles and plastic surgery, it's about being open and adventurous.* (Frank)

An exercise below, based on the television series *One Day at a Time* (Kellett et al., 2017) and a character named Lydia, helps students explore older-adult sexual stereotypes. Interestingly, Lydia, a grandmother role, was not intended to be a sexual being until the actress Rita Moreno, who plays Lydia, insisted that this dimension be integrated into the scripts. According to Moreno,

> *I did ask a favor [of the producer]. I know she [Lydia] is a grandmother and I know she's supposed to be in her late 70s, but she has to be sexual ... I think it is because it's not seen enough on television and because people have an odd notion of what a woman of 80 – well, actually, I'm 87 I'm playing younger. She's supposedly about 77, 78, something like that. And you don't see that but it exists. And that's why I insisted that she be a sexual being.* (Kennedy, 2019)

Prior to class, students can also retrieve the newspaper article interview with Moreno and clips from the television show. Questions in the classroom can focus on older adults being depicted as asexual or hypersexual and how "Lydia" fits or does not fit with these stereotypes.

Birthday Card Example

Aging and sexuality presented in birthday cards and cartoons provide another opportunity for discussion and learning about sexuality and aging. Except for very old age (centenarians), birthday cards for middle-aged and older adults tend to focus on losses (e.g., hair, teeth, beauty, and physical, cognitive, social, and sexual abilities) and overlay a dark humour on these losses. Almost any card shop will have examples of sexual stereotypes of older adults that can be studied in the classroom. Probing questions can be asked, such as "Is this card funny? Why is it funny or not funny? What is the underlying societal message about sexuality and aging? Have we, as citizens of society, integrated these messages into our belief and values?"

A United Kingdom company (TRACKS Publishing Ltd.) produces general (blank inside) greeting cards under themes, one of which is called "naughty by nature." These particular cards primarily use nude older adult models (without full-frontal view) in various playful, enjoyable, or routine activities (e.g., a man and woman riding together on a motorcycle, dancing on the beach, fishing and camping, and doing chores). The visual images of older adults on these cards will elicit varied responses from students and will stimulate students to compare their beliefs and values with those depicted on the cards. Suggested questions are "What ideas of aging and sexuality are expressed in these images? How do these ideas fit with what you have learned in class and from your own life experiences?"

Conclusion

Sexuality is about our identity, our relationship with others, and the sociocultural influences that contribute to our thinking and behaviour. In addition, sexuality is an inclusive concept, broadly defined, and subject to individual interpretation. Clearly, there is evidence that as people age, their sexual interest and activities continue on a consistent basis (Brestschneider & McCoy, 1988). It is also accurate to say that age-related changes in health and functional ability, as well as loss of partners and ageist attitudes, have an impact on the continuity of sexual interest and activities. Thus, acknowledging and learning more about sexuality and aging is important, complicated, and currently lacking breadth and depth. Teaching the topic of sexuality and aging requires that, as educators, we work interprofessionally to expand our perspectives and our knowledge base. We must introduce future healthcare and helping professionals to theoretical perspectives, concepts, and discussions that equip them to link classroom learning to their life experiences, and go beyond individual interpretation to broader understandings of diversity, choice, and sexual expression among older adults. Also, teachers and students should reflect on their own values because "it is important to remember that we all hold sexual attitudes and beliefs that we embrace as truths" (Brandon, 2016, p. 54). Finally, we would be wise to consider the caution that while we acknowledge older adults as sexual beings, "care must be taken not to over-sexualize the ageing process nor to over-medicalize declining sexual function and interest" (Taylor & Gosney, 2011, p. 541).

REFERENCES

AARP. (2005). *Sexuality at midlife and beyond*. Washington, DC.

Araujo, A. B., Mohr, B. A., & McKinlay, J. B. (2004). Changes in sexual function in middle aged and older men: Longitudinal data from the Massachusetts male aging study. *Journal of the American Geriatrics Society, 52*, 1502–1509. https://doi.org/10.1111/j.0002-8614.2004.52413.x

Archibald, C. (2002). Sexuality and dementia in residential care: Whose responsibility? *Sexual and Relationship Therapy, 17*, 301–309. https://doi.org/10.1080/14681990220149103

Baker, H. E., Kruger, T. M., & Karasik, R. J. (2018). *A hands-on approach to teaching about aging: 32 activities for the classroom and beyond*. New York: Springer Publishing Company.

Benbow, S., & Beeston, D. (2012). Sexuality, aging, and dementia. *International Psychogeriatrics, 24*(7), 1026–1033. https://doi.org/10.1017/s1041610212000257

Bentrott, M. D., & Margrett, J. A. (2011). Taking a person-centered approach to understanding sexual expression among long-term care residents: Theoretical perspectives and research challenges. *Ageing International, 36,* 401–417. https://doi.org/10.1007/s12126-011-9110-7

Brandon, M. (2016). Psychosocial aspects of sexuality with aging. *Topics in Geriatric Rehabilitation, 23*(30) 151–153. https://doi.org/10.1097/tgr.0000000000000116

Brestschneider, J. G., & McCoy, N. L. (1988). Sexual interest and behavior in healthy 80–102-year-olds. *Archives of Sexual Behavior 15,* 109–129. https://doi.org/10.1007/bf01542662

Casta-Kaufteil, A. (2004). The old and the restless: Mediating rights to intimacy for nursing home residents with cognitive impairments. *Journal of Medicine and Law, 8,* 69–86.

Chen, Y., Jones, D., & Osborne, D. (2017). Exploratory study of Australian aged care staff knowledge and attitudes of later life sexuality. *Australasian Journal of Ageing, 36*(2), 35–38. https://doi.org/10.1111/ajag.12404

Clarke, L. H., & Korotchenko, A. (2011). Aging and the body: A review. *Canadian Journal on Aging, 30*(3), 495–510. https://doi.org/10.1017/s0714980811000274

Cort, E. M., Attenborough, J., & Watson, J. P. (2001). An initial exploration of community mental health nurses' attitudes to and experience of sexuality related issues in their work with people experiencing mental problems. *Journal of Psychiatric and Mental Health Nursing, 8*(6), 489–499. https://doi.org/10.1046/j.1351-0126.2001.00425.x

DeLamater, J., & Karraker, A. (2009). Sexual functioning in older adults. *Current Psychiatry Reports, 11*(1), 6–11. https://doi.org/10.1007/s11920-009-0002-4

Di Napoli, E. A., Lauren Breland, G., & Allen, R. S. (2013). Staff knowledge of sexuality and dementia of older adults in nursing homes. *Journal of Aging and Health, 25*(7), 1087–1105. https://doi.org/10.1177/0898264313494802

Elder, G. H., Johnson, M. K., & Crosnoe, R. (2003). The emergence and development of life course theory. *Handbook of the life course.* NY: Springer.

Elias, J., & Ryan, A. (2011). A review and commentary on the factors that influence expression of sexuality by older people in care homes. *Journal of Clinical Nursing 20,* 1668–1676. https://doi.org/10.1111/j.1365-2702.2010.03409.x

Eyler, A. E. (1997). Sexuality issues and common sexual dysfunctions: Evaluation and management in the primary care setting. In D. J. Knesper, M. B. Riba, & T. L. Schwenk (Eds.), *Primary care psychiatry.* Philadelphia: W.B. Saunders Co.

Fisher, L. (2010). *Sex, romance and relationships: AARP survey of midlife and older adults.* Washington, DC: AARP.

Fostaty Young, S., & Wilson, R.J. (2000). *Assessment and learning: The ICE approach.* Winnipeg: Portage & Main Press.

Gatling, M., Mills, J., & Lindsay, D. (2017). Sex after 60? You've got to be joking! Senior sexuality in comedy film. *Journal of Aging Studies 40,* 23–28. https://doi.org/10.1016/j.jaging.2016.12.004

George, N. (2015). *The little Paris book shop.* New York: Crown Publishing.

Gott, M., & Hinchliff, S. (2003). How important is sex in the later life? The views of older people. *Social Science and Medicine, 56,* 1617–1628. https://doi.org/10.1016/s0277-9536(02)00180-6

Gray, P., & García, J. (2012). Ageing and human sexual behavior: Biocultural perspectives – A mini-review. *Gerontology, 58,* 446–452. https://doi.org/10.1159/000337420

Haesler, E., Bauer, M., & Fetherstonhaugh, D. (2016). Sexuality, sexual health and older people: A systematic review of research on the knowledge and attitudes of health professionals. *Nursing Education Today, 40,* 57–71. https://doi.org/10.1016/j.nedt.2016.02.012

Hajjar, R. R., & Kamel, H. K. (2003a). Sexuality in the nursing home, part 1: Attitudes and barriers to sexual expression. *Journal of the American Medical Directors Association, 4,* 152–156. https://doi.org/10.1016/s1525-8610(04)70091-2

Hajjar, R. R., & Kamel, H. K. (2003b). Sexuality in the nursing home, part 2: Managing abnormal behavior – legal and ethical issues. *Journal of the American Medical Directors Association, 4,* 203–206. https://doi.org/10.1016/s1525-8610(04)70093-6

Hinchliff, S., Gott, M., & Ingelton, C. (2010). Sex, menopause and social context: A qualitative study with heterosexual women. *Journal of Health Psychology, 15,* 724–733. https://doi.org/10.1177/1359105310368187

Im, E., & Meleis, A. (2000). Meanings of menopause to Korean immigrant women. *Western Journal of Nursing Research, 22*(1), 84–102. https://doi.org/10.1177/019394590002200107

Jen, S. (2018) Sexuality of midlife and older women: A review of theory use. *Journal of Women & Aging, 30*(3), 204–226. https://doi.org/10.1080/08952841.2017.1295680

Kasif, T., & Band-Winterstein, T. (2017). Older widows' perspectives on sexuality: A life course perspective. *Journal of Aging Studies, 41,* 1–9. https://doi.org/10.1016/j.jaging.2017.01.002

Kellett, G. C., Royce, M., Lear, N., Miller, B., & Signer, D. (2017). *One day at a time* [television broadcast]. United States: Netflix.

Kennedy, M. (2019, February 22). Rita Moreno on playing a sassy grandma, "West Side Story." Associated Press News. Retrieved from https://www.apnews.com/e459db7aa67f4947bdfc26ab4724dcf4

Kwon, S., & Schafer, M.H. (2017). Obesity and sexuality among older couples: Evidence from the National and Social Life, Health and Aging Project. *Journal of Aging and Health, 29*(5), 735–768. https://doi.org/10.1177/0898264316645541

Lindau, S. T., & Gavrilova, N. (2010). Sex, health, and years of sexually active life gained due to good health: Evidence from two US population based cross sectional surveys of ageing. *British Medical Journal* Advance online publication. https://doi.org/10.1136/bmj.c810

Loring, S. (2014). *Age of love* [motion picture]. United States: Free Play Pictures.

Marshall, B. L. (2014). Sexualizing the third age. In C. L. Harrington, D. D. Bielby, & A. R. Bardo (Eds.), *Aging, media and culture* (pp. 169–180). NY: Lexington Books.

Marshall, B. L (2018). Happily ever after? "Successful ageing" and the heterosexual imaginary. *European Journal of Cultural Studies, 21*(3), 363–381. https://doi.org/10.1177/1367549417708434

McInnis-Dittrich, K. (2020). *Social work with older adults, fifth edition*. Boston: Pearson.

Meleis, A., Sawyer, L. M., Im, E., Hilfinger Messias, D. H., & Schumacher, K. (2000). Experiencing transitions: An emerging middle-range theory. *Advances in Nursing Science, 23*(1), 12–28. https://doi.org/10.1097/00012272-200009000-00006

Morrissey Stahl, K. A., Gale, J., Lewis, D. C., & Kleiber, D. (2019). Pathways to pleasure: Older adult women's reflections on being sexual beings. *Journal of Women & Aging, 31*(1), 30–48. https://doi.org/10.1080/08952841.2017.1409305

Mulligan, T., & Palguta, R. F. (1991). Sexual interest, activity and satisfaction among male nursing home residents. *Archives of Sexual Behaviour, 20*, 199–204. https://doi.org/10.1007/bf01541944

Nicolosi, A., Laumann, E. O., Galsser, D. B., Moreira Jr., E. D. Paik, A., & Gingell, C. (2004). Sexual behavior and sexual dysfunctions after age 40: The Global Study of Sexual Attitudes and Behaviors. *Urology, 64*(5), 991–997. https://doi.org/10.1016/j.urology.2004.06.055

Novak, M., Northcott, H., & Campbell, L. (2018). *Aging and society: Canadian perspectives*. 8th edition. Toronto: Nelson Education.

Polley, S. (2006). *Away from her* [motion picture]. Canada: Capri Releasing; Echo Lake Productions; Foundry Films; Gabway Films; The Film Farm.

Price, J. (2015). *The ultimate guide to sex after fifty: How to maintain – or regain – a spicy, satisfying sex life*. Cleis Press.

Price, J. (2011). *Naked at our age: Talking out loud about senior sex*. Seal Press.

Pslacios-Cena, D., Martinez-Piedrola, R. M., Perez-de-Heredia, M., Huertas-Hoyas, E., Carrasco-Garrido, P., & Fernandez-de-las-Penas, C. (2016). Expressing sexuality in nursing homes: The experience of older women: A qualitative study. *Geriatric Nursing, 37*, 470–477. https://doi.org/10.1016/j.gerinurse.2016.06.020

Reingold, D., & Burros, N. (2004). Sexuality in the nursing home. *Journal of Gerontological Social Work, 43*(2–3), 175–186. https://doi.org/10.1300/j083v43n02_12

Roney, L., & Wallace Kazar, M. (2015). Geriatric sexual experiences: The seniors tell all. *Applied Nursing Research 28*, 254–256. https://doi.org/10.1016/j.apnr.2015.04.005

Sadovsky, R., Alam, W., Enecilla, M., Cosiquien, R., Tipu, O., & Etheridge-Otey, J. (2006). Sexual problems among a specific population of minority women aged 40–80 years attending a primary care practice. *Journal of Sexual Medicine*, *3*(5), 795–803. https://doi.org/10.1111/j.1743-6109.2006.00288.x

Simpson, P., Brown Wilson, C., Brown, L., Dickinson, T., & Horner. M. (2018). "We've had our sex life way back": Older care home residents, sexuality and intimacy. *Ageing & Society*, *38*, 1478–1501. https://doi.org/10.1017/s0144686x17000101

Skultety, K. M. (2007). Addressing issues of sexuality with older couples. *Generations*, *31*(3), 31–37.

Syme, M. L. (2014). The evolving concept of older adult sexual behavior and its benefits. *Generations*, *38*(1), 35–41.

Taylor, A., & Gosney, M. (2011). Sexuality in older age: Essential considerations for healthcare professionals. *Age and Ageing*, *40*, 538–543. https://doi.org/10.1093/ageing/afr049

Tiefer, L. (1996). The medicalization of sexuality: Conceptual, normative, and professional issues. *Annual Review of Sex Research*, *7*, 252–282.

Wada, M., Clarke, L. H., & Rozanova, J. (2015). Construction of sexuality in later life: Analyses of Canadian magazine and newspaper portrayals of online dating. *Journal of Aging Studies*, *32*, 40–49. https://doi.org/10.1016/j.jaging.2014.12.002

Watson, W. K., Stelle, C., & Bell, N. (2017). Older women in new romantic relationships: Understanding the meaning and importance of sex in later life. *The International Journal of Aging and Human Development*, *85*(1), 33–43. https://doi.org/10.1177/0091415016680067

World Health Organization (2010). *Measuring sexual health: Conceptual and practical considerations and related indicators (Report No. WHO/RHR/10.12)*. Retrieved from http://whqlibdoc.who.int/hq/2010/who_rhr_10.12_eng.pdf

12 Uncertain Subjects: (Un)Teaching Pain(ful) Sexualities, Power, and Pedagogy

RENEE DUMARESQUE

As a graduate student in a master of social work program, I conducted autoethnographic research to deconstruct my experiences as a white non-binary settler with chronic vulvar pain, also known as vulvodynia. The contents of the research, as well as this chapter, were lived and written in Toronto/Tkaronto, on land that, while commonly referred to as "Canada," is contested by the sovereignty of Indigenous nations, communities, and peoples who refuse settler occupation and dispossession (Simpson, 2014). The research revealed the ways in which not only my experiences but also my mad/crip subjectivity was generated, fractured, and shifting according to my positionality within the historical and contemporary processes, dominant discourses, and power relations of (Canadian) white supremacist settler colonial sanist/ableist heteropatriarchy (Arvin, Tuck, & Morrill, 2013; Ben-Moshe, 2020; Lugones, 2007). In this chapter, I resource the knowledge acquired through my encounters with, and inquiries of, vulvar pain to propose that queer-critical autoethnography is a tool that can contribute to mad and crip pedagogies for teaching sexuality in higher education.

Within education, autoethnography is typically suggested as a methodology to reflect on one's own teaching practice rather than as a pedagogical tool in and of itself (Barr, 2019). Hickey and Austin (2007), however, have demonstrated its usefulness in encouraging students to reflect on how the self is socially constructed within relations of power. Similarly, Barr (2019) identified autoethnography as a tool that allows students to more deeply appreciate complexity, multiplicity, and relationality, while also encouraging student meta-reflection regarding their writing and learning processes. An autoethnography of vulvodynia in particular demonstrates its effectiveness as a pedagogical method in that it supports self-study that theorizes beyond the self – a method that engages the self in asking "questions like 'How has the world taken the shape that it has?,' but also 'Why is it that power relations are so difficult to transform?,' 'What does it mean to be invested in the conditions of subordination as well as dominance?'" (Ahmed, 2004, p. 182).

In this chapter, my central argument is that autoethnography, implemented within an ethics of "wonder" (Ahmed, 2004, p. 179), can disrupt totalizing epistemologies; contribute to the intelligibility of mad, crip, and pain(ful) sexualities; and attend to the relations of "power/knowledge" (Foucault, 1980) that produce sexual subjects and sexuality education. I approach wonder, as framed by Sara Ahmed (2004), as an analytic of uncertainty that moves us to historicize what we read as familiar and finds us "questioning our own investments" (p. 178), including our epistemic, disciplinary, pedagogical, and for white settlers, especially, investments in land and place (Tuck & McKenzie, 2015; Smith, Tuck, & Yang, 2019). As I have argued elsewhere (Dumaresque, 2020), autoethnography methodology, deployed from a transdisciplinary orientation, provides the tools to support layered analysis in service to intersectional mad/crip coalitions. Autoethnography also directs the writer's attention to detail and nuance, allowing for new critiques to emerge, as Thomas (2008) advocates that it is within sites of "micro-political" (p. 156) engagement that resistance can be enacted.

Ultimately, this chapter advocates for an approach to pedagogy that centres the "self-subject" (Adams & Holman Jones, 2014, p. 9) as a site of inquiry, embodied within broader discussions of how sex(uality), sexual subjectivity, and stories about (sex)uality emerge in accordance with historically specific regimes of governance and processes of normalization (McWhorter, 1999), which, as Indigenous scholars of education (Smith, Tuck, & Yang, 2019; Tuck & McKenzie, 2015) make clear, are always lived on, and thus must be engaged in relation to, "place" – an element that is crucial to the project of making visible the violent underpinnings of settler colonial scholarship and curricula (Tuck & Yang, 2012). Lastly, autoethnography as pedagogy is dependent here not on "fixed content, … [or] a set of guidelines" (Britzman, 1995, p. 155) but, in line with other proponents of queer pedagogy in higher education (Alexander, 2012; Kumashiro, 2002), on a method for asking questions (Britzman, 1995), which necessarily, involves analysis of the pedagogical process itself.

A Maddened/Cripped Schooling on Vulvar Pain and Sex

I locate this writing within larger projects of maddening (LeFrançois & Voronka, in press) and cripping (McRuer, 2006) knowledge and interventions related to pain (Patsavas, 2014), sex(uality) (Erickson, 2016), and education (Loutzenheiser & Erevelles, 2019; Snyder et al., 2019).

My intervention into vulvodynia, sex, and pedagogy is informed by "crip/ mad of color critique" (Ben-Moshe, 2020, p. 10; see also Kim, 2017); mad studies (Menzies, LeFrançois, & Reaume, 2013); and Black, queer (Bell, 2011; Dunhamn et al., 2015; Ejiogu & Ware, 2018), transnational, and feminist disability thought (Erevelles, 2011; Kafer, 2013; Price, 2015). Madness, crip, and disability operate here as historically-contingent and context-specific identities, experiences (Gorman, 2017; Gorman & LeFrançois, 2018), unruly sites of community and knowledge production (LeFrançois & Voronka, in press). When deployed as analytics, they support an accounting of how madness, disability, and sexuality have been produced and governed within systems of white supremacy, (settler) colonialism, and neoliberalism (Schalk, 2017). In relation to vulvodynia, this lens helps, for example, to interrogate the gender, racial, and colonial logics that inform diagnostic patterns, as well as the psychiatric and sexual production of vulvar pain subjects (Dumaresque, 2020).

A mad/crip-of-colour–informed approach to sex education is developed, here, from an understanding that sites of education are active in processes of normalization (McWhorter, 1999) and in upholding white settler narratives in standard approaches to both queer and disability studies in Canada (Ejiogu & Ware, 2018). It is grounded in a commitment to centre mad/crip pedagogies and epistemologies, or "cripistemologies" (Johnson & McRuer, 2014) in curricula. In the classroom, a "cripistemology of chronic pain" (Sheppard, 2018, p. 56) can unpack discourses of vulvodynia and sexuality, whether they be rooted in health and pathology or emergent forms of "settler sexuality" (Morgensen, 2011, p. 31), by "defamilariz[ing]" (Siebers, 2012, p. 38) their referents in (a)sexual moments and biomedical, psychiatric, and alternative understandings of pain, disability, and distress. Doing so exposes the role of "white rationality" and "anti-Black sanism" (Meerai, Abdillahi, & Poole, 2016, p. 24) in shaping "racialized medical imaginaries" of vulvar pain (Labuski, 2017, p. 166), along with seemingly radical alternatives. In addition to working as an analytic, mad and crip pedagogies offer practices that can challenge enlightenment logics and "compulsory able-bodymindedness" (Sheppard, 2018, p. 59) in sex education through accessible, creative approaches to knowledge production and curricular engagement (Snyder et al., 2019).

Queer-Critical Autoethnography for Mad/Crip Pedagogy

Autoethnography is a creative and critical methodology that situates the self at the centre of sociopolitical inquiry (Allen-Collinson, 2013). In this chapter, I work with queer, critical, and poststructural applications of autoethnography (Adams & Holman Jones, 2011, 2014; Holman Jones, 2016;

Gannon, 2006) that encourage a reading of theory, story, self, and the body as co-constituting and shifting. A queer-critical approach is in alignment with mad and crip modes of knowledge production by supporting unruly, "irrational" forms of inquiry.

The poststructural emphasis on power and knowledge positions queer-critical autoethnography as well suited to support intersectional mad/crip movements to disrupt sanist/ableist discourse and colonial modes of authorization that shape settler sites of higher education (Castrodale, 2017; LeFrançois & Voronka, in press). In a discussion of poststructural and postcolonial praxis, Blackman (2017) emphasizes that "the subjective nature of knowledge [and] stories … lead us to ask how are some stories more 'right' than others and accepted as truth" (p. 9). Educators can engage a poststructural understanding of power/knowledge and subject formation (Foucault, 1980, 1994) to support students in attending to how the self-subject and the "Other" (Blackman, 2017, p. 2) are both produced in relation to dominant knowledges of sexuality, madness, and disability.

Agitating Codes of Erotic Intelligibility

"What do you think about visiting a sex club?"

I feel my chest heat up and sense redness crawl up to eat my neck. My partner and I sit across from one another on a rug in the living room of our west-end apartment. We're separated by low light and a coffee table spattered with lit candles, half-empty glasses, and a pack of rolling papers. Our attention is locked but our bodies don't touch. Sex is everywhere – all over and around us.

Before my partner and I first visited a sex club together, we had a series of discussions that were *about* sex and sexuality; however, I failed to identify the moments we shared as sex or sexual themselves. That failure of identification is the result of "compulsory able-bodiedness" and "compulsory heterosexuality" (McRuer, 2006, p. 1; see also Rich, 1980), which naturalizes the "regimes of truth" (Foucault, 1980) that render sex(uality) (un)intelligible in relation to disability. In a discussion of queer pedagogy, Britzman (1995) argues that education ought to engage processes that examine the limits of "thinkability," to ask about "the unmarked criteria that work to dismiss as irrelevant or valorize as relevant a particular mode of thought, field of study, or insistence upon the real" (p. 156).

Tobin Siebers's (2012) discussion of sex as the ultimate enactment of humanness and the "ideology of ability [as] determin[ing] how we think about sex" (p. 40) reflects the co-constitutive relationship between sex and sexuality, disability (Schalk, 2017), madness (Pickens, 2019), and Eurocentric notions of the human, which as Sylvia Wynter (2003) demonstrates is over-determined by anti-Blackness and coloniality. Siebers (2012) also assists in identifying the signifiers through which sex(uality) is made legible and governed. In the moment referenced above, rigid definitions and spatial-temporal codes that distinguish sex from unsexed spaces obstructed me from recognizing that talking about sex was itself a form of sex.

Queer and crip theorists have, however, demonstrated that in making visible the mechanics of ableist sexuality, it is possible to conceptualize "sex and sensuality in denaturalized, new and potentially queer forms" (Groner, 2012, p. 275; see also Erickson, 2016). As Mollow and McRuer (2012) argue,

> If we understand sex as more than penetration that occurs in the bedroom, then we can perceive sex and disability coming together in many places we might have otherwise missed them: a heated exchange in a parking lot, a caress on the back of a neck, an online chat mediated by voice-recognition software. (p. 24)

This crip reckoning with sexuality alerts me to the operation of sex in new sites, rendered, for example, by the clutch of anticipation and movements of temperature, tone, and dress that animated the space between me and my partner. It is, however, crucial to recognize, both when engaging in and when teaching autoethnography, that there is never access to an absolute, essential, or innocent truth (Butler, 2005). Rather, "The (autoethnographic) researcher questions how 'experience [is] structured, how what [is] constituted as experience [is] reminiscent of ... available and normative discourses'" (Britzman, 2000, as cited in Gannon, 2006, p. 491).

Medicine, Psychiatry, and White Supremacist Settler Colonial Sanist/Ableist Heteropatriarchy: (Re)reading the Production of Sex, Gender, and Vulvodynia

Vulvodynia is a broad diagnostic category that problematizes unexplained chronic vulvar pain (Bornstein et al., 2016). Rather than being regarded as a coherent pathology, vulvodynia is classified, via the collaboration of several international "authorities" on pain, as having "potential associated factors," including "other pain syndromes," "Generics," "Hormonal factors," "Neurological mechanisms," and "Psychosocial factors" (ibid., p. 128). The prevalence rate of vulvar pain in so-called Canada is undocumented; however, in the so-called United States, it is estimated to be around 16% (Harlow & Stewart, 2003). Despite studies that suggest comparable rates of vulvar pain, regardless of sexuality, race, and ethnicity (Armstrong & Reissing, 2012; Reed et al., 2012), vulvar pain remains commonly imagined as a condition that primarily impacts white cis-heterosexual women (Labuski, 2017).

A mad/crip approach to vulvodynia (Dumaresque, 2020) makes it necessary to attend to the parallels between the logics that underpin vulvodynia, on the one hand, and both nineteenth- and twentieth-century anti-Black and colonial metrics of pain perception and the construction of hysteria, on the other (Briggs, 2000; Labuski, 2015). Hysteria was a disease developed and largely applied to wealthy white women to explain their sensitivity to pain, "frigidity," and "infertility" as a result of "overcivilization" (Briggs, 2000, p. 246). The discursive construction of white women as sexually frigid and their pain as a form of "nervous illness" (Briggs, 2000, p. 258) must be traced relative to the construction of Black, Indigenous, and racialized women as "hyper-sexual" and, correlatively, to the relegation of their pain to a state of incomprehensibility (Cooper Owens, 2017). Vulvodynia research suggests that chronicity is often correlated with hyper-reactivity of the nervous system (Sadownik, 2014), a correlation that is paralleled in hysteria (Labuski, 2015).

The relationship between medicine, psychiatry, and white supremacist settler colonial sanist/ableist heteropatriarchy is explicitly reflected in the articulation of vulvar pain as a sexual dysfunction (Dumaresque, 2020), included under "genito-pelvic pain/penetration disorder" (GPPPD). This diagnosis is situated in the fifth edition of the *Diagnostic and Statistical Manual of Mental Disorders (DSM-5)* (American Psychiatric Association, 2013). GPPPD is produced through the "ideology of ability" to secure colonial categories of race, sexuality, gender, and madness (Tosh & Carson, 2016) and fuel self-governance by reproducing compulsory heterosexuality and compulsory able-bodymindedness (Dumaresque, 2020).

A mad/crip approach to sex education requires that we go beyond learning *about* vulvar pain sex(uality), or even the marginalization of vulvar-pain sexual subjects, and engage students in "how questions" (Petersen, 2015, as cited in Blackman, 2017) to ask "how knowledge has been constructed, and the way truths are created as discourse is circulated and widely shared, creating social realities" (p. 8). Autoethnography can help students to examine how the "personal" is never *solely* personal and to discern "how ... [a] story [has] become one that is less mobile, less circulated, less known, in comparison to other ... stories and narratives" (Blackman, 2017, p. 10).

Grappling with Pain(ful) Sexualities

A friend and I sit on his leather couch, eat leftover spaghetti, and watch results of the election creep in on the TV in front of us. The newscast hauls up a map of "Canada" and zooms in on Newfoundland, peppered red.

"Least it's not blue," I say, placing a forkful of red sauce in my mouth. "It's still early. Mom said the lines were still long after 8 p.m."

I continue to eat but my stomach is sour with anticipation, the origin of which I locate in two seemingly unrelated sites: the election unfolding on the TV in front of us and the confession I'm braced to make.

I sit stiff, stare toward the TV, and silently school myself. "Come on, Renee. Spit it up, you'll feel better. 'Come out' already."

The words roll out sticky, at first – caked onto my esophagus like a sore throat.

***

I throw my weight against the front door of my friends building to leave. As I step outside, November air strikes my face, shaving the heat from my cheeks.

A rush soon hits me, followed by a gnawing feeling in my guts. "I felt 'seen,'" I say, reassuring myself.

Not only was my vulvar pain experience governed through explicit pathologization, but also through the "healthicization of sex" (Cacchioni, 2007, p. 306). This process is further contextualized by Siebers (2012), such that "when disability is linked to sex, it becomes a clinical matter in which each disability betrays a particular limitation of sexual opportunity, growth, or feeling" (p. 42). Reflecting on the above encounter through autoethnography reveals, however, that "visibility" alone does not necessarily constitute a form of refusal. In fact, the pressure to "come out," or "compulsory coming out," as Masoumi (2018) has named it, is always produced through the racialized politics of in/hyper-visibility (ibid.), and is entangled with compulsory heterosexuality and compulsory able-bodymindedness (Sheppard, 2018). Containing pain(ful) sexuality through language renders pain, and the pain-subject sexually intelligible (ibid.), such that promises of "recovery" spawn "compulsory confession" (Gannon, 2006, p. 479) and are implicated in the formation of emergent queer and crip normativities.

On the evening referenced above, I recall noting that the Canadian federal election served as an odd backdrop to the intimate conversation that my friend and I were having about my experience of pain and crip sexuality; I only later realized just how *intimately* the two were connected. My speech and behaviour were governed by a longing to find recuperation within "(sexual) citizenship" (Dryden & Lenon, 2015, p. 7). Yet engaging the encounter through the scholarship of Jose Muñoz (2009) allows for an additional reading, where I locate the "gnawing feeling in my guts" as a disruptive affect that constituted a performative act of refusal alongside the "politics of failure ... which is not so much a failure to succeed as it is to participate in a system of valuation that is predicated on exploitation and conformity" (pp. 173–174). The sense of unease that struck me while walking home revealed my continued displacement from, and facilitated my sidestepping of, normative sexuality.

When queer, crip, and mad knowledge production takes places through compulsory confession, then the result is often a further inscription of settler sexuality (Morgensen, 2011) and the settler nation state that thrives off of one's attachment to being "queerly Canadian" (Dryden & Lenon, 2015, p. 4). Reflecting on the interaction above through queer-critical autoethnography, however, helps to "emphasize discontinuities ... disjunctures and jarring moments" (Gannon, 2006, p. 480) in epistemological, affective, and relational configurations. Despite my being motivated to speak by a desire to be recuperated into sexual intelligibility, and indeed, my feeling of being "seen" after doing so, I also faced a persistent sense of displacement that resulted in a deeper questioning of the terms that constitute normative queer and crip (be)longing. This questioning, when enacted in dialogue with queer and mad/crip-of-colour scholarship, can map movement toward forms of queer, mad/crip "national (un)belonging" that advance intersectional queer, mad/crip coalitions (Dryden & Lenon, 2015, p. 13). Like queerness, crip sexuality is "illegible and therefore lost in the straight minds' mapping of space ... to accept loss is to accept queerness – or more accurately, to accept the loss of heteronormativity, authorization and entitlement" (p. 173).

Un/Mapping Power, Knowledge, and Sex in Higher Education: Toward a Pedagogy of Wonder

Biomedical and colonial frameworks for understanding vulvar pain are maintained and reproduced through the structures and practices of education. In relation to vulvodynia, Boyer, Chamberlain, and Pukall (2017) have called for a greater emphasis on sexuality in medical school curricula in Canada, suggesting that resident attitudes about sex correlate with quality of vulvodynia patient care. However, the situating of sex and gender education within conceptual geographies of health, across disciplines, de-contextualizes and de-historicizes sexuality education (Marshall, 2012), obscuring the role played by medical and psychiatric knowledge in producing and governing sex, gender, and desire (Foucault, 1978) through racial logics and colonial power relations (Stoler, 1995). As Gupta and Cacchioni (2013) demonstrate, the healthicization of sex across professionalized sites of "care" does not reflect a break from medical power so much as a shift in governance strategies and the "(re)medicalization of sex" (p. 445) in relation to neoliberal rationalities of "personal responsibility" and "optimization."

Interventions based on tolerance and inclusion have been heavily challenged in the field of education (Ahmed, 2004; Allen, 2015), and more broadly (Bannerji, 2000; Thobani, 2007), for not only failing to disrupt but ultimately serving their intended function in concealing, while reproducing, relations of power and domination. The mainstream trend toward inclusion plays an integral function in the mechanics through which some subjects, bodies are produced as belonging and others as abject (Greteman, 2013; Schippert, 2006). Educational approaches therefore must promote queer interventions that query and interrupt how technologies of diversity and inclusion generate new norms of civility that are indicative of and productive of new forms of violence (Britzman, 1995; see also Goldberg, 2009).

Education around vulvodynia and sexuality ought to grapple not only with the production of heteronormativity and compulsory able-bodymindedness, but also be informed by an understanding of sexual citizenship as mobile (Dryden & Lenon, 2015) and as connected to medicine and "psychiatry [which does] not exist outside of the political economy and global socio-political relations shape its development and operationalization" (Snyder et al., 2019, p. 496). Reckoning with sexual citizenship under neoliberal democracy requires attention to ongoing articulations of settler colonialism, anti-Blackness, and white supremacy (Smith, 2006), and requires grappling with the question, "How does neoliberalism create conditions for or demand conformity to particular forms of sexual identity … and presentations of gender identity?" (Wesling, 2013, p. 296).

Categories of sex and gender, along with madness and disability, have been crucial to separating the national subject and citizen from the outsider (Chadha, 2008; Chapman & Withers, 2019). At times, deviance and pathology have, in accordance with the specificities of gender and class, operated as fundamental signifiers of settler subjectivities (Stoler, 1995). The surge in tactics born of "Canadian homonationalisms" (Dryden & Lenon, 2015; see also Puar, 2007) and "crip" McRuer & Markotic, 2012, p. 166) or "Mad nationalism" (Gorman, 2013, p. 269) reveals the positioning of settler mad, crip, and queer subjects within contemporary projects of settler colonialism, dependent not on marginalization from but on identification with, and inclusion into, the state. Considering that sexual citizenship is activated by both deviancy and "pride," in relation to the white diagnostics of histories of hysteria and contemporary currents of vulvodynia, then, we might understand the mad and sexual subjectivities surrounding vulvar pain as fulfilling their intended functions in reinforcing regimes of race and gender for the Canadian settler state, not only through marginalization but also "liberation" (Dumaresque, 2020). In other words, it remains necessary to be attentive in sexuality education to the subversive power effects produced within strides toward the queering of vulvar pain.

In a discussion of "unlearning through mad positive pedagogies," Snyder et al. (2019, p. 492) suggest that students "interrogate how violent practices have been repackaged in sanitized and modernized ways" (p. 495), as a tactic to expose the normalized forms of violence enacted by professions taken for granted as offering benevolent "care" (see also Chapman & Withers, 2019). We might consider this here in relation to discourses of "sex as health" (Gupta & Cacchioni, 2013). Just as LeFrançois (2013) demonstrated autoethnography as a means to unzip the guise of benevolence that is cast over the colonial and genocidal practices of "child protection" in the Canadian context, autoethnography is a means for students to interrogate the power effects and morphing faces of sexuality, mad, and crip knowledges.

It is imperative that sexuality education facilitate processes that historicize harm to defamiliarize what and who is subjugated according to deviance and dysfunction. Intersectional analysis can support students to unpack how medical and psychiatric categories of sexuality, madness, and disability, as well as queer, mad and crip political movements, are formed in relation to white supremacist settler colonial sanist/ableist heteropatriarchy. By analyzing the autoethnographic excerpt above, I can locate my own "coming out" in the reproduction of complex networks of power. In the final section, I turn to a closer discussion of how autoethnography, by inverting the researcher's gaze, can propel students to read themselves in and through reading critical scholarship.

Autoethnographic Uncertainty

The theoretical orientation of the autoethnographer is crucial to the type of knowledge generated (Gannon, 2006) – a principle that remains when deploying autoethnography as pedagogy. For example, while Hickey and Austin (2007) engage students in understanding the self as socially constructed, the approach that they offer, wherein students ought to "interrogate rigorously the social construction of their identities via three principal axes of identity: race, class and gender" (p. 26) falls short of identifying the simultaneous operation of multiple subjectivities or the power-effects produced from the pedagogical activity itself. The risk, here, is a supposition of mastery based on "identity, authenticity, and resistance," as identified by Heidi Zhang (2018, p. 128).

In a Foucauldian poststructural critique of anti-oppressive practice (AOP), Zhang (2018) problematizes AOP as a discursive technology that essentializes and governs students toward occupying "moral subjectivities" (p. 134), which effectively reconfigures but fails to disrupt power:

> There is a strong desire in anti-oppressive teachings to see social issues as complex and deeply embedded within structures of dominance, but solvable. Therefore, resistance is returned to a hypernormative status since the foundations of AOP subjectivity do not become troubled in the process, except in the form of confessionals, responding to personal shame or guilt whenever "failure" occurs within micro settings of individual practice. (p. 137)

Zhang (2018) demonstrates that failing to consider the generative products of AOP enables a belief that one can exist outside power and, for white students, this often accompanies a claim to innocence. We can infer from Zhang's analysis the importance of not only transmitting critical knowledges, but also engaging students in interrogating pedagogy as enveloped within structures of power. This is critical to autoethnography: the practice of "self-writing" has long been identified by Michel Foucault (1994) as a technology through which one renders themselves knowable in relation to dominant forms of knowledge and power (Gannon, 2006); and by Andrea Smith (2014), who, in emphasizing the relational production of subjects, further problematizes white settler confessions – even those confessing privilege – for simultaneously fixing racialized subjects as knowable and the white self-subject as self-determining.

Teresa Macias (2012) offers an approach to reading, informed by Foucauldian ethics, that can be applied to autoethnography to support students in moving toward "self-making in ways that remain in full view of the power/knowledge regimes that determine subjectification" (p. 15). Macias emphasizes that like writing, the act of reading is situated in assumptions, discourse, and regimes of practice that merge to co-constitute the "reader-text relationship" (p. 1). Macias's articulation can inform students' entry into autoethnographic inquiry by offering prompts for students to reflect on how they read themselves in and through the sexuality knowledges taken up in class. It can also work as a framework for students to analyse their own autoethnographic entries once completed. In other words, as students read texts – both autoethnographic and otherwise – they should be encouraged to ask questions such as, "Who am I as I read this text? What kind of subject does this text allow me to become? What are the social and political implications of this act of becoming? … How does this text allow me to imagine different ways of being?" (p. 15).

When conducting autoethnography, students should be instructed to interface with a range of critical literature and "imagine the text as a temporary port in which [they] set anchor" (Macias, 2012, p. 14). They ought to analyse their everyday moments and those moments more apparently productive, locate themselves within the subject under critique, and through layered analysis of critical scholarship, explore how the self is produced through power and knowledge. Practically, this might be advanced through nonlinear approaches to learning, such as those forwarded by Snyder et al. (2019) in their discussion of mad pedagogy, whereby students are encouraged to enter the course outline from the point of their choosing and move between topics. This approach is suited to disrupting compulsory able-bodymindedness and establishing innovative connections (Snyder et al., 2019) in sexuality education.

Difficult emotions or other feelings generated through "intellectual wandering [in] … practices of subject making and reading" (Macias, 2012, p. 15) all exist within the configurations of power and knowledge that have been placed under examination (Ahmed, 2004). Embracing a pedagogy of wonder requires, then, that we also embrace what Megan Boler (1999) has termed a "pedagogy of discomfort": an ethical orientation toward uncertainty and attunement with "what it is that one doesn't want to know" (p. 176). Alexander (2012) affirms that "prompt-ing uncomfortable moments in the queer classroom can … give the classroom a sense of texture – and risk – such that students become more aware of the normative structures which condition their readings of, and identifications with, course texts" (p. 65). Queer-critical autoethnography allows us to value this knowledge and to engage it in transformative learning by asking *how* I have come to feel like this.

In/Conclusive

Multiple and diffuse relations of power are present in higher education, generating explicit knowledge and quiet rationalities that shape content, pedagogy, material conditions, and student and educator subjectivities (Macias, 2012; Thomas, 2008). The subversive character of power becomes especially dangerous in sexuality education, where sexuality knowledge and pedagogy emerged as, and continue to operate as, a feature of race and nation formation. A mad/crip approach to queer-critical autoethnography offers a transdisciplinary intervention that can register the inexplicabilities of categories of sexuality, madness, and disability in broad (settler) colonial networks by embracing the analytic potential of unruly inquiry and an ethics of unlearning and, equally, a practice of (un)teaching.

Autoethnography offers a frame through which to hold in balance the epistemological, experiential, and relational, as co-constituting and as tools to unhook the functions of normalizing discourses within colonial relations. This chapter pushes back against compulsory reason, compulsory confession, and the neoliberal standardization of knowledge production in education (Goedl, 2016), by leaning into the what Greteman (2013) details as "risky-sex education (as opposed to safer-sex education)." A risk approach to sex education constitutes an ethics that centres questions and modes of critique that inquire as to how the self and Other are produced and erased; it mingles with learning as a necessary risk to self; and, ultimately, situates risk as a relationality akin to pedagogy.

REFERENCES

Adams, T., & Holman Jones, S. (2011). Telling stories: Reflexivity, queer theory, and autoethnography. *Cultural Studies – Critical Methodologies, 11*(2), 108–116. https://doi.org/10.1177/1532708611401329

Adams, T., & Holman Jones, S. (2014). Autoethnography is queer. In N. K. Denzin, Y. S. Lincoln, & L. T. Smith (Eds.), *Handbook of critical and Indigenous methodologies* (pp. 373–390). Thousand Oaks: SAGE Publications, Inc.

Ahmed, S. (2004). *The cultural politics of emotion.* Abingdon, Oxon: Routledge.

Alexander, K. B. C. (2012). Teaching discomfort? Uncomfortable attachments, ambivalent identifications. *Transformations: The Journal of Inclusive Scholarship and Pedagogy, 22*(2), 57–71.

Allen, L. (2015). Queer pedagogy and the limits of thought: Teaching sexualities at university. *Higher Education Research & Development, 34*(4), 763–775, https://doi.org/10.1080/07294360.2015.1051004

Allen-Collinson, J. (2013). Autoethnography as the engagement of self/other, self/culture, self/politics, selves/futures. In S. H. Jones, T. E. Adams, & C. Ellis (Eds.), *Handbook of autoethnography* (pp. 281–299). Walnut Creek, CA: Left Coast Press.

American Psychiatric Association. (2013). *Diagnostic and statistical manual of mental disorders* (5th ed.). Arlington, VA: Author.

Armstrong, H., & Reissing, E. D. (2012). Chronic vulvo-vaginal pain in lesbian, bisexual and other sexual minority women. *Journal of Sexual Medicine, 9*, 166–167.

Arvin, M., Tuck, E., & Morrill, A. (2013). Decolonizing feminism: Challenging connections between settler colonialism and heteropatriarchy. *Feminist Formations, 25*(1), 8–34. https://doi.org/10.1353/ff.2013.0006

Bannerji, H. (2000). *The dark side of the nation: Essays on multiculturalism, nationalism, and gender*. Toronto, ON: Canadian Scholars Press.

Barr, M. (2019). Autoethnography as pedagogy: Writing the "I" in IR. *Qualitative Inquiry, 25*(9–10), 1106–1114. https://doi.org/10.1177/1077800418792940

Ben-Moshe, L. (2020). *Decarcerating disability: Deinstitutionalization and prison abolition*. Minneapolis, MN: University of Minnesota Press.

Bell, C. M. (Ed.). (2011). *Blackness and disability: Critical examinations and cultural interventions*. East Lansing, MI: Michigan State University Press.

Blackman, T. (2017). Using poststructuralism and postcolonialism in education praxis: An exploration of teaching about the "developing Other" in an Australian high school. *The International Education Journal: Comparative Perspectives, 16*(4), 1–12.

Boler, M. (1999). *Feeling power: Emotions and education*. New York, NY: Routledge.

Bornstein, J., Goldstein, A. T., Stockdale, C. K., Bergeron, S., Pukall, C., Zolnoun, D., & Coady, D. (2016). 2015 ISSVD, ISSWSH and IPPS consensus terminology and classification of persistent vulvar pain and vulvodynia. *Journal of Lower Genital Track Disease, 20*(2), 126–130. https://doi.org/10.1097/aog.0000000000001359

Boyer, S., Chamberlain, S., & Pukall, C. (2017). Vulvodynia attitudes in a sample of Canadian post-graduate medical trainees. *The Canadian Journal of Human Sexuality, 26*(3), 249–301. https://doi.org/10.3138/cjhs.2017-0019

Briggs, L. (2000). The race of hysteria: "Overcivilization" and the "savage" woman in late nineteenth-century obstetrics and gynecology. *American Quarterly, 52*(2), 246–273. https://doi.org/10.1353/aq.2000.0013

Britzman, D. P. (1995). Is there a queer pedagogy? Or, stop reading straight. *Educational Theory, 45*(2), 151–165. https://doi.org/10.1111/j.1741-5446 .1995.00151.x

Britzman, D. P. (2000). "The question of belief": Writing poststructural ethnography. In E. St. Pierre & W. Pillow (Eds.), *Working the ruins: Feminist poststructural theory and methods in education* (pp. 27–40). New York, NY: Routledge.

Butler, J. (2005). *Giving an account of oneself.* New York, NY: Fordham University Press.

Cacchioni, T. (2007). Heterosexuality and "the labour of love": A contribution to recent debates on female sexual dysfunction. *Sexualities, 10*(3), 299–320. https://doi.org/10.1177/1363460707078320

Castrodale, M. A. (2017). Critical disability studies and mad studies: Enabling new pedagogies in practice. *Canadian Journal for the Study of Adult Education, 29*(1), 49–66.

Chadha, E. (2008). "Mentally defectives" not welcome: Mental disability in Canadian immigration law. *Disability Studies Quarterly, 28*(1), 1857–1927.

Chapman, C., & Withers, A. (2019). *A violent history of benevolence: Interlocking oppression in the moral economies of social working.* Toronto, CA: University of Toronto Press.

Cooper Owens, D. B. (2017). *Medical bondage: Race, gender, and the origins of American gynecology.* Athens, GA: University of Georgia Press.

Dryden, O. H., & Lenon, S. (Eds.). (2015). *Disrupting queer inclusion: Canadian homonationalisms and the politics of belonging.* Vancouver, BC: UBC Press.

Dumaresque, R. (2020). Vulvodynia, it's in my head: Mad methods toward crip coalition. *Journal of Feminist Scholarship, 17*(17), 81–105. https://doi.org/10.23860/jfs.2020.17.06

Dunhamn, J., Harris, J., Jarrett, S., Moore, L. Nishida, A., Price, M., Robinson, B., & Schalk, S. (2015). Developing and reflecting on a Black disability studies pedagogy: Work from the National Black Disability Coalition. *Disability Studies Quarterly, 35*(2). https://doi.org/10.18061/dsq.v35i2.4637

Ejiogu, N., & Ware, S. M. (2018). Calling a shrimp a shrimp: A Black queer intervention in disability studies. In J. Haritaworn, G. Moussa, & S. M. Ware (Eds.), *Queering urban justice: Queer of colour formations in Toronto* (pp. 187–201). Toronto, ON: University of Toronto Press.

Erevelles, N. (2011). *Disability and difference in global contexts: Enabling a transformative body politic.* New York, NY: Palgrave Macmillan.

Erickson, L. (2016). Transforming cultures of (un)desirability: Creating cultures of resistance. *Graduate Journal of Social Science, 12*(1), 11–22.

Foucault, M. (1978). *The History of Sexuality.* New York, NY: Pantheon Books.

Foucault, M. (1980). *Power/knowledge: Selected interviews and other writings, 1972–1977.* New York, NY: Pantheon Books.

Foucault, M. (1994). Technologies of the self. In P. Rabinow (Ed.), *Michel Foucault: Ethics, subjectivity and truth* (pp. 223–254). New York, NY: The New York Press.

Gannon, S. (2006). The (im)possibilities of writing the self-writing: French poststructural theory and autoethnography. *Cultural Studies – Critical Methodologies, 6*(4), 474–495. https://doi.org/10.1177/1532708605285734

Goedl, D. (2016). Decolonizing dominant knowledge and knowledge production: Special issue editorial introduction. *Postcolonial Directions in Education, 5*(2) 163–171.

Goldberg, D. T. (2009). *The threat of race: Reflections on racial neoliberalism.* Malden, MA: Wiley-Blackwell.

Gorman, R. (2013). Mad nation? Thinking through race, class, and mad identity politics. In B. A. LeFrançois, R. J. Menzies, & G. Reaume (Eds.), *Mad Matters: A Critical Reader in Canadian Mad Studies* (pp. 269–280). Toronto: Canadian Scholars Press.

Gorman, R. (2017). Quagmires of affect: Labor, whiteness, and ideological disavowal. *American Quarterly, 69*(2), 309–313. https://doi.org/10.1353/AQ.2017.0025

Gorman, R., & LeFrançois, B.A. (2018). Mad studies. In B.M.Z. Cohen (Ed.), *Routledge international handbook of critical mental health* (Routledge international handbooks). London: Routledge.

Greteman, A. J. (2013). Fashioning a bareback pedagogy: Towards a theory of risky (sex) education. *Sex Education, 13*(sup 1), S20–S31. https://doi.org/10.1080/14681811.2012.760154

Groner, A. (2012). Sex as "spock": Autism, sexuality, and autobiographical narrative. In R. McRuer & A. Mollow (Eds.), *Sex and disability* (pp. 263–280). Durham, NC & London, UK: Duke University Press.

Gupta, K., & Cacchioni, T. (2013). Sexual improvement as if your health depends on it: An analysis of contemporary sex manuals. *Feminism & Psychology, 23*(4), 442–458. https://doi.org/10.1177/0959353513498070

Harlow, B. L., & Stewart, E. G. (2003). A population-based assessment of chronic unexplained vulvar pain: Have we underestimated the prevalence of vulvodynia? *Journal of the American Medical Women's Association, 58*(2). 82–88.

Hickey, A., & Austin, J. (2007). Pedagogies of self: Conscientising the personal to the social. *International Journal of Pedagogies and Learning, 3*(1), 21–29. https://doi.org/10.5172/ijpl.3.1.21

Holman Jones, S. (2016). Living bodies of thought: The "critical" in critical autoethnography. *Qualitative Inquiry, 22*(4), 228–237. https://doi.org/10.1177/1077800415622509

Johnson, M. L., & McRuer, R. (2014). Cripistemologies: Introduction. *Journal of Literary & Cultural Disability Studies, 8*(2), 127–147. https://doi.org/10.3828/jlcds.2014.12

Kafer, A. (2013). *Feminist, queer, crip.* Bloomington, IN: Indiana University Press.

Kim, J. B. (2017). Toward a crip-of-color critique: Thinking with Minich's "enabling whom?" *Lateral: Journal of the Cultural Studies Association, 6*(1). https://doi.org/10.25158/l6.1.14 Retrieved from: https://csalateral.org/issue/6-1/forum-alt-humanities-critical-disability-studies-crip-of-color-critique-kim/

Kumashiro, K. K. (2002). *Troubling education: "Queer" activism and anti-oppressive pedagogy*. New York, NY: RoutledgeFalmer

Labuski, C. (2015). *It hurts down there: The bodily imaginaries of female genital pain*. Albany, NY: New York Press.

Labuski, C. (2017). A black and white issue? Learning to see the intersectional and racialized dimensions of gynecological pain. *Social Theory & Health*, *15*(2), 160–181. https://doi.org/10.1057/s41285-017-0027-4

LeFrançois, B. A. (2013). The psychiatrization of our children, or, an autoethnographic narrative of perpetuating First Nations genocide through "benevolent" institutions. *Decolonization: Indigeneity, Education & Society*, *2*(1), 108–123.

LeFrançois, B. A., & Voronka, J. (in press). Mad epistemologies and the ethics of knowledge production. In T. Macias (Ed.), *Un/Ethical un/knowing: Ethical reflections on methodology and politics in social science research*. Toronto: Canadian Scholars Press Inc.

Loutzenheiser, L. W., & Erevelles, N. (2019) "What's disability got to do with it?": Crippin' educational studies at the intersections. *Educational Studies: A Journal of the American Educational Studies Association*, *55*(4), 375–386. https://doi.org/10.1080/00131946.2019.1630131

Lugones, M. (2007). Heterosexualism and the colonial/modern gender system. *Hypatia*, *22*(1), 186–209.

Macias, T. (2012). In the world: Toward a Foucauldian ethics of reading in social work. *Intersectionalities: A Global Journal of Social Work Analysis, Research, Polity, and Practice*, *1*(1), 1–19.

Marshall, D. (2012). Historicizing sexualities education. *Review of Education, Pedagogy, and Cultural Studies*, *34*(1–2), 23–34. https://doi.org/10.1080/10714413.2012.643730

Masoumi, A. (2018). Compulsory coming out and agentic negotiations: Toronto QTPOC narratives. In J. Haritaworn, G. Moussa, & S. M. Ware (Eds.), *Queering urban justice: Queer of colour formations in Toronto* (pp. 187–201). Toronto, ON: University of Toronto Press.

McRuer, R (2006). *Crip theory: Cultural signs of queerness and disability*. New York, NY & London, UK: New York University Press.

McRuer, R., & Markotic, N. (2012). Leading with your head: On the borders of disability, sexuality, and the nation. In R. McRuer & A. Mollow (Eds.), *Sex and disability* (pp. 165–183). Durham, NC & London, UK: Duke University Press.

Meerai, S., Abdillahi, I., & Poole, J. (2016). An introduction to anti-Black sanism. *Intersectionalities: A Global Journal of Social Work Analysis, Research, Polity, and Practice*, *5*(3), 18–35.

Menzies, R., LeFrançois, B. A., & Reaume, G. (Eds.). (2013). Introducing mad studies. In B. A. LeFrançois, R. Menzies, & G. Reaume (Eds.), *Mad matters: A critical reader in Canadian mad studies*. Toronto: CSPI.

McWhorter, L. (1999). *Bodies and pleasures: Foucault and the politics of sexual normalization*. Bloomington, IN: Indiana University Press.

Mollow, A., & McRuer, R. (2012). Introduction. In R. McRuer & A. Mollow (Eds.), *Sex and disability* (pp. 1–34). Durham, NC & London, UK: Duke University Press.

Morgensen, S. L. (2011). *Spaces between us: Queer settler colonialism and Indigenous decolonization*. Minneapolis, MN: University of Minnesota Press.

Muñoz, J. E. (2009). *Cruising utopia: The then and there of queer futurity*. New York, NY: New York University Press.

Patsavas, A. (2014). Recovering a cripistemology of pain: Leaky bodies, connective tissue, and feeling discourse. *Journal of Literary & Cultural Disability Studies, 8*(2), 203–218. https://doi.org/10.3828/jlcds.2014.16

Petersen, E. B. (2015). Education policies as discursive formations: A Foucauldian Optic. In K. N. Gulson, M. Clarke, & E. B. Petersen (Eds.), *Education policy and contemporary theory: Implications for research* (pp. 63–72). New York, NY: Routledge.

Pickens, T. A. (2019). *Black madness:: Mad blackness*. Durham, NC: Duke University Press.

Price, M. (2015). The body mind problem and the possibilities of pain. *Hypatia, 30*(1), 268–284. https://doi.org/10.1111/hypa.12127

Puar, J. K. (2007). *Terrorist assemblages: Homonationalism in queer times*. Durham, NC: Duke University Press.

Reed, B. D., Harlow, S. D., Sen, A., Legocki, L. J., Edwards, R. M., Arato, N., & Haefner, H. K. (2012). Prevalence and demographic characteristics of vulvodynia in a population-based sample. *American Journal of Obstetrics and Gynecology, 206*(2), 170.e1–9. https://doi.org/10.1016/j.ajog.2011.08.012

Rich, A. (1980). Compulsory heterosexuality and lesbian existence. *Signs: Journal of Women in Culture and Society, 5*(4), 631–660. https://doi.org/10.1086/493756

Sadownik, L. A. (2014). Etiology, diagnosis, and clinical management of vulvodynia. *International Journal of Women's Health, 6*, 437–449. https://doi.org/10.2147/ijwh.s37660

Schalk, S. (2017). Critical disability studies as methodology. *Lateral: Journal of the Cultural Studies Association, 6*(1). https://doi.org/10.25158/l6.1.13 Retrieved from: http://csalateral.org/issue/6-1/forum-alt-humanities-critical-disability-studies-methodology-schalk/

Schippert, C. (2006). Critical projection and queer performativity: Self-revelation in teaching/learning otherness. *Review of Education, Pedagogy, and Cultural Studies, 28*(3–4), 281–295. https://doi.org/10.1080/10714410600873191

Sheppard, E. (2018). Using pain, living with pain. *Feminist Review, 120*(1), 54–69. https://doi.org/10.1057/s41305-018-0142-7

Sheppard, E. (2019). Chronic pain as fluid, BDSM as control. *Disability Studies Quarterly, 39*(2). https://doi.org/10.18061/dsq.v39i2.6353 Retrieved from: https://dsq-sds.org/article/view/6353

Siebers, T. (2012). A sexual culture for disabled people. In R. McRuer & A. Mollow (Eds.), *Sex and disability* (pp. 37–53). Durham, NC & London, UK: Duke University Press.

Simpson, A. (2014). *Mohawk interruptus: Political life across the borders of settler states.* Durham, NC: Duke University Press.

Smith, A. (2014). Native studies at the horizon of death: Theorizing ethnographic entrapment and settler self-reflexivity. In A. Simpson & A. Smith (Eds.), *Theorizing native studies* (pp. 203–233). Durham, NC & London, UK: Duke University Press.

Smith, A. (2006). Heteropatriarchy and the three pillars of white supremacy: Rethinking women of color organizing. In INCITE! Women of Color Against Violence (Ed.), *Color of violence: The INCITE! Anthology* (pp. 66–72). Cambridge, MA: South End Press.

Snyder, S. N., Pitt, K., Shanouda, F., Voronka, J., Reid, J., & Landry, D. (2019). Unlearning through mad studies: Disruptive pedagogical praxis. *Curriculum Inquiry, 49*(4), 485–502. https://doi.org/10.1080/03626784.2019 .1664254

Stoler, A. L. (1995). *Race and the education of desire: Foucault's history of sexuality and the colonial order of things.* Durham, NC: Duke University Press.

Thobani, S. (2007). *Exalted subjects: Studies of the making of race and nation in Canada.* Toronto, ON: Toronto University Press.

Thomas, N. (2008). Pedagogy and the work of Michel Foucault. JAC: *A Journal of Composition Theory, 28*(1–2), 151–180.

Tosh, J., & Carson, K. (2016). A desire to be "normal"? A discursive and intersectional analysis of "penetration disorder." *Intersectionalities: A Global Journal of Social Work Analysis, Research, Polity, and Practice, 5*(3), 151–172. https://doi.org/10.2307/j.ctt20d87xh.12

Tuck, E., & McKenzie, M. (2015). Relational validity and the "where of inquiry": Place and land in qualitative research. *Qualitative Inquiry, 21*(7), 633–638. https://doi.org/10.1177/1077800414563809

Tuck, E., & Yang, W.K. (2012). Decolonization is not a metaphor. *Indigeneity, Education & Society, 1*(1), 1–40.

Tuhiwai Smith, L., Tuck, E., & Yang, K. W. (Eds.). (2019). *Indigenous and decolonizing studies in education: Mapping the long view.* New York, NY: Routledge.

Wesling, M. (2013). Epistemologies of empire: Sexuality and knowledge within the neoliberal academy. *American Quarterly, 65*(2), 291–302. https://doi.org /10.1353/aq.2013.0031

Wynter, S. (2003). Unsettling the coloniality of being/power/truth/freedom: Towards the human, after man, its overrepresentation – An argument. *CR: The New Centennial Review, 3*(3), 257–337. https://doi.org/10.1353/ncr.2004.0015

Zhang, H. (2018). How "anti-*ing*" becomes mastery: Moral subjectivities shaped through anti-oppressive practice. *British Journal of Social Work, 48*(1), 124–140. https://doi.org/10.1093/bjsw/bcx010

PART THREE

Practical Applications and Recommendations

SUSAN HILLOCK

Part 3, "Practical Applications and Recommendations," integrates current theories, concepts, and methods, applies them to everyday teaching and skills development, and suggests ways to improve sex education in higher education. Based on their teaching expertise, these last contributors share their insights and wisdom about how higher education can more effectively incorporate sexuality(ies) content and sex positive/well-being approaches, including useful recommendations on how to best teach sexuality(ies), as well as how to provide ethical care and support. For instance, social work professor Heather Peters critically thinks about her own teaching of a sex education course in Chapter 13, "Sex and Gender in the Classroom: Lessons from (and for) the Front Lines," to discuss methods for teaching about reproductive anatomy and genitalia, sexual activities, and health. Her approach and methods challenge a binary approach by exploring sexuality, sexual and gender identity, and sexual orientation on an intersectional continuum and as a complex and dynamic interplay of aspects of identity, and demonstrate the value of student presentations in building leadership skills to share important sexuality information with others. Furthermore, Peters highlights the importance of professionals being trained in content related to sex, sexuality(ies), and identity, as well as in skills on how to talk with service users about these topics, especially as they are relevant to everyone and are often brought up by service users in interactions with social work and healthcare professionals. Despite its importance, Peters reports that faculty members in professional disciplines struggle to prepare students to adequately address the sex and sexuality concerns of service users. Furthermore, she states that it is essential to teach sex education courses for many reasons, not only because service users need professionals who can talk about sex and sexuality, but also because structures of power and privilege are interwoven into what passes for fundamental truths about sex. In her teaching, Peters has found that the creativity of students and their willingness to talk about and present challenging sexual topics offers hope that it is possible to successfully prepare students for discussions of sex, sexuality, and gender in professional practice. She presents teaching strategies, discusses issues that come up, and shares her course outline as an exemplar (Appendix A). Peters recommends that instructors who teach these topics need to be prepared to share their experiences and ideas with colleagues, as well as with other disciplines, in the hope that together, over time, we will become better at ensuring that our students are prepared for professional practice and activism in the area of sex, sexuality, and gender.

Next, Chapter 14, "The Pitch: Teaching Sexuality at Multiple Levels," by queer activist and social work professor Nick J. Mulé, offers interesting insights into the intersections that students bring into the classroom – their social locations to their affiliated studies, the subjective positioning on gender, sex, and sexuality to societal normative notions – and how these often impact the classroom and discussion of issues that are framed as controversial, such as abortion, asexuality, BDSM, intergenerational relationships, polyamoury, pornography, sex trafficking, and sex work. Furthermore, Mulé examines the added pressures and tensions that come with teaching sexuality-based courses. Given the sensitive nature of the content of sexuality-based courses, he considers all the variables, identities, and social locations that students bring to such courses. He argues that this intersectional view is important, as external conceptions and perspectives on sexuality tend to dominate course content and class discussions, with little taken up at the subjective level. At the same time, he acknowledges that addressing sexuality-based issues at a subjective level within a university class environment has its own challenges.

If one is to be true to the subject matter, an interesting balance must be struck in pitching topics, content, and material when teaching gender, sex, and sexuality, regardless of the positioning and shifting of individual students or the class as a collective body. Moreover, Mulé posits that the complexities, perspectives, and sensitivities involved in teaching a sexuality course require constant reflexivity. Therefore, he recommends that a multilevel pitch is necessary to do justice to a subject matter of such complexity and fluidity. Further, to help students gain knowledge about gender, sex, and sexuality, instructors must rise to the challenges of managing varying theoretical approaches without succumbing to the domination of one; allowing for an open and engaging learning environment that encourages students to bring in and explore varying perspectives – theirs and that of others; and not shying away from controversial issues but rather embracing them in service of education, the furthering of knowledge, and the development of students who are applying themselves to it.

Chapter 15, "Sexual Health Education for Individuals with Intellectual and Developmental Disabilities," written by occupational therapy professor Shaniff Esmail, and master's students Meg Tronson and Sheena Churla, critically examines the individual, structural, and attitudinal barriers that mire healthy sexual expression in misinformation and shame. Esmail, Tronson, and Churla describe how general education related to sexuality with those living with disability has largely been homogenous, centring on sexual safety and harm reduction. However, the authors explain that for individuals with intellectual and developmental disability (IDD), there exist significant gaps that remain unaddressed, including meaningful conceptualization of consent, adoption of sex-positive frameworks, and delivery methods tailored to individuals' learning needs. The authors present a case for the need to develop sex education programming and content based on the desire for the IDD population to be able to develop meaningful and intimate relationships (if they so choose). Additionally, the authors highlight the support, information, and sex education that neurotypical individuals receive and compare those to what is received or missing for IDD individuals. For instance, they explain that neurotypical individuals receive formal and informal education and support, navigating intimacy through conversations, advice, and emotional validation from community networks. For individuals with intellectual disabilities, this support is often framed as dependency, making invisible the support neurotypical relationships receive. In contrast, the authors suggest that stakeholders in the lives of individuals with intellectual disabilities require a shift of perspective regarding sexuality that recognizes structural and societal barriers and moves away from dependency toward community responsibility. To start this dialogue, the authors articulate an educational framework that provides specific strategies to promote healthy sexual expression for individuals living with intellectual and developmental disability(ies).

Correspondingly, disabilities studies and women's and gender studies' expert Michelle Owen and Baden Gaeke-Franz, autistic self-advocate and Manitoba chapter president of Autistics United Canada, contribute a fascinating Chapter 16, "Teachable Moments: The Intersections of Disabilities and Sexualities," based upon Owen's experience of developing and teaching a course entitled "Sexualities, Disabilities, and Rights." The authors highlight key theories and ideas about the intersection of disability, sexuality, gender, and sex education and present important recommendations about which content, curriculum, and methods can be used to discuss disability and sexuality in higher education. Owen (instructor) and Gaeke-Franz (student from the inaugural class) also share and critically reflect on their experiences in Owen's course "Disabilities, Sexualities, and Rights," a second-year undergraduate course cross-listed between disability studies and women's and gender studies. This course has no prerequisites and has the word "sex" in it, so it attracts a diverse range of students. Owen discusses the history of the course's development and describes teaching moments that stood out for them. Baden troubles Michelle's account by adding their perspective. They maintain that instructors should always include disability perspectives. In terms of teaching sexuality, their aim is for instructors to create and support a dynamic pedagogical experience that goes far beyond learning the facts. Moreover, they believe that if instructors want students to learn about sexuality, they must feel at ease with the topic themselves and demonstrate that they are comfortable with the topic, especially when confronted with something new that pushes their boundaries. Furthermore, they must be open to students who challenge them.

Next, in Chapter 17, "Developing a Sexual Education Workshop: Addressing a Gap in Social Work Education," social work doctoral student Christopher Sterling-Murphy and social work professor Rick Csiernik propose that the social work profession has the potential to influence sex research, education, and training in a manner that is less pathologizing and more service-user focused. They suggest that examining sexuality from a person-in-environment lens is advantageous compared to traditional approaches, as it can provide more accurate descriptions of sexual behaviours as well as their implications and origins. This can not only ease service users' anxiety regarding sex and their sexuality(ies) but also enrich their lives, given the importance that sex plays in the human condition. The authors summarize Sterling-Murphy's experiences and reflections about teaching a required three-hour professional development social work workshop on human sexuality. They also evaluate the results of a needs' assessment survey (included in Appendix B) and the implementation of the workshop itself in terms of assessing which theories and skills related to sexuality that students had been previously taught, identifying students levels of knowledge and competence in responding to service users' sexuality, highlighting topics students stated that they needed to know, and discovering best practices that correlate to what students stated were their preferred methods of instruction when learning about sexually orientated material. They make the case that social work students are currently inadequately trained in the area of sexuality(ies) practice and do not know how to discuss sex and issues of sexuality with service users, despite most expressing an interest in obtaining more knowledge and training in this area. From their work, they identify a need for the social work profession to better educate new social workers about sexuality(ies) and suggest ongoing workshops, such as this one, as a possible solution.

In conclusion, Chapter 18, "Can We Just Stop Faking It: Real Talk about Sex and Sexualities in the Classroom," highlights key themes that are interwoven across the book. From my point of view, the book contributors have demonstrated that coverage of sex education should be added and increased in higher education, particularly in the helping professions and professional programs; outlined the merits of multidisciplinary approaches to teaching sex; and emphasized the need to utilize inclusive approaches that interrogate heteronormativity, monogamy, and cisgenderism, while also celebrating diversity. For this final chapter, I further expand on three other significant themes: recommendations for the continued development of sex-positive versus sex-negative approaches; examination of common barriers to teaching sex education; and the need for instructors to develop comfort with sexuality(ies). Based on the preceding chapters, as well as my own experiences and research, I present recommendations regarding which sex education content should be taught in higher education (e.g., KAS), suggest helpful sources and models that readers can source for their teaching and practice (Appendix C), and explore how best to teach sexuality(ies) in higher education.

13 Sex and Gender in the Classroom: Lessons from (and for) the Front Lines

HEATHER PETERS

Sex, sexuality, and related identity topics are relevant to everyone and are often brought up by service users in interactions with social and health-care professionals; thus, it is important that professionals be trained not only in content related to these topics, but also in how to talk with service users about them (Murphy, 2019). Unfortunately, from elementary school through high school and into university, the teaching of these topics continues to be haphazard (Murphy, 2019), debated (Shipley, 2014), and often vilified (Fahs, Plante, & McClelland, 2018). Irvine (2014) argues that even inside universities with mandates of academic freedom, sexuality research is "an occupation simultaneously socially necessary and stigmatized" (p. 632) and that "the production of sexuality research as dirty work affects not only the researchers themselves but shapes the broad production of sexual knowledge" (p. 653). In this context, faculty members in professional disciplines struggle to prepare students to adequately address the sex and sexuality concerns of service users. It is essential to teach these courses for many reasons, not only because service users need professionals who can talk about sex and sexuality, but "also because the sexual ideas, laws, and practices of a society embody fundamental "truths" about it, particularly about interlacing structures of power and privilege" (Davis, 2005, p. 29).

During my years of front-line social work practice, including work with youth and volunteering with HIV/AIDS organizations, I learned the importance of having professionals in every community and discipline who can talk openly with service users about sex, gender identity, sexual health, sexual identity, sexual orientation, and gender expression. However, I did not feel prepared for teaching these topics myself. For years, I waited for someone else to teach such a course; then I realized that if I wanted it to happen, I had to step up. I decided to rebuild an already existing fourth-year undergraduate social work elective course called "Gender and Sexuality" from the ground up. I spent much time researching the topics, reading potential textbooks and articles, watching videos, and talking with any colleague or friend who did not shy away from the topics. The first time I taught the course I was nervous, but the interest and engagement of the students allayed my fears. As an elective, the course is open to students from any discipline; in my experience, most students have been in social work and nursing, although other disciplines, including dental hygiene and women's studies, have been represented. The course, as presented here, can be taught across disciplines. This chapter shares my challenges, fears, learning opportunities, and successes in teaching the course. I also identify the goals I hoped to accomplish, as well as specific methods, activities, and topics that helped me achieve the goals. Additionally, I share examples from the classroom and from my experiences in preparing for and teaching the course.

SOCW 449 Gender and Sexuality: Course Goals

Here are the objectives for the course: (1) develop a critical awareness of the social construction of gender, sexuality, sexual relations, and oppression; (2) base this understanding in an examination of the historical character and social construction of gender and sexualities; (3) understand how this "common sense" and socially constructed knowledge of gender and sexuality influence professional practice and policy; (4) examine the interaction of personal perspectives, values and beliefs with behaviour and actions on personal, professional, and societal levels; and (5) develop an ability to talk openly and appropriately with service users and others about these topics. See Appendix A for full course outline. Overall, the course is divided into three sections. The first section is an introduction including anatomy, norms, and social constructions. The second section explores sexual orientation, sexual and gender identities, and sexuality. The last section examines the policing, politicizing, and pathologizing of sexuality and identifies ways to challenge these in the classroom and in professional practice (see Appendix A).

The course begins by acknowledging that much of our societal and cultural knowledge of sexuality is based on historical social constructions that hide, ignore, or malign the sexuality and related identity realities for many people (Kimmel & Holler, 2013; Rutter & Schwartz, 2012). In the course, the starting point is to challenge any preconceived notions about sexuality, sexual health, and identity, and to support students in interrogating their assumptions. Although the course includes readings, lectures, and discussions on theories of sexuality and sexual health (Ferber, Holcomb, & Wentling, 2013; Rutter & Schwartz, 2012), one of the main goals of the course is to assist students in becoming comfortable with talking about sex and sexuality with service users. To get to this point, they first need to be comfortable talking about it with each other, with people they know, and in class.

Class Structure

The classes are structured in a way to allow for maximum participation in various ways, including discussions, exercises, and student presentations. In my experience, smaller class sizes of 10 to 15 students are more conducive to this process; however, the course can be taught to larger numbers with a slight restructuring of assessment methods. I work to create a safe and relaxed environment, where students are comfortable talking about the topics without fear of reprisal, while maintaining space for us to respectfully challenge each other. In my school, there are other courses that focus on issues of abuse and trauma. While I did not want to minimize these issues, one of the goals of the course was to acknowledge that sex and sexuality are not always about risk or violence; that they can be, indeed should be, fun and enjoyable. As such, we explore topics of healthy sexuality and sex, and ways to talk about these with each other and with service users.

The Missing Links

Stigma related to talking about sexual health and sexuality information is not just a problem of the past (Rutter & Schwartz, 2012). Having moved through the sexual revolution of the 1960s and 70s, we may assume that the current era is more open to these topics, but this is not necessarily so (Irvine, 2014). In British Columbia, reproductive and sexual health is included in the required school curricula from elementary through high school. In spite of this, teachers can be worried about delivering this content. In preparing for this course, I heard two stories from teachers who experienced pushback when they tried to include this material in their classrooms.

The first story is from someone who taught introductory information to early elementary school students, covering curriculum requirements. The next day, a parent accosted her and, in an angry voice and manner, expressed outrage that the teacher had taught this topic in the classroom. The teacher was shaken by the experience and felt unsupported by the school. The second story is of a high school teacher who also taught required material as per the provincial curriculum. One of his students, during the class, asked if sex was enjoyable. The teacher's answer was "yes." This was couched in a much broader conversation of sexual health and was not in any way an endorsement of students rushing out to try it. The teacher had also talked about ways to stay safe and the option of abstinence, but was trying to answer the student's question honestly. A few days later, a parent of one youth in the classroom wrote a letter to the school complaining about the teacher's choice of response to this question. The teacher was given little opportunity to defend himself and the letter of complaint from the parent went on his file. Both teachers seriously considered not teaching sexual-health material again.

I bring these stories into the classroom to make a point about the reality of continued resistance to sexual-health discussions, and to initiate a dialogue with university students about whether or not sexual-health topics were addressed in their grade school experiences. Most say they had little or no such information in their elementary or high school years; this is true even for younger students who are more recent high school graduates. Over and over again, they say they wish that they had been taught this information. This leads to a broader discussion of how society can and should ensure that everyone has access to accurate information.

Course Delivery

Setting the Stage in the First Class

Students can be nervous coming into a gender and sexuality course. The first class is the time to talk about goals for the course, set boundaries to create some safety, introduce terms and definitions, and get people talking. Congruent with Hillock in Chapter 1, setting boundaries related to sensitive topics requires a balancing act. I can request that everyone keep what they hear in the class confidential, but I cannot guarantee it. A discussion of boundaries includes that acknowledgment, along with a discussion of why confidentiality is important, and how it is equally important to be comfortable with the information students choose to reveal in case it does get disclosed elsewhere. I am clear at this point that choosing what to share and what not to share is up to each individual and no one will be pressured to talk about personal information. At the same time, I explain that all of us will benefit if there is space to be honest, and everyone in the room has a responsibility to keep that space safe by being respectful, open, and keeping personal information disclosed by others confidential. I point out that I do not want people feeling tense and uncomfortable, but I do want people to be challenged; each person has to figure out what the boundary is between those two for him/her/

themselves. Discussion of boundaries includes not permitting oppressive comments such as those that are racist, sexist, classist, ageist, homophobic, heterosexist, or other types of oppression.

Getting Comfortable with Sex-Talk Exercises

The second half of the first class is designed to support students in becoming more comfortable talking about sex and sexuality. I use three exercises to start this process, and they intentionally build from safer to more challenging. The first is a small group discussion of what stereotypes, norms, and societal values exist about gender roles and about sex. This question asks for external information – in other words, for stereotypes that others or society as a whole tends to believe – but does not ask about students' beliefs. Likewise, the first question about gender roles is more comfortable for people than the second question related to stereotypes about sex, but both questions are couched as about others, not themselves. This leads to discussions of how stereotypes and societal norms or expectations create narratives about groups of people that can limit them, or us, in terms of how we see ourselves, and our identities.

The second exercise builds on this and asks students to identify a narrative or story that was developed about them, and whether they agreed with it or not. These stories do not have to be about sex, gender, or sexuality. I start with an example from my family of origin, where one of the family narratives became about how I could not cook. I was fine with the narrative, as I did not enjoy cooking. However, years later when my partner and I moved in together, I found that I did enjoy cooking with him and I realized I was ready for that story to change. The stories shared are generally equally safe, but students say that this does get them thinking about the effects of narratives on them and how problematic they can be to change.

The third exercise explores slang and verbal slurs related to gender, sex, and sexuality. When someone's sexual and gender identity does not fit with social constructions, this clash often results in stigma and otherness, including verbal slurs and denigrations. In addition, for uncomfortable topics, we sometimes develop slang to make things easier to talk about. Thus, this is a brainstorming exercise to share as many slang words and slurs as they can, about anything related to gender, gender roles, sex acts, genitals, and sexual orientation. This exercise can be challenging for students as they end up saying words out loud that are normally not spoken in classrooms or with one's instructor. I repeat each word as I write it on the board pausing at times for me, or someone else in class, to explain what a word or term means. I find that humour can make difficult topics more comfortable, so this exercise combines the serious and humorous. It is also important to note that, similar to Hillock's description in Chapter 1, service users often do not use scientific or "proper" language for body parts or sex acts. As professionals, we need to be familiar or comfortable with the terms they use, even if the terms are disquieting. This practical reality becomes part of the classroom discussion. A survey of all the words on the board also leads to a discussion about which groups of people are overrepresented in sex and gender slurs – typically women and people with sexual orientations other than heterosexual. These are the people who face the most pressure to co-opt their identities to fit with societal norms.

Reproductive Anatomy and Physiology

The next section of the course brings in a health professional, complete with life-size mannequins with removable body parts, to provide basic information on reproductive anatomy and genitalia. The nurse who teaches for me is someone who is comfortable and relaxed with the topic. In addition to the mannequins, he has pictures of genitalia and incorporates a discussion of the diversity and complexities of bodies. Later on, he comes back to class, to talk about sexually transmitted infections (STIs) and contraception.

Readings to support this topic include one on sexual anatomy (Hyde, DeLamater, & Byers, 2012), as well as one that discusses intersex people and blurring of gender chromosomes (Fausto-Sterling, 2017). It would be easy to slip from a discussion of reproductive anatomy into the assumption that sex and gender are binary. This additional article, along with another that comes later (Preves, 2017), challenges a binary perspective.

Students can ask questions throughout the anatomy and physiology presentation, but there is also space for anonymous questions on slips of paper. Students become bolder, asking direct questions about sex by this point, but there are always a few anonymous questions. They have included "What is the size of a clitoris?" "Do women ejaculate during sex?" "Is anal sex safe for women, and how can you prepare so it doesn't hurt?" In my experience, the reluctance to talk about sex in our society means many people arrive at adulthood and enter relationships still being unsure about their own bodies and with a sense of guilt about what they are doing. The healthcare professional and I both need to feel comfortable and be prepared to answer any sex question in a matter-of-fact way, just as we hope students will do with service users when they are working in the field.

On one occasion, nursing students in the course told me that in their required nursing course on anatomy and physiology, the instructor skipped the chapter on reproductive anatomy, saying there was not enough time to cover it! This is consistent with the literature. One study at a medical school in the United States found that although faculty agreed that education about sex and sexuality are important elements of medical training and practice, they were not mandated components of the curriculum so faculty members could include it or not as they wished (Murphy, 2019). Murphy also stated that "teachings about sexuality were fragmented and did not produce a consistent set of messages about what sexuality means or how it might matter to practice" (p. 203). Another faculty member in the Murphy study stated that there are medical students who complete their degrees who do not know how to have basic conversations with patients about sexual activity.

Additional Topics and Activities

In addition to the topics already mentioned, I cover a variety of topics that periodically change, including social construction of masculinity, femininity, and gender roles; a brief historical perspective of sex and sexuality with a focus on women's orgasms; diversity of sexual orientation and gender identity (SOGI) and the concept of these on a continuum or gender spectrum; gender fluidity and nonbinary gender identity; as well as heterosexism, homophobia, transphobia, and related forms of discrimination; gender and sexual behaviour; sexual relationships, activities, and setting boundaries while being open to new experiences; how to talk with others about safer sexual practices; policing of sex and sexuality; racism, ableism, and other oppressions and their intersection with sex, sexuality, and gender; effects of moral and legal discourses about sex; sex work and discussions of legalization; politics of sexuality; talking with children about sex and sexuality; eroticism and sexual variations; and talking with service users about sex, sexual and gender identity, and sexual orientation (see the course outline in Appendix A, for references for these topics).

Another guest speaker I invite is a local person who is a teacher and identifies as gay. He is known locally as someone who speaks eloquently about SOGI and the gender and sexual identity spectrum. His presentation is a skilled weaving of his own personal experiences, with information on identity, oppression, and some history of LGBTQ+ movements and successes. He discusses all of this in the context of the local community in which the course takes place, which brings much of what he says home for the students.

I show a variety of DVDs in class, and three stand out. One documentary, titled *The Mask You Live In* (The Representation Project, 2016), is on the social construction of masculinity and effects on both women and men. Among other topics related to this DVD is the discussion that even dominant groups in society – typically young white heterosexual males – face pressure to live up to societal expectations around gender and sex. A second documentary, *Assume Nothing* (Films Media Group, 2009), is both beautiful and thought provoking as it explores the diversity of gender and sexuality through the work of a photographer and interviews with the people she photographs. In an effort to bring humour into the classroom, the third DVD is a British comedy movie titled *Hysteria* (Becker, Cairo, & Curtis, 2011). It is a fictional re-enactment of the invention of the vibrator in the 1880s in Britain for physicians to use to treat hysteria, which was then thought of as a woman's disease. We then examine historical views of women's sexuality generally, and orgasms specifically, during this era and over time (Bolackledge, 2013). The DVD has a special feature: a one-hour documentary on women's sexuality and vibrators, including mention of legal cases in Texas where women have been charged (though not brought to trial) for owning more than six vibrators, which is (or was at the time) illegal and is considered to be possession for the purpose of trafficking (Becker, Cairo, & Curtis, 2012). Aspects of this are relevant to the topic of the policing of sexuality. Although it is not particularly focused on the aspect of sexual health, another resource is a book, edited by Murphy and Ribarsky (2013), called *Activities for Teaching Gender and Sexuality in the University Classroom.*

A number of other exercises and group discussions are also utilized during the course. During the discussion of gender and sexual identity and sexual orientation spectrums, I draw different continuums for each of these on the board. I ask students to think about their identities and where they may fit on the continuums. They do not have to disclose personal information, but it does provide an opportunity to think about and connect the readings and discussions to their own lives. One academic who teaches a sexuality course writes,

> I think it is fair to claim that those who teach courses in gender, race, ethnicity, and other similar topics seek to encourage students to see the connections between academic knowledge and everyday life, and to use those connections to help make sense of ourselves, the lives we live, and the worlds we inhabit … The same objectives should equally apply to sexualities courses. (Waskul, 2009, p. 660)

Thus, providing students with the space to understand the course material in the context of their own lives is important.

Another thought-provoking exercise from the course is the Gingerbread Person exercise. Everyone in the class gets a piece of paper with the outline of a gingerbread figure on it. Independently, everyone circles or writes on the places of the body where each person believes the concepts of sex, gender, and sexuality are located; locations that come up are typically genitals, heart, and brain. There are no right or wrong answers, and the exercise leads to an interesting discussion of the interrelatedness of emotions, social constructions, beliefs, and identities.

Near the end of the course I return to a discussion of healthy sexuality and how this can be defined. I also ask, what sexual activities can be considered to be healthy? Students are typically much more talkative by this time, and there is a robust discussion of various sexual activities, including those considered to be variant or alternative. The class usually comes to the conclusion that all activities are healthy as long as they occur in the context of consent, a lack of power imbalance, and within the age and related limitations set out in Canadian law (see Government of Canada, *Age of Consent to Sexual Activity*, n.d.). Students also talk about the importance of being able to set boundaries with one's partner(s) and what this, and consent, may or should look like. On one occasion, an older student spoke up during this part of the discussion and pointed out that setting boundaries is good, but trying new things is also important and that partners should also be able to negotiate potential new activities, trying new things out before deciding that an activity is outside one's area of interest.

Student Presentations and Workshop Development

One of the most interesting parts of the course is student presentations (a description of all student assessment tools in the course is found in Appendix A). Perhaps it is the topic, how the course progresses, or the personalities of the students who sign up for the course, but these are the best student presentations I have ever seen. The assignment is described as the development of a workshop that they could actually give in professional practice to teach services users or other professionals about a topic related to sex, sexual orientation, and/or sexual and gender identity. As professionals we are often asked to present information on a variety of topics and so this assignment reflects the reality of a workshop they could actually give in practice. Students work individually or in pairs, selecting a topic and identifying a target audience. They are required to develop a workshop on their topic appropriate to their audience. Although students hand in a written outline for a one-hour workshop, they present only a portion of that in class; a one-student presentation is a 15-minute piece of the larger workshop and a two-student presentation is a 30-minute piece. The assignment becomes a tool they can take with them into their practice. As well, I hope that students take ideas and activities from each other into their professional practice. Indeed, I often use their presentation activities and ideas in later deliveries of the course.

Some of the presentations are serious, including topics such as sex positivity; teaching disabled service users about sex, sexuality, and boundaries; exploring sex and sexuality with teens in a group setting; sexual activity while pregnant; and maintaining a sex life through menopause and aging. One student who was studying dental hygiene did a demonstration of an oral exam where something in the person's mouth necessitated a conversation about oral sex activities. Two students acted out a skit of how a newly together same-sex couple could negotiate a difficult conversation about sex if one of them had an STI. Some of the presentations, while being serious, also prove to be quite humorous. But through all of the presentations, the rest of the students watch and participate with rapt attention.

Course readings about sharing sexual health and sexual anatomy information with children (Hickling, 2005; Hickling, 2002; Noon & Hickling, 2016) led to two students teaching a sexual-health class to 6-year-olds. The presentations are all delivered to the rest of the class as if we are the intended target audience. This requires participation by the audience as well, and in this latter case, we all pretended to be 6-year-olds. That presentation was done with a considerable attention to detail, including skits with cutout dolls demonstrating conversations about what constitutes a private body part. They also demonstrated a skilled handling of questions from the supposed 6-year-old audience members at the end.

Two very confident students in my first delivery of the course introduced themselves to the owner of a local sex shop and worked with her to develop a workshop on types of sex toys and how to use them. The 30-minute presentation included passing around numerous items that the store owner had loaned to them and talking about how they could be used to enhance one's sexual experience while discussing how to stay safe during activities. As a part of their workshop, they also developed a four-page pamphlet on the topic and made copies for the sex-store owner to share with customers.

Conclusion

The creativity of students and their willingness to talk about and present challenging topics offers hope that it is possible to successfully prepare students for discussions of sex, sexuality, and gender in professional practice. They are eager learners in this course, and that helps make the course easier to teach, and I enjoy being a part of the learning process. I want to add that in sharing my way of teaching the course, I am not intending to suggest that this is the only way it can be done. I think the options, activities, and topics are endless and I appreciate opportunities to learn new ideas from others in the field. Tiefer (2018) points out that as academics, we are willing to theorize about sex and sexuality, yet "little is written about activism and advocacy how-to, why and what-for" (p. 1246). I think that those of us teaching these topics need to be prepared to share our experiences and ideas with each other in the hope that together, over time, our disciplines will become better at ensuring that our students are prepared for professional practice and activism in the area of sex, sexuality, and gender.

REFERENCES

Becker, T., Cairo, J., & Curtis, S. (Producers). (2011). *Hysteria* [DVD]. Toronto: Entertainment One.

Bolackledge, C. (2013). The function of the orgasm. In A. L. Ferber, K. Holcomb, & T. Wentling (Eds.),*Sex, gender, and sexuality: The new basics.* 2nd ed. New York & Oxford: Oxford University Press.

Davis, N. J. (2005). Taking sex seriously: Challenges in teaching about sexuality. *Teaching Sociology, 33*(1), 16–31. https://doi.org/10.1177/0092055x0503300102

Fahs, B., Plante, R. F., & McClelland, S. (2018). Working at the crossroads of pleasure and danger: Feminist perspectives on doing critical sexuality studies. *Sexualities, 21*(4), 503–519. https://doi.org/10.1177/1363460717713743

Fausto-Sterling, A. (2017). Dueling dualisms. In A. L. Ferber, K. Holcomb, & T. Wentling (Eds.), *Sex, gender, and sexuality: The new basics.* 3rd ed. New York and Oxford: Oxford University Press.

Ferber, A. L., Holcomb, K. & Wentling, T. (Eds.). (2013). *Sex, gender, and sexuality: The new basics.* 2nd ed. Oxford: Oxford University Press.

Films Media Group. (Producer). (2009). *Assume nothing* [DVD]. Hamilton, N.J.

Government of Canada. (n.d.) *Age of consent to sexual activity.* Retrieved on Sept. 26, 2019 from https://www.justice.gc.ca/eng/rp-pr/other-autre/clp/faq.html

Hickling, M. (2002). *Boys, girls & body science: A first book about facts of life.* Madeira Park, BC: Harbour Publishing Co. Ltd.

Hickling, M. (2005). *The new speaking of sex: What your children need to know and when they need to know it.* Kelowna, BC: Northstone.

Hyde, J. S., DeLamater, J. D., & Byers, E. S. (2012). *Chapter 4: Sexual anatomy. Human sexuality.* 5th Canadian ed. Toronto: McGraw-Hill Ryerson.

Irvine, J. M. (2014). Is sexuality research "dirty work"? Institutionalized stigma in the production of sexual knowledge. *Sexualities, 17*(5/6), 632–656. https://doi.org/10.1177/1363460713516338

Kimmel, M. S., & Holler, J. (2013). *The gendered society*. 2nd Canadian ed. Don Mills, ON: Oxford University Press.

Murphy, M. (2019). Everywhere and nowhere simultaneously: The "absent presence" of sexuality in medical education. *Sexualities, 22*, 203–223. https://doi.org/10.1177/1363460717708147

Murphy, M. J., & Ribarsky, E. N. (Eds). (2013). *Activities for teaching gender and sexuality in the university classroom*. Lanham, MD: Rowman & Littlefield Education.

Noon, S., & Hickling, M. (2016). *Talk sex today: What kids need to know about how adults can teach them*. Kelowna, BC: Wood Lake Publishing, Inc.

Preves, S. E. (2017). Intersex narratives: Gender, medicine, and identity. In A. L. Ferber, K. Holcomb, & T. Wentling (Eds.), *Sex, gender, and sexuality: The new basics*. 3rd ed. New York and Oxford: Oxford University Press.

The Representation Project. (Producer). (2016). *The mask you live in* [DVD]. Ross, California.

Rutter, V., & Schwartz, P. (2012). *The gender of sexuality: Exploring sexual possibilities*. 2nd ed. Lanham, MD: Rowman & Littlefield Publishers, Inc.

Shipley, H. (2014). Religious and sexual orientation intersections in education and media: A Canadian perspective. *Sexualities, 17*(5/6), 512–528. https://doi.org/10.1177/1363460714526115

Tiefer, L. (2018). More about sexualities activisms please, we need it! *Sexualities, 21*(8), 1246–1250. https://doi.org/10.1177/1363460718770449

Waskul, D. D. (2009). "My boyfriend loves it when I come home from this class": Pedagogy, titillation and new media technologies. *Sexualities, 12*(5), 654–661. https://doi.org/10.1177/1363460709340374

14 The Pitch: Teaching Sexuality at Multiple Levels

NICK J. MULÉ

Teaching has long been considered an honourable profession, based on its sharing knowledge for the growth and development of others, with the expectation that they in turn will contribute positively to society. The work of teaching is not an easy process; it is made that much more challenging when focused on the sensitive subjects of gender and sexual diversity. This chapter will reflect on my experiences teaching sexuality-based courses for two programs. At the graduate level, I have taught the Social Work Perspectives on Gender and Sexual Diversity course to master of social work (MSW) students, and at the undergraduate level, I both codeveloped and have taught the Sexual Activism, Movements, and Politics course to students in the Sexuality Studies program.

Of primary concern when teaching sexuality-based courses at the post-secondary level is who is being taught. Whether at the undergraduate or graduate levels, it must be recognized that the students are adults, on an age spectrum, with a diversity of backgrounds and experiences. Their previous education, learning styles, and life experiences all need to be taken into consideration, with flexibility being a key component of teaching such student bodies (Lederer, 2016; Sanders, 2001a). Context also plays a role: for example, teaching a sexuality-based course in a professional program such as social work, a discipline that has not been at the forefront of issues of gender and sexual diversity (Hillock, 2016). Apart from known social issues faced by LGBTQ people, it has been only in the last few years that the literature has challenged the profession to become more responsive theoretically (Mulé, 2016; Pyne, 2016); pedagogically in areas such as race (Mullings, 2016), relationships, and ethics outside of social norms (Idems, 2016); and in field-placement experiences (Swan & McConnell, 2015). Social work, often stereotyped as an open-minded and accepting discipline, has its challenges, whether teaching mixed sex and sexualities classes at the undergraduate level (Profitt, 2015), graduate level (taken up in this chapter), as well as geographical locales such as rural settings (Yorke, Byrch, Ham, Craggs, & Shute, 2016). The experiences of LGBTQ-identified students within social work program settings on campuses across the country indicate climates needing improvements at the systemic, programmatic, and physical levels (Craig, McInroy, & Doiron, 2016).

Teaching sexuality on a more general level outside a discipline-specific context also introduces many of its own challenges. The course I have taught in the interdisciplinary Sexuality Studies program attracts undergraduate students from a number of disciplines, including equity studies, gender and women's studies, geography, history, political science, psychology, religion, social sciences, social work, and sociology. Therefore, students bring myriad perspectives into such a course, not to mention varying degrees of comfort (Lederer, 2016; Sanders, 2001a, 2001b). Because the subject matter is not limited to gender and sexual diversity but also includes activism, movements, and politics of gender, sex, and sexuality issues in general, it is a course that is less structured within disciplinary and social location frameworks (James, 2001). Additionally, although both cohorts may differ, both courses feature similar theories, explored later in this chapter, that highlight intersectionalities across numerous social locations.

Correspondingly, this chapter reviews the added pressures and tensions that come with teaching sexuality-based courses, beyond those already experienced in teaching other types of courses. Given the sensitive nature of the content of sexuality-based courses, what students bring to such courses is also of value. This is important as external conceptions and perspectives of sexuality tend to dominate course content and class discussions, with little uptake at the subjective level. Yet addressing sexuality issues at a subjective level within a university class environment has its own challenges. Another challenge is how to address sexuality at the broader sociosystemic level, given the structural paradoxes that exist regarding this issue. To explore these challenges in more detail, I begin by describing my university setting and the students that I teach in these courses. I then outline the two sexuality-based courses that I teach at the postsecondary educational level, along with their respective objectives. From there, a number of challenges unique to teaching sexuality-based courses are discussed before I provide some concluding thoughts.

University Setting and Student Descriptions

For contextual purposes, before discussing the experience of teaching sexuality-based courses, it is important to have an understanding of the setting in which these courses are taught.

York University is the second largest university in the province of Ontario and the third largest in the country and has approximately 56,000 students: 6,000 graduate students, and 8,500 international students from 178 countries. The two courses discussed above are in academic units that are part of the country's largest liberal arts faculty program – the Faculty of Liberal Arts and Professional Studies – as well as the largest of York's 11 faculties (York University, 2019). I have taught both these courses on the large Keele campus located in the upper northwest section of Toronto. This campus is situated in the North York division of the amalgamated City of Toronto, an area that has tremendous growth, with large numbers of immigrants settling there (City of Toronto, 2019). As a result, many students that enrol at York University from this area are "first-generation university students," meaning they are the first in their families to pursue postsecondary education at the university level. Their parents, aunts, uncles, or grandparents have not attended university. These kinds of students bring a special dynamic to the pedagogical experience on numerous fronts: diaspora; being immigrants or the children of immigrant parents; a desire to shape their futures differently than their parents; a high level of curiosity; a sociopolitical awareness of settler struggles; and a serious commitment to their studies, so as not to disappoint their families as "first-generation university students." These dynamics are further manifested by sociocultural, economic, religious, and spiritual differences that may influence these students' perspectives on sexuality studies. With both these courses being electives, taking them outside their respective family involvement speaks to the students' desire to learn in this area, yet openness to the content may vary.

From this broad student body, there is always a mix of students who elect to enrol in the two sexuality-based courses. The intersections that students bring into the classroom – their social locations to their affiliated studies, the subjective positioning on gender, sex, and sexuality to societal-normative notions – often impact the courses. The diversity of their sociocultural backgrounds and their social locations brings both a level of inquiry and life experience that enrich the learning environment. Examples of this include how sex and sexuality is taken up in other cultures; the paradoxical means by which sex and sexuality is taken up here in North America; a deconstruction of sex and sexuality "norms" and "mores"; and a question of how to approach sex and sexuality through a professional social work lens or an activist lens in relation to the two respective courses.

Maturity, as well as where students are at in their own journeys of identity development and sexual experience, can contribute greatly to the learning process. Also, the degree to which students are open to being challenged on issues of gender, sex, and sexuality is often predicated on the dominant narrative society has imposed and can make for some interesting and animated discussions in the classroom. Reading about, studying, and discussing a topic that we are socialized to categorize as private in and of itself can prove a challenge to some students who are internally still trying to make sense of it all (not that any of us really ever do), while other students bring a more confident and inquisitive disposition to their approach to the course work.

About the Courses

To provide context for the discussion later in this chapter, descriptions for each of the two sexuality-based courses are presented here, along with their respective objectives.

Course One: Social Work Perspectives on Gender and Sexual Diversity

The Social Work Perspectives on Gender and Sexual Diversity course has two versions, one at the undergraduate level and the other at the graduate level. As I have taught only the latter, the focus here is on the graduate-level teaching of this course. Both versions are electives, and the graduate course is open to graduate social work students, either from the advanced stream (students doing a one-year MSW due to having an undergraduate social work degree [BSW]), and the post-degree stream (students doing a two-year MSW as their undergraduate degree is not a BSW). Graduate students outside of the social work program may also take the course with permission of the professor.

The intent of this course is to highlight varying social work perspectives on gender and sexually diverse populations (e.g., lesbian, gay, bisexual, transsexual, transgender, Two spirit, intersex, queer, questioning, and others). The perspectives regarding these populations encompass theory, sociopolitical, cultural, health, and well-being issues within the diversified populations of gendered and sexualized communities inclusive of intersectional identities, varying expressions of gender and sexuality, identity formation, assertion strategies, and age-related concerns. Multiple levels of social work intervention are studied and discussed regarding these populations, including ethics, practice, and policy and the need to sustain resistance and maintain social action on the gender and sexual diversity front. The specific course content is contextualized within an anti-oppression theoretical framework utilizing a critical perspective that highlights the intersecting and interlocking structural forms of oppression, and challenges current neoliberal influences in the queer movement (Allan, Briskman, & Pease, 2009; Fook, 2012; Mullaly, 2007).

COURSE OBJECTIVES

- To offer an advanced graduate seminar in which students can consider, explore, discuss, and debate issues related to social work perspectives on gender and sexually diverse populations and communities.
- To use an anti-oppression framework and critical perspective to understand the social context within which the daily lives of gender and sexually diverse people are situated. Therefore, the focus is on social oppression and the problematic treatment of these populations as a central issue, challenging notions of individual pathology. Highlighted are the connections between personal experiences and social forces and their resulting sociopolitical implications.
- To explore multiple hegemonic organizations of oppression and privilege and the multiple identity groups who exist and intersect within gender and sexually diverse communities.
- To position social work practice as a multilevel phenomenon and to explore issues related to practice with gender and sexually diverse people at multiple levels of intervention, encompassing ethics, clinical work, and policy.
- To consider student-raised particular needs and issues facing gender and sexually diverse people within specific topic areas and their related interventions.

To assist students in meeting the learning objectives of this course, I have singularly assigned the only two books utilizing Canadian content that link social work to sexuality: *LGBTQ People and Social Work: Intersectional Perspectives* (O'Neill, Swan, & Mulé, 2015) and *Queering Social Work Education* (Hillock & Mulé, 2016). Assessment of student learning has been undertaken by having students present in seminar style their topic for the final assignment, introducing their preliminary questions, and expressing their interest in the topic and research completed to date. They are also expected to facilitate a discussion on the topic with the class. This is then followed up by writing a full-fledged essay on this topic, providing a critical analysis as their final assignment. Allowing students to choose topics of their choice (within the parameters of the course) provides them with the freedom to explore areas of interest to them and encourages them to excel in that area. In essence, this course exposes social work students to the diversity of genders and sexualities, society's response or lack thereof toward this diversity, issues faced by gender and sexually diverse populations, and practice-based responses to them.

Course Two: Sexual Activism, Movements, and Politics

The Sexual Activism, Movements, and Politics course is an undergraduate elective in a small interdisciplinary Sexuality Studies program, housed within the School of Gender, Sexuality, and Woman's Studies at York University. It is one of the few specialized courses developed for this program, as many courses that make up the curriculum are from Gender and Women's Studies. I was one of three faculty members who collaborated in the development of this course. Being an interdisciplinary program, undergraduate students from varying faculties are welcome to enrol in the course, provided they have completed a prerequisite six credits in the Sexuality Studies core or primary courses.

This course examines twentieth- and twenty-first-century sexual activism, movements, and politics, focusing on everyday resistance, organized protest, and mobilizations for reform and revolution. Depending on the expertise of the instructor, the course concentrates on Canada, North America, or other regions of the world. There is significant attention devoted to bisexual, gay, intersex, lesbian, Two-Spirit People, queer, transgender, and transsexual activism, but the course may also deal with movements focused on abortion, birth control, interracial sex, pornography, sex work, sex education, sexually transmitted infections, sexual slavery, sexual tourism, sexual violence, and sterilization. It introduces students to sexual activism in labour unions, professional associations, religious institutions, and grassroots movements; highlights diverse forms of activism centred on sexual liberation, sexual equality, sexual expression, sexual privacy, sexual publicity, sexual space, and sexual citizenship; focuses on sexual rights as these relate to the politics of relationship recognition, marriage, reproduction, and childcare; and emphasizes a range of activist skills, tactics, strategies, and theories. All these subjects are explored with attention to intersections of sexual politics with the politics of ability, colonialism, class, ethnicity, gender, gender identity and expression, race, sexual orientation, religion, age, and other social formations.

COURSE OBJECTIVES
- To develop theoretical understandings of sexuality, how it is taken up in society, and how individuals, groups, organizations, and movements have influenced these.

- To gain insights into the conceptual frameworks of sexuality and how they have shifted over time.
- To learn the key stages involved in social advocacy work from various contexts related to developing practice skills to undertake such activism.
- To develop awareness of the complexity, including intersectionality, of sex activism and analytical skills as a means of addressing sexual hegemony, regulation, repression, and oppression at multiple levels, locally to globally.

Readings for this course have been drawn from the anthology *Canadian Perspectives in Sexualities Studies: Identities, Experiences, and the Context of Change* (Naugler, 2012). Once again, Canadian content is prioritized and is updated based on available Canadian literature on the topic of sexual activism. Given that so much sexual activism is carried out by social movements, the assignments are based on group work with the first focused on submitting a preparatory group paper that outlines a sexuality-based issue and how it is being taken up by an advocacy group. The topic itself is researched and plans provided for a group presentation, which becomes the final assignment. This final assignment – group presentation to the class – outlines the sexuality-based issue of the midterm assignment and features a review of the group or organization engaged in activism regarding the issue. The presentation is expected to provide a summation of the sexuality issue, what the problems are, and an outline of the students' strategic responses to further advocacy work done to date. Ultimately, this course is designed to provide students with an understanding and knowledge of sexual activism as an important means of addressing a fundamental part of human existence – society's uptake of sexuality – and the varied impact activism and advocacy can have on sexuality and its role in society.

Teaching about Sex: The Challenges

In this section, I discuss a number of challenges associated with teaching sexuality-based courses, made that much more interesting due to the diversity of the students who enrol. Returning to the title of this chapter, my experience of teaching both these courses has had me questioning what pitch to take, given the diversity of students who enrol, the complexity of the subject matter, and the sensitivity that tends to surround it. Herein, I discuss the theoretical foundations that undergird the courses, the student subjectivities that are brought into the course, and the controversial issues that inevitably arise with regard to gender, sex, and sexuality issues. I then close the section by highlighting the importance of a multivariate approach, given the importance of these three areas of pedagogical challenge in teaching sexuality.

As a means of anchoring both courses, I base them on a similar set of theories from which to examine and explore sexuality(ies), as well as help students flourish as a class (Adem, 2001). The theories highlighted in this section are utilized in the course to deconstruct traditional notions of sexuality such as male licence to sexuality over female interest and desires in or for it; heterosexist notions of normative sexuality contrasted with the abnormality of sexual proclivities outside it; and moralistic valuing of sexuality (postmarital sex for procreation) versus the valuing of sexual pleasure (promiscuity, BDSM, role playing, etc.). Affect theory looks at sexuality issues from social and cultural perspectives, touching on biological and physical issues (Ahmed, 2014). Feminist theory steers the discourses away from the more dominant gendered perspectives, such as cis and male genders, to ensure insights from the more disempowered genders, such as trans and female (Anderson, 2001; McPherson, 2001). Critical race theory diversifies the learnings by recognizing not only the experiences of racialized people but also how colonialism narrows our understanding of the topic (Bell, 1995). A postmodern discourse is brought to bear by queer theory, which questions the social construction of gender and sexuality by highlighting the fluidity of each (Jagose, 1996). Imagining an emancipatory existence in terms of our gender and sexuality and the means of developing it is the challenge put forth by queer liberation theory (Mulé, 2015, 2016). In addition to social construction is the structuring of our society, which creates opportunities for gender and sexual expression with the able bodied and sane minded and not necessarily for those whose abilities vary from these (Dewsbury et al., 2010). The eclecticism of these theories is deliberate in that they collectively provide an important underscoring of the complexity of issues in gender and sexuality studies. Importantly, each is drawn from the critical school of thought allowing for a deconstruction (Sanders, 2001b) of what we have been heavily socialized to believe regarding gender and sexuality.

As described earlier, the York University student body is a highly diversified one, and this is reflected in the students who enrol in these two courses. Some bring cultural perspectives from outside Western views while simultaneously developing their own understanding through the teachings, readings, and class discussions. For example, some students are born and raised in countries where "homosexuality" is illegal, with various penalties, including charges, incarceration, torture, and sometimes execution. This provides an opportunity to review such socialization, which includes its past existence here in North America and its evolution from a lens of colonization into a normative discourse of cisgenderism and heterosexuality. Some students will take up the content of these courses at a very personal level and disclose (usually through their written essays, not necessarily in class discussions) having been sexually abused as a child or that they are currently engaging in sex work to help pay their tuition fees. The extent to which, or even whether, students take up such issues in class is left up to them, yet sometimes they do arise on a general level. Such issues raise concerns regarding safety in engaging in classroom discussions on such topics. As the instructor for these courses, I must carefully navigate addressing such issues for pedagogical reasons, while not breaking the confidences of those students who have disclosed in other forums. I have tended to handle such circumstances by focusing on the issue itself, while simultaneously monitoring the comfort level in the room. I neither call upon nor direct the discussion toward a student who has previously disclosed related information. It is left up to that student to participate to the extent that they choose or not to participate.

Apart from student disclosure, controversy inevitably arises and becomes most apparent when discussing issues that are framed as controversial in daily discourse, such as abortion, asexuality, BDSM, intergenerational relationships, polyamoury, pornography, promiscuity, sex trafficking, and sex work. Questions or learning needs can arise from students as basic as "I've heard of bathhouses through the media and such, but no one seems to explain what they are. I don't even know what a bathhouse is," to students intricately describing the machinations of sex trafficking and how it so often eludes the law. When faced with the decisions some porn companies have made to film barebacking sex scenes, I have witnessed students quickly resorting to the normative and uncontroversial narrative of the importance of engaging in safer sex practices and contraception, coupled with the latest science regarding sexually transmitted infections. This response tends to arise in the one class of the undergraduate Sexual Activism, Movements, and Politics course in which I show porn to discuss its place in the realm of sexual discourse. Rather than consider the multitude of reasons individuals choose to bareback, students often resort to a blanket response of labelling such behaviour as unsafe and wrong. On the other hand, I have also witnessed mature and carefully balanced responses to scenarios in the literature in which women who had had abortions question the pro-choice option. Impressively, students have shared being open to a woman's feelings about abortion with regard to where she is at, at a given point in time. Hence, this recognizes the fluidity of feelings and respects a woman's choice, even if her position changes, rather than getting caught up in the abortion debates. These examples illustrate varying learning processes regarding controversial issues around sexual activism.

Recommendations and Insights

Both these elective courses provide interesting insights from students who enrol based solely on their individual interests. However, there are limits to the pedagogical tools available, from the minimal Canadian-based readings of the Sexual Activism, Movements, and Politics course, to shifting theoretical approaches with some, such as queer theory, dominating over others (Hicks, 2008; Mulé, 2016), depending on the course. As professors know, any class into which we walk will present its own dynamics, partly due to the content of the course and often due to the constitution of students enrolled in the course, which can be quite unpredictable (Briskin, 2001). Add to this a highly diversified student population and the critical approach taken at both the School of Gender, Sexuality & Women's Studies and School of Social Work, not to mention in general at York University, and determining the appropriate pitch for teaching these sexuality-based courses is truly a challenge.

To address this, I have borrowed (with a degree of success) from the social work practice skill of being "where the client is at" (Fook, 2012). Despite the preparation that goes into each of these courses, I begin with a check-in at the beginning of the respective courses and engage in a discussion regarding the students' interest in the course, what they hope to learn, and their expectations. For example, in the Sexual Activism, Movements, and Politics course, I have received requests for teachings on opportunities to engage in actual activism, on dealing with sexuality issues, and on activist and advocacy skills. In the Social Work and Sexual Diversities course, students have requested information on intervention skills in cases of sensitive sexuality issues such as disclosures related to sexuality, gender identity and expression, abuse, and abortion. They have also wanted to discuss how to navigate sexual diversity issues in traditional mainstream social service settings, some of which are faith-based, and how to navigate policy and procedures therein. Their feedback is noted and used to guide the direction of the course content and their work in it. This generalized approach is also utilized more specifically with course teachings; for example, taking direction from students on which porn to watch (beyond this, observing and discussing various forms of pornography, such as feminist porn, racialized porn, amateur porn, and bareback porn) and allowing students to choose their own course-related subject for their final essay.

As a result, there is no one pitch that I can recommend, but I do believe that what is best are multiple pitches dependent on a balance between the interests of the students, the knowledge I believe is of value to impart, and the importance of facilitating reflexive critical dialogues that become a process of knowledge exchange for everyone's learning, including my own (Lederer, 2016; McGrath, 2014). This involves being cognizant of the needs, differences, and expectations of undergraduate versus graduate students (Lederer, 2016), not shying away from difficult and sometimes uncomfortable issues such as privilege (Kirby, 2016) and consent (deFur, 2016), and being open to ongoing evaluation of the values that typically arise in sexuality-based courses (Lederer, 2016). Specific to the students in these two courses, there is a felt difference between the undergraduate and graduate levels, based on their respective ages and life experiences (albeit these can vary within the courses). The undergraduate students are slower to question and trouble normative tropes; but this comes more naturally for the graduate students, who are prepared to decontextualize what many of us have been socialized to regard as normative sexual orientations, gender identities and expressions, interests and desires for varying sexual activities and how these can be gendered, classed, and culturally defined. Gender, sex, and sexuality are important topics that all of us live with, and with which we grapple. Whether the learnings are applied to being future social workers (Hillock & Mulé, 2016; O'Neill, Swan, & Mulé, 2015) or to one's life and eventual occupation(s), teaching and learning about sex at the postsecondary level allows for an in-depth exploration into the research and knowledge produced on a topic that society, still to this day, struggles with.

Conclusion

If one is to be true to the subject matter, an interesting balance must be struck in pitching topics, content, and material when teaching gender, sex, and sexuality, regardless of the positioning and shifting of individual students or the class as a collective body. Whether teaching a sexuality-based course in a specialized profession such as social work or more generically in sexuality studies, the complexities, perspectives, and sensitivities involved require constant reflexivity. My experience has taught me that a multilevel pitch is necessary to do justice to a subject matter of such complexity and fluidity. For students to gain knowledge about gender, sex, and sexuality, we must rise to the challenges of managing varying theoretical approaches without succumbing to the domination of one; allowing for an open and engaging learning environment that encourages students to bring in and explore varying perspectives (theirs and those of others); and not shying away from controversial issues but rather embracing them in service of education, the furthering of knowledge, and the development of students who are applying themselves to it.

REFERENCES

Adem, T. (2001). The university classroom: From laboratory to liberatory education. In J. Newton, J. Ginsburg, J. Rehner, P. Rogers, S. Sbrizzi, & J. Spencer (Eds.), *Voices from the classroom: Reflections on teaching and learning in higher education* (pp. 40–44). Toronto: Garamond Press and Centre for the Support of Teaching, York University.

Ahmed, S. (2014). *The cultural politics of emotion.* (2nd Ed.). Edinburgh: Edinburgh University Press.

Allan J., Briskman, L., & Pease, B. (2009). *Critical social work: Theories and practice for a socially just world.* (2nd Ed.). Crows Nest, NSW: Allen and Unwin.

Anderson, R. (2001). Empowering students through feminist pedagogy. In J. Newton, J. Ginsburg, J. Rehner, P. Rogers, S. Sbrizzi, & J. Spencer (Eds.), *Voices from the classroom: Reflections on teaching and learning in higher education* (pp. 68–74). Toronto: Garamond Press and Centre for the Support of Teaching, York University.

Bell, D.A. (1995). "Who's afraid of critical race theory?" *University of Illinois Law Review, 1995*(4): 893ff.

Briskin, L. (2001). Power in the classroom. In J. Newton, J. Ginsburg, J. Rehner, P. Rogers, S. Sbrizzi, & J. Spencer (Eds.), *Voices from the classroom: Reflections on teaching and learning in higher education* (pp. 25–39). Toronto: Garamond Press and Centre for the Support of Teaching, York University.

City of Toronto. (2019). Neighbourhood profiles. Toronto. Accessed from: https://www.toronto.ca/city-government/data-research-maps/neighbourhoods-communities/neighbourhood-profiles/

Craig, S. L., McInroy, L. B., & Doiron, C. (2016). Oh Canada: LGBTQ students and campus climates in Canadian social work programs. In S. Hillock & N. J. Mulé (Eds.), *Queering social work education* (pp. 163–184). Vancouver, BC: UBC Press.

deFur, K. (2016). Selections from unequal partners: Teaching about power, consent, and healthy relationships. *American Journal of Sexuality Education, 11*(2), 149–159. https://doi.org/10.1080/15546128.2016.1174025

Dewsbury, G., Clarke, K., Randallb, D., Rouncefield, M., & Sommerville, I. (2010). The anti-social model of disability. *Disability & Society, 19*(2), 145–158. https://doi.org/10.1080/0968759042000181776

Fook, J. (2012). *Social work: A critical approach to practice* (2nd Ed.). Los Angeles, CA: Sage.

Hicks, S. (2008). Thinking through sexuality. *Journal of Social Work*, *8*(1), 65–82. https://doi.org/10.1177/1468017307084740

Hillock, S. (2016). Social work, the academy and queer communities: Heteronormativity and exclusions. In S. Hillock & N. J. Mulé (Eds.), *Queering social work education* (pp. 73–92). Vancouver, BC: UBC Press.

Hillock, S., & Mulé, N. J. (Eds.). (2016). *Queering social work education*. Vancouver, BC: UBC Press.

Idems, B. (2016). Opening theory: Polyamorous ethics as a queering inquiry in the social work classroom. In S. Hillock & N. J. Mulé (Eds.), *Queering social work education* (pp. 185–204). Vancouver, BC: UBC Press.

Jagose, A. (1996). *Queer theory: An introduction* (Reprint. ed.). New York: New York University Press.

James, C. E. (2001). Diversity in the classroom: Engagement and resistance. In J. Newton, J. Ginsburg, J. Rehner, P. Rogers, S. Sbrizzi, & J. Spencer (Eds.), *Voices from the classroom: Reflections on teaching and learning in higher education* (pp. 45–53). Toronto: Garamond Press and Centre for the Support of Teaching, York University.

Kirby, E. L. (2016). Encountering my privilege (and others' oppression). *Communication Teacher*, *30*(3), 172–178. https://doi.org/10.1080/17404622.2016.1192659

Lederer, A. M. (2016). Implementation and evaluation of a values clarification activity for a large undergraduate human sexuality course. *American Journal of Sexuality Education*, *11*(1), 92–105. https://doi.org/10.1080/15546128.2016.1142407

McGrath, K. (2014). Teaching sex, gender, transsexual, and transgender concepts. *Communication Teacher*, *28*(2), 96–101. https://doi.org/10.1080/17404622.2013.865764

McPherson, K. (2001). Feminist pedagogy: Paradoxes in theory and practice. In J. Newton, J. Ginsburg, J. Rehner, P. Rogers, S. Sbrizzi, & J. Spencer (Eds.), *Voices from the classroom: Reflections on teaching and learning in higher education* (pp. 58–62). Toronto: Garamond Press and Centre for the Support of Teaching, York University.

Mulé, N. J. (2015). The politicized queer, the informed social worker: Dis/re-ordering the social order. In B. J. O'Neill, T. A. Swan, & N. J. Mulé (Eds.), *LGBTQ people and social work: Intersectional perspectives* (pp. 17–36). Toronto, ON: Canadian Scholars' Press Inc.

Mulé, N. J. (2016). Broadening theoretical horizons: Liberating queer in social work academe. In S. Hillock & N. J. Mulé (Eds.), *Queering social work education* (pp. 36–53). Vancouver, BC: UBC Press.

Mullaly, B. (2007). *The new structural social work*. (4th Ed.). Don Mills, ON: Oxford University Press.

Mullings, D. (2016). Social work education: Exploring pitfalls and promises in teaching about Black queer older adults. In S. Hillock & N. J. Mulé (Eds.), *Queering social work education*. Vancouver, BC: UBC Press, pp. 205–226.

Naugler, D. (Ed.) (2012). *Canadian perspectives in sexualities studies: Identities, experiences, and the context of change*. Don Mills, ON: Oxford University Press.

O'Neill, B. J., Swan, T. A., & Mulé, N. J. (Eds.). (2015). *LGBTQ people and social work: Intersectional perspectives*. Toronto, ON: Canadian Scholars' Press Inc.

Profitt, N. J. (2015). Somewhere over the rainbow: Reflections on teaching a LGBT-S bachelor of social work course. In B. J. O'Neill, T. A. Swan, & N. J. Mulé (Eds.), *LGBTQ people and social work: Intersectional perspectives* (pp. 297–316). Toronto, ON: Canadian Scholars' Press Inc.

Pyne, J. (2016). Queer and trans collisions in the classroom: A call to throw open theoretical doors in education. In S. Hillock & N. J. Mulé (Eds.), *Queering social work education* (pp. 54–72). Vancouver, BC: UBC Press.

Sanders, L. (2001a). Adult students. In J. Newton, J. Ginsburg, J. Rehner, P. Rogers, S. Sbrizzi, & J. Spencer (Eds.), *Voices from the classroom: Reflections on teaching and learning in higher education* (pp. 93–94). Toronto: Garamond Press and Centre for the Support of Teaching, York University.

Sanders, L. (2001b). Responsibility and respect in critical pedagogy. In J. Newton, J. Ginsburg, J. Rehner, P. Rogers, S. Sbrizzi, & J. Spencer (Eds.), *Voices from the classroom: Reflections on teaching and learning in higher education* (pp. 54–57). Toronto: Garamond Press and Centre for the Support of Teaching, York University.

Swan, T.A., & McConnell, S.M. (2015). Transformative engagement in LGBTQ student/field instructor relationships. In B. J. O'Neill, T. A. Swan, & N. J. Mulé (Eds.), *LGBTQ people and social work: Intersectional perspectives* (pp. 339–360). Toronto, ON: Canadian Scholars' Press Inc.

Yorke, J., Byrch, L., Ham, M., Craggs, M., & Shute, T. (2016). Queering space in social work: How Simcoe County has moved from queerful to queerious. In S. Hillock & N. J. Mulé (Eds.), *Queering social work education* (pp. 227–245). Vancouver, BC: UBC Press.

York University. (2019). About York University. Toronto. Accessed from: http://about.yorku.ca/

15 Sexual Health Education for Individuals with Intellectual and Developmental Disabilities

SHANIFF ESMAIL, MEG TRONSON, AND SHEENA CHURLA

Intellectual and developmental disability (IDD) is defined by the American Association of Intellectual and Developmental Disability as "characterized by significant limitations in both intellectual functioning and in adaptive behaviour, which covers many everyday social and practical skills ... [and] originates before the age of 18" (AAID, 2019, p. 1). Common diagnoses include autism, Down syndrome, and fetal alcohol spectrum disorder; however, there is not a unified definition within all disability communities. Within the United Kingdom, self-advocates identify as having learning difficulties (Goodley, 2001), while other self-advocates, particularly within the autism community, use the term neurodiverse to describe individuals whose intellectual functioning differs (rather than deviates) from their neurotypical counterparts (Silberman, 2015). This chapter combines contributions from both self-advocates and rehabilitation professionals; therefore, we use these terms interchangeably.

The varied definitions ascribed to this population suggest a diversity of experience. Education related to sexuality, however, has primarily been homogenous, centring on sexual safety and harm reduction in recent decades (Craft, 1994; Frawley & Wilson, 2016). Although programming for sexual health education tends to orient around harm-reduction, significant aspects of sexuality within this population remain unaddressed. Notably, individuals with IDD report poorer self-esteem (Ailey, Marks, Crisp, & Hahn, 2003) and unsatisfying social lives (Downs & Craft, 1996; Emerson & Hatton, 2008; Landman, 2014) compared to neurotypical populations. This is in spite of increased societal uptake of inclusion-based programs in response to segregation-based histories (see Campbell, 2017 for eugenics histories). The evolution of sexual health education for populations with IDD demands meaningful conceptualization of consent, adoption of sex-positive frameworks, and delivery methods tailored to individuals' learning needs. Thus, the intention of this chapter is to inform educators on the unique barriers and challenges related to teaching populations with IDD. Also discussed are specific sexual-health content and effective delivery strategies that educators may use when supporting this population.

Defining Healthy Sexual Expression for Individuals with IDD

Sexuality is a component of human intimacy that informs identity as well as comprises "physical, mental, and social well-being" (WHO, 2006, p. 4). Sexuality embodies different definitions for many people, but advocates mutually agree that individuals with IDD have the right to decisions regarding their own lives, as well as to experience positive, safe, and healthy relationships free of coercion and abuse (Ailey et al., 2003; Esmail, Esmail, & Munro, 2001; Friedman, Arnold, Owen, & Sandman, 2014; WHO, 2006). Expressions of disabled sexuality are modelled by many in the disability movement (e.g., Clare, 2015; Esmail, Darry, Walter, & Knupp, 2010; Gurza, 2019; Trace, 2014; Williams, 1999); however, many individuals with intellectual disabilities still lack positive representation within mainstream media (Parsons, Reichl, & Pedersen, 2016). Sexual health educators are tasked with both understanding and addressing personal, attitudinal, and societal barriers that prevent individuals from attaining healthy sexuality.

Barriers

Personal

At the individual level, several factors can limit people with IDD in meaningfully expressing their sexuality. For instance, people in this population may experience impairments in daily functioning, as well as difficulties in the social, behavioural, and cognitive domains. Difficulties with "reasoning, problem-solving, planning, thinking abstractly, comprehending complex ideas, judgment, [...] and learning from experience" (APA, 2013, p. 33) can all impact the ability of an individual to learn and practice healthy sexuality. In many cases, there are also deficits in social skills important to developing and maintaining healthy relationships, such as assertiveness, understanding boundaries, and recognizing social cues (Travers & Tincani, 2010). Each individual is unique and will have his/her/zer own combination of strengths and challenges (Barnard-Brak et al., 2014). Fortuitously, research indicates that these skills can improve with education and ongoing practice (Hayashi, Arakida, &

Ohashi, 2011; Whitehouse & McCabe, 1997). The ability to generalize sexual health information to daily living is important as it helps to ensure learned material is translated to sexual safety and healthy relationships (Blanchett & Wolfe, 2002, Dixon, Bergstrom, Smith, & Tarbox, 2010).

Physical and developmental factors can also negatively impact individuals' sexual functioning and limit their ability for sexual expression. Sexual needs are the same as neurotypical peers, but individuals with IDD can also experience a later onset of sexual development (Kijak, 2011). Adolescence and puberty may be an especially distressing time for these individuals due to a lack of education on what to expect (Kijak, 2011) and limited social interaction with peers (Ailey et al., 2003; Gougeon, 2009).

Attitudinal

The literature demonstrates that individuals with IDD often mirror the attitudes and beliefs of their caregivers (Löfgren-Mårtenson, 2009, McCabe & Schreck, 1992), even when those attitudes are negative (Cuskelly & Bryde, 2004). In the last decade, a positive shift relating to acceptance and openness toward sexuality of populations with IDD has been observed in parents (Cuskelly & Bryde, 2004; Karellou, 2003; Swango-Wilson, 2008), teachers (Fader Wilkenfeld & Ballan, 2011; Wolfe, 1997), and community members (Cuskelly & Gilmore, 2007). Despite positive attitudinal shifts, sexual health education continues to be limited as stakeholders identify feeling unqualified to deliver sexual health education to this population (Ballan, 2001). When asked, "Whose job is it to teach sexual health education to individuals with IDD?", all parties point to one another, absconding personal responsibility (Fader Wilkenfeld & Ballan, 2011).

Parents are fearful that teaching sex to their children with IDD will lead to their children becoming sexually active (Fader Wilkenfeld & Ballan, 2011), despite the literature revealing this is not the case (Doyle, 2008). When interviewed, parents identified discussing sex with their neurotypical children and avoiding sex conversations with their children with intellectual disabilities, preferring to delay the advent of sexual activity (Jahoda & Pownall, 2014). Research within the field of sex and disability, however, reveals that individuals within the intellectual disability community are already sexually active (Wolfe, 1997), debunking the belief that they are asexual. Despite self-advocacy that challenges notions that intellectual disability negates adult status (e.g., Goode, 2011), the belief that adults with intellectual disabilities are perpetual children continues to proliferate (Aunos & Feldman, 2002; Esmail et al., 2010; Parchomiuk,

2013). These attitudes pose the risk of becoming a self-fulfilling prophecy as those responsible for sexual health education refuse to support populations with IDD with the knowledge necessary to make adult choices regarding sex and sexuality.

Structural

Social isolation: A study originating from London, UK, suggests that "only 30 percent of people with learning disabilities have any friends at all" (Dept of Health, 2001 as cited in Landman, 2014, p. 359). Those with friends largely identify having friends exclusively from their mother's social networks (Downs & Craft, 1996). For individuals with IDD, a lack of social networks often limits dating pools to small ponds (Löfgren-Mårtenson, 2009) and denies models of healthy relationships informing communication and intimacy skills (Bates, Terry, & Popple, 2016). Tools necessary to form healthy relationships cannot be taught exclusively in the classroom but require the lived experience of reciprocal and supportive relationships within the community. Additionally, loving relationships set a positive foundation for future intimacy (Bates et al., 2017; Eastgate, Van Driel, Lennox, & Scheermeyer, 2011; Walter-Brice, Cox, Priest, & Thompson, 2012), including exposing abusive patterns as problematic rather than normal and natural (Bates et al., 2017).

Privacy: Within school systems, individuals with IDD are often paired with educational aids, disallowing peer interactions without an adult presence (Ailey et al., 2003; Pownall, 2010; Watson, Shakespeare, Cunningham-Burley, & Barnes, 1999). Some scholars have suggested that this constant supervision deprives students of informal sexual-health education that occurs between peers during leisure and work activities (Gougeon, 2009). Also, lack of privacy extends into the home context, where many individuals who live in group homes lack spaces that are not simultaneously accessible to other roommates and/or care providers (Fader Wilkenfeld & Ballan, 2011).

Sexualized Abuse and Violence: Estimates within Canada suggest that women with IDD are 40% more likely to experience sexual abuse than their neurotypical counterparts (Brownridge, 2006) and are more likely to report multiple sexual assaults (Eastgate et al., 2011, p. 229). Women with IDD reported higher rates of assault and more sadistic experiences than their neurotypical counterparts (Brownridge, 2006; Hassouneh-Phillips & Curry, 2002, Landman, 2014; Saxton, Curry, Powers, Maley, Eckels, & Gross, 2001). In contrast, research relating to sexualized violence experienced by men with IDD is sparse. Some suggest men with IDD experience sexualized violence at rates similar to those experienced by females (Dunne & Power, 1990; Buchanan & Wilkins, 1991), but sample sizes in these studies were small (McCarthy, 1996).

At times, the prevalence of sexual abuse has been erroneously attributed to characteristics intrinsic to IDD, rather than addressing the cultural landscape that makes such abuse possible. Research shows that perpetrators target individuals with intellectual disabilities, believing a trusting demeanour and lack of societal support will translate into partners who are easier to manipulate and isolate (Plummer & Findley, 2012). Landman (2014) suggests that individuals with IDD are more likely to experience community members who befriend them for the purposes of exploitation rather than for reciprocal and respectful relationships. Perpetrators often build a trusting relationship with individuals with IDD before sexual abuse occurs, which can lead to challenges for individuals with IDD to "correctly identify specific partner betrayal later in development" (Gobin & Freyd, 2009, as cited in Houdek & Gibson, 2017, p. 13). Therefore, sexual-health educators need to support individuals in delineating between healthy relationships and abusive ones in which abuse is often naturalized.

Moreover, if the experience of having an IDD is characterized by a lack of positive relationships within the community, then sexual-health education must expand beyond an individualized approach to address the social nature of this problem. Individuals with IDD need not only education related to healthy versus abusive behaviour, but also community members committed to relationships of reciprocity. At present, the public response to the disproportionate rates of sexualized violence has been characterized by apathy and inaction (McCarthy, 2014, 2017).

Sexual Orientation: Historically, sex education designed for individuals with disabilities (specifically, physical disabilities) exclusively taught heterosexual sex (Campbell, 2017). Many individuals with IDD remain ignorant of the diversity of sexual expression and come to understand homosexuality as odd or wrong (Löfgren-Mårtenson, 2009). Additionally, studies conducted on the intersection between LGBTQ* and intellectual disability show a consistent theme of exclusion from both communities (McRuer & Mollow, 2012; McRuer & Wilkerson, 2003). Voices within the self-advocacy movement, in contrast, request that sexual health curriculum for individuals with IDD cover topics relating to sexual orientation and trans* identities (Friedman, Arnold, Owen, & Sandman, 2014).

Consent

Within definitions of healthy sexuality, the ability to consent is a necessary component and often the most difficult for all parties involved to navigate. At times, individuals with IDD experience organic brain dysfunction (such as impairments in judgment and impulse control) that disinhibits sexual behaviours and sparks conduct that is inappropriate to context (Kellerman, 2002; Ryan & Lane, 1997). Even when individuals can identify appropriate and inappropriate behaviour, sexual behaviour that is consensual and appropriate to the context does not always follow. Mere regurgitation of rules is insufficient. Instead, a meaningful demonstration of consent must be attained. Niederbuhl and Morris (1993) outline "consent-ability" as a threefold process (p. 296). Niederbuhl and Morris suggest that an individual's ability to consent to sex is informed by "the person's ability to make a decision based on knowledge of the nature of sexual contact, its possible consequences; and the social and moral context in which it occurs" (p. 296). In cases where one or both parties do not have all three consent-ability markers, consensual sex has not been achieved; however, the ability to consent is not static. Denying sexual expression from individuals with intellectual disabilities is never the conclusion of any sexual-health intervention. Rather, stakeholders need to collaborate around enabling sex and sexuality within populations with IDD who have not yet attained a meaningful understanding of consensual sex.

The ability to give consent increases with sexual knowledge, level of intellectual ability, and having participated in sexual-health education courses (Niederbuhl & Morris, 1993). Therefore, supporting individuals with IDD to understand the nature, consequences, and social context of sex improves their capacity for autonomous sexual decision-making. Sexual decision-making capacity is contextual to the individual and may be present even when other decision-making capacities (such as financial independence or choosing where to live) are absent (AAP, 1996). In addition to equipping individuals with skills to consent to sexual activity, stakeholders may also support individuals through situational competency or the belief that while some forms of sexual contact may not be accessible to all individuals with IDD, sexual expression should not be denied across the board (Bonnie, 1992). For example, if individuals fail to understand the consequences of sexual intercourse, sex educators may promote other forms of intimacy (e.g., hand holding, snuggling, massage, and mutual masturbation). In one study, interviews with women with intellectual disabilities found that despite many engaging in sexual intercourse, their actual preference for sexual touch was kissing and cuddling (Bates et al., 2016). Teaching consent requires a broadened understanding of the needs, desires, and consent capacity of participants with IDD.

Approaches to Sexual-Health Education

Harm Reduction Model

The Western context of sex and disability has largely been characterized by fear, sparking a history of forced sterilization with the aim of preventing individuals with disabilities from having sex, from becoming parents, and from passing genetic inheritance to subsequent generations (Campbell, 2017; Malacrida, 2015). The harm reduction model of sexual-health education stems, in part, from this context of increased rates of negative life experiences such as unplanned pregnancies and sexually transmitted infections (Erickson, Riley, Cheung, & O'Hare, 1997; Harrison & Inciardi, 2000). Harm reduction curriculum intends to build greater sexual decision-making capacity but continues to resonate with societal fears from previous generations. Although these fears no longer translate into forced sterilization and segregation, intended outcomes continue to orient toward preventing unplanned pregnancies and sexually transmitted infections. Bernert and Ogletree (2013) suggest that sexual-health education provides a narrative for individuals with intellectual disabilities characterized by "sexual suppression rather than sexual expression, procreation rather than pleasure, and marital context rather than mutual exchange" (p. 247).

Sex-Positive Model

In contrast, sex positivity is a holistic approach involving an inherent recognition that sexuality is unique to each individual and can be expressed in countless ways (Ailey et al., 2003; Bernert & Ogletree, 2013). A sex-positive model leads from a position of providing examples of healthy sexuality for students to follow. In addition to informing individuals about risks and consequences inherent in sex, this model also speaks to the ways sex can inform someone's sense of self, build self-esteem and confidence, empower a sense of agency, provide pleasure, and promote intimacy (Doyle, 2008; East & Orchard, 2014). This approach recognizes the importance of education that is free of shame and judgment (Ailey et al., 2003).

The benefits of sexual-health education include a decreased risk for negative sexual consequences such as sexually transmitted infections and unplanned pregnancy (Blanchett & Wolfe, 2002), improved communication (Hayashi et al., 2011; Maurer, 2007; Sweeney, 2007) and decision-making skills (Dukes & McGuire, 2009), greater capacity to recognize healthy relationships and sexually appropriate behaviour (Doyle, 2008; Swango-Wilson, 2008), and the opportunity to develop a positive sexual identity that includes confidence, self-esteem, pleasure, and safe healthy relationships (East & Orchard, 2014; Maurer, 2007; Noonan & Taylor Gomez, 2011; Swango-Wilson, 2008, 2011; Sweeney, 2007; Whitehouse & McCabe, 1997).

Often, due to the neurodiverse needs of individuals with IDD, "cookie-cutter" classroom curriculum is not effective (Gougeon, 2009). Instead, a flexible and adaptive approach is required when working with this population. Materials should be customizable to participants' needs (Dukes & McGuire, 2009) and provide a range of options to accommodate the degree of cognitive ability (Barnard-Brak et al., 2014; Blanchett & Wolfe, 2002). There are several important questions to answer regarding effective delivery, including who should be providing education, what content should be taught, when and where this education should occur, and how this information is best delivered.

Who?

Teachers, parents, paid care staff, health professionals, and peers are all potential sources of education and support, and all bring diverse experience and expertise to the table. A single population is not best equipped to teach individuals with IDD; however, attributes that contribute to effective sexual-health education have been observed. Fegan, Rauch, and McCarthy (1993) outline as important educator traits such as confidence in one's knowledge of sexuality, an ability to discuss sensitive topics, having access to relevant and current information, challenging educators' own personal biases and assumptions, being open and straightforward about material, using a variety of strategies and tools, and knowing when to refer to someone with greater training and expertise (as referenced in Travers & Tincani, 2010).

With this in mind, each demographic of people supporting individuals with IDD is uniquely equipped to fulfil educational roles. Parents and care staff are important for promoting and reinforcing sex-positive knowledge, attitudes, and behaviour in tandem with classroom instruction. Teachers are qualified to provide formal education, especially in terms of fact-based mechanics of sex, such as anatomy and physiology. Healthcare professionals can educate and provide interventions, including suggesting and applying specific therapies or approaches, as with the case of concerning behaviours. Peer mentors, whether neurotypical or neurodiverse, can be strong sources of information and experience (Frawley & Bigby, 2014; Gougeon, 2009), make realistic role-play partners (Graff et al., 2018; Hayashi et al., 2011), and contribute valuable and relatable content to group discussions (Blanchett & Wolfe, 2002; Frawley & Bigby, 2014). Indeed, some have argued for peer-led teaching as a way to reduce power dynamics; however, at this time there is a lack of research on the effectiveness of this approach (Frawley & Bigby, 2014; Gougeon, 2009). Whether peer support and mentorship takes place in small or large group settings, it is important that an educator be present to act as a facilitator and to correct any inaccurate information discussed.

What?

Throughout their lives, individuals with IDD often accumulate misinformation about sexuality that has the potential to be harmful if left uncorrected (Blanchett & Wolfe, 2002). Assessing the current level and accuracy of knowledge of the individual student, whether formally or informally, is important before delivering sexual-health education. This approach establishes a baseline of knowledge, while also providing the opportunity to correct any misinformation learned over time (Blanchett & Wolfe, 2002; Grieveo, McLaren, & Lindsay, 2007; Whitehouse & McCabe, 1997). Measuring progress at regular intervals also helps to ensure that individuals understand the information they are learning and provides opportunities for ongoing support and feedback (Blanchett & Wolfe, 2002; Smith, Wheeler, Pilecki, & Parker, 1995). Informally incorporating questions into conversation throughout lessons (Blanchett & Wolfe, 2002) or having students demonstrate skills (Smith et al., 1995) are simple means to assess the attainment of materials while decreasing anxieties associated with testing and evaluation.

The inclusion of skills training has become a significant piece of comprehensive sexual-health education programs, including areas such as social skills (Swango-Wilson, 2011; Travers & Tincani, 2010), decision-making (Dukes & McGuire, 2009), and assertiveness training (Grieveo et al, 2007; Hayashi et al., 2011). Informed sexual decision-making has been shown to be central in navigating the complexities of all relationships, whether platonic or romantic (Dukes & McGuire, 2009; Healy, McGuire, Evans, & Carley, 2009; Swango-Wilson, 2011). Skill development is a gradual process that requires educators' willingness to use ongoing repetition and situation-specific rules to help the individual with IDD to form prosocial habits.

Motivation is necessary for individuals to be successful in applying sexual-health knowledge and skills to daily life and is best encouraged through ensuring that content is meaningful to individuals with IDD and their context (Dixon et al., 2010; Smith et al., 1995; Swango-Wilson, 2011). Education should be relevant to the individuals' lived experience. For instance, examples should be based on true stories or relate closely to real-life scenarios (Blanchett & Wolfe, 2002; Smith et al., 1995). Where possible, visuals chosen should be "explicit and life-like" (Blanchett & Wolfe, 2002, p. 53) for individuals to translate materials to real-world contexts, such as using photos to assist in body part identification (Lindsay et al., 1992).

When?

Sexuality evolves over time. Consequently, sexual-health education must accommodate this dynamic nature of sexual identity. Sexual-health education shows greater efficacy when generalized across the lifespan, from reinforcing proper terminology of body parts in early childhood to promoting skills relating to friendship, intimacy, and consent into adolescence (Ailey et al., 2003; Travers & Tincani, 2010). Thus, it is important to begin education early to better prepare individuals for the barriers that often accompany living with an intellectual disability and further prevent knowledge disparities (Doyle, 2008; O'Callaghan & Murphy, 2007). Additionally, the use of booster sessions could be helpful to maintain knowledge over time (Dukes & McGuire, 2009).

Where?

Individuals benefit from having the opportunity to learn sexual-health education in classrooms alongside their neurotypical peers (Katz, Mirenda, & Auerbach, 2002), as peers are an important source of sexual information during adolescence (Gougeon, 2009) and can act as role models for healthy relationships (Frawley & Bigby, 2014). To enhance classroom learning, individuals should also receive individualized multi-session, one-on-one support to promote the understanding of important topics and mastery of skills (Dukes & McGuire, 2009; Harader, Fullwood, & Hawthorn, 2009). This could occur in a variety of settings such as in the individual's home, community, day programs, and general health clinics or clinics that specialize in sexual health. Any setting could be appropriate so long as the space is safe and respectful for the individual (Craft, 1994).

How?

Knowing how to deliver information effectively to individuals is one of the most challenging aspects of sex education. Educators should incorporate a variety of strategies and media that emphasize student strengths and offset challenges (Harader et al., 2009). The following means of delivering information have been found to be effective for adults with IDD: Verbal information should be "presented concretely, simply, matter of factly, and repeatedly" (Ailey et al., 2003, p. 247), and should be well-paced and engaging, while avoiding abstract concepts (Ramage, 2015; Smith et al., 1995). When abstract concepts must be discussed, a scaffolding approach should be utilized. Scaffolding involves teaching information in a step-by-step manner, beginning with simple ideas and language and building on them through repetition, purposeful planning, ongoing evaluation, and review to ensure understanding. (Blanchett & Wolfe, 2002; Smith et al, 1995). Other interactive strategies could include group discussions (Katz et al., 2002), question and answer sessions (Blanchett & Wolfe, 2002), theatre (Munro, Selman, Esmail, & Ponzetti Jr., 2007), as well as music and singing (Knight, 2009).

Written materials should be colourful, visually appealing, and modern (Graff et al., 2018) while accounting for the reading abilities of the individual and can include handouts, pamphlets, books, slides, workbooks, and activity sheets (Blanchett & Wolfe, 2002). Pictorial support, such as photos and illustrations, has been found to be useful for individuals with IDD of all levels and can help enhance understanding of written and verbal materials presented (Grieveo et al., 2007). Drawings (Blanchett & Wolfe, 2002; Grieveo et al., 2007), models (Dixon et al., 2010), and "anatomically correct dolls" are also viable options (Ailey et al, 2003, p. 247)

Skills, such as assertiveness and decision-making, are best developed through practice that mimics real-world conditions, and role play is an effective strategy to support this (Blanchett & Wolfe, 2002; Carter, 1999; Graff et al., 2018; Hayashi et al., 2011). Practicing with a variety of people in different contexts can also increase the likelihood that skills will generalize to daily life (Blanchett & Wolfe, 2002; Harader et al., 2009). Other functional approaches include visually demonstrating with models to represent places (Dixon et al., 2010), objects, or anatomy (Hayashi et al., 2011; Whitehouse & McCabe, 1997), such as using a 3D model of an anatomically correct penis to let individuals practice using condoms appropriately (Whitehouse & McCabe, 1997).

Technology such as computer-delivered education programs, animation (Delaine, 2012; Wells, Clark, & Sarno, 2012), games, videos (Gougeon, 2009), and virtual reality (Dixon et al., 2010) all show potential as accessible and entertaining resources for individuals with IDD. Interactive computer-based programming is sometimes utilized as a tool to teach sexual health topics to individuals with IDD (Delaine, 2012; Wells, Clark, & Sarno, 2012). Unfortunately, even in neurotypical youth populations, these programs and individual techniques are limited and not well studied, despite the huge potential for accessibility (Holstrom, 2015). With the increasing number of online resources, it can be difficult to decide which sexual health resources are evidence based. Many online resources, such as diagnosis-specific organizations or government health agencies, have begun to provide information and resources to make this task less daunting.

Conclusion

"How do I teach sexual-health education to my student with intellectual disability?" might be a lingering question, even after reading this chapter. The best answer is to get your head out of the books and start taking cues from your students. The individuals before you, alongside their support networks, are the richest source of information that you can draw on, when creating sexual-health curriculum. If the prospect of educating individuals with intellectual disabilities appears intimidating, that is because it is. Life is messy, so we must use our flexibility, creativity, and common sense in working with this population. Rather than following a rigid curriculum, educators are more effective if they incorporate all the tools in their repertoire to find the best means of teaching and supporting individuals. This includes expecting challenges relating to boundaries, safety, sexual orientation, public versus private behaviour, and unconventional sexual compensations. We also need to recognize that the sexuality of individuals with disabilities is often denied or characterized by exploitation.

However, despite the many barriers that individuals with disabilities face, a growing body of literature reveals respectful and satisfying relationships between individuals with IDD (Bates et al., 2017; Healy et al., 2009; Friedman et al., 2014; Löfgren-Mårtenson, 2009; Stoffelen et al., 2017; Turner & Crane, 2016). For example, Bates and colleagues capture expressions of love and intimacy between two lovers who both identify with IDD: "Joe: She's [current partner] a great person in my life, friendly, kind, funny and fun to be with [turning to (partner)]. I love you so much. So happy about the person I am married to and also she is my soulmate" (pp. 606–607). Thus, the desire for meaningful and intimate relationships is both a realistic and attainable goal for individuals with intellectual disabilities.

Neurotypical individuals receive formal and informal education and support navigating intimacy through conversations, advice, and emotional validation from community networks. For individuals with intellectual disabilities, this support is often framed as dependency, making invisible the support neurotypical relationships receive (Friedman et al., 2014). In contrast, stakeholders in the lives of individuals with intellectual disabilities require a shift in perspective regarding sexuality that recognizes structural and societal barriers and moves away from a discourse of dependency and toward community responsibility.

REFERENCES

Ailey, S. H., Marks, B. A., Crisp, C., & Hahn, J. E. (2003). Promoting sexuality across the lifespan for individuals with intellectual and developmental disabilities. *The Nursing Clinics of North America, 38*, 229–252. https://doi.org/10.1016/s0029-6465(02)00056-7

American Academy of Pediatrics (AAP). (1996). Sexuality education of children and adolescents with developmental disabilities. *Pediatrics, 97*, 275–278.

American Association of Intellectual Disability (AAID). (2019, September 15). *Definition of intellectual disability.* Retrieved from: https://aaidd.org/intellectual-disability/definition.

APA (American Psychiatric Association). (2013). *Diagnostic and statistical manual of mental disorders.* 5th ed. Washington, DC: APA.

Aunos, M., & Feldman, M. A. (2002). Attitudes towards sexuality, sterilization and parenting rights of persons with intellectual disabilities. *Journal of Applied Research in Intellectual Disabilities, 15*(4), 285–296. https://doi.org/10.1046/j.1468-3148.2002.00135.x

Ballan, M. (2001). Parents as sexuality educators for their children with developmental disabilities. *SIECUS Report, 29*(3), 14–19.

Barnard-Brak, L., Schmidt, M., Chesnut, S., Wei, T., & Richman, D. (2014). Predictors of access to sex education for children with intellectual disabilities in public schools. *Intellectual and Developmental Disabilities, 52*(2), 85–97. https://doi.org/10.1352/1934-9556-52.2.85

Bates, C., Terry, L., & Popple, K. (2016). Partner selection for people with intellectual disabilities. *Journal of Applied Research in Intellectual Disabilities.* https://doi.org/10.1111/jar.12254

Bates, C., Terry, L., & Popple, K. (2017). Supporting people with learning disabilities to make and maintain intimate relationships. *Tizard Learning Disability Review, 22*(1), 16–23. https://doi.org/10.1108/tldr-03-2016-0009

Bernert, D. J., & Ogletree, R. J. (2013). Women with intellectual disabilities talk about their perceptions of sex. *Journal of Intellectual Disability Research, 57*(3), 240–249. https://doi.org/10.1111/j.1365-2788.2011.01529.x

Blanchett, W. J., & Wolfe, P. S. (2002). A review of sexuality education curricula: Meeting the sexuality education needs of individuals with moderate and severe intellectual disabilities. *Research and Practice for Persons with Severe Disabilities*, *27*(1), 43–57. https://doi.org/10.2511/rpsd.27.1.43

Bonnie, R. J. (1992). Defendants with mental retardation. In R. W. Conley, R. Luckasson, & G. N. Bouthilet, *Criminal justice system and mental retardation: Defendants and victims*. Baltimore, MD: Paul H. Brookes.

Brownridge, D. A. (2006). Partner violence against women with disabilities: Prevalence, risk, and explanations. *Violence Against Women*, *12*(9), 805–822. https://doi.org/10.1177/1077801206292681

Buchanan, A., & Wilkins, R. (1991). Sexual abuse of the mentally handicapped: Difficulties in establishing prevalence. *Psychiatric Bulletin*, *15*, 601–605 https://doi.org/10.1192/pb.15.10.601

Campbell, M. (2017). Disabilities and sexual expression: A review of the literature. *Sociology Compass*, *11*(9): 1–19. https://doi.org/10.1111/soc4.12508

Carter, J. C. (1999). Sexuality education for students with specific learning disabilities. *Intervention in School and Clinic*, *34*(4), 220–223. https://doi.org/10.1177/105345129903400404

Clare, E. (2015). *Exile and pride: Disability, queerness and liberation*. Durham: Duke University Press.

Craft, A. (1994). Issues in sex education for people with learning disabilities in the united kingdom. *Sexual and Marital Therapy*, *9*(2), 145–157. https://doi.org/10.1080/02674659408409577

Cuskelly, M., & Bryde, R. (2004). Attitudes towards the sexuality of adults with an intellectual disability: Parents, support staff, and a community sample. *Journal of Intellectual and Developmental Disability*, *29*(3), 255–264. https://doi.org/10.1080/13668250412331285136

Cuskelly, M., & Gilmore, L. (2007). Attitudes to Sexuality Questionnaire (individuals with an intellectual disability): Scale development and community norms. *Journal of Intellectual/Developmental Disability*, *32*, 214–221. https://doi.org/10.1080/13668250701549450

Delaine, K. (2012). A computer-based interactive multimedia program to reduce HIV transmission for women with intellectual disability. *Journal of Intellectual Disability Research*, *56*, 371–381. https://doi.org/10.1111/j.1365-2788.2011.01482.x

Department of Health. (2001). *Valuing people: A new strategy for intellectual disability for the 21st century*. Department of Health, London

Dixon, D. R., Bergstrom, R., Smith, M. N., & Tarbox, J. (2010). A review of research on procedures for teaching safety skills to persons with developmental disabilities. *Research in Developmental Disabilities*, *31*, 985–994. https://doi.org/10.1016/j.ridd.2010.03.007

Downs, C., & Craft, A. (1996). Sexuality and profound and multiple impairment. *Tizard Learning Disability Review*, *1*, 17–22, https://doi.org/10.1108/13595474199600015

Sexual Health Education for Individuals with Disabilities 265

Doyle, J. (2008). Improving sexual health education for young people with learning disabilities. *Paediatric Nursing, 20*(4), 26–28. https://doi.org /10.7748/paed.20.4.26.s23

Dukes, E., & McGuire, B. E. (2009). Enhancing capacity to make sexuality-related decisions in people with an intellectual disability. *Journal of Intellectual Disability Research, 53*(8), 727–734. https://doi.org/10.1111/j.1365-2788.2009 .01186.x

Dunne, T., & Power, A. (1990). Sexual abuse and mental handicap: Preliminary findings of a community-based study. *Journal of Applied Research in Intellectual Disability, 3*(2), 111–125. https://doi.org/10.1111/j.1468-3148.1990 .tb00031.x

East, L., & Orchard, T. (2014). Somebody else's job: Experiences of sex education among health professionals, parents and adolescents with physical disabilities in southwestern Ontario. *Sexuality and Disability, 32*(3), 335–350. https://doi.org/10.1007/s11195-013-9289-5

Eastgate, G., Van Driel, N., Lennox, & Scheermeyer, E. (2011). Women with intellectual disabilities: A study of sexuality, sexual abuse and protection skills. *Australian Family Physician, 40*(4), 226–230.

Emerson, E., & Hatton, C. (2008). People with intellectual disabilities in England, research report 2008:1 (May). Lancaster University, Lancaster: Centre for Disability Research.

Erickson, P. G., Riley, D., Cheung, Y., & O'Hare, P. A. (1997). *Harm reduction: A new direction for drug policies and programs.* Toronto: University of Toronto Press.

Esmail, S., Darry, K., Walter, A., & Knupp, H. (2010). Attitudes and perceptions towards disability and sexuality. *Disability & Rehabilitation, 32*(14), 1148–1155. https://doi.org/10.3109/09638280903419277

Esmail, S., Esmail, Y., & Munro, B (2001). Sexuality and disability: The role of health care professionals in providing options and alternative for couples. *Sexuality and Disability, 19*(4), 267–282. https://doi.org/10.1023/a:1017905425599

Fader Wilkenfeld, B., & Ballan, M. (2011). Educators' attitudes and beliefs towards the sexuality of individuals with developmental disabilities. *Sexuality & Disability, 29*(4), 351–361. https://doi.org/10.1007/s11195-011-9211-y

Fegan, L., Rauch, A., & McCarthy, W. (1993). *Sexuality and people with intellectual disability* (2nd ed.). Baltimore, MD: Paul H. Brookes.

Frawley, P., & Bigby, C. (2014). "I'm in their shoes": Experiences of peer educators in sexuality and relationship education. *Journal of Intellectual & Developmental Disability, 39*(2), 167–176. https://doi.org/10.3109/13668250.2014.890701

Frawley, P., & Wilson, N. (2016). Young people with intellectual disability talking about sexuality education and information. *Sexuality and Disability, 34*(4), 469–484. https://doi.org/10.1007/s11195-016-9460-x

Friedman, C., Arnold, C. K., Owen, A. L., & Sandman, L. (2014). "Remember our voices are our tools:" Sexual self-advocacy as defined by people with intellectual and developmental disabilities. *Sexuality and Disability, 32*(4), 515–532. https://doi.org/10.1007/s11195-014-9377-1

Gobin, R., & Freyd, J. (2009). Betrayal and revictimization: Preliminary findings. *Psychological Trauma: Theory, Research, Practice, and Policy, 1*(3), 242–257. https://doi.org/10.1037/a0017469

Goode, B. (2011). *The Goode life: Memoirs of disability rights activist Barb Goode*. Vancouver, BC: Spectrum Press.

Goodley, D. (2001). "Learning difficulties," the social model of disability and impairment: Challenging epistemologies. *Disability & Society, 16*(2), 207–223. https://doi.org/10.1080/09687590120035816

Gougeon, N. A. (2009). Sexuality education for students with intellectual disabilities, a critical pedagogical approach: Outing the ignored curriculum. *Sex Education, 9*(3), 277–291. https://doi.org/10.1080/14681810903059094

Graff, H., Moyher, R., Bair, J., Foster, C., Gorden, M., & Clem, J. (2018). Relationships and sexuality: How is a young adult with an intellectual disability supposed to navigate? *Sexuality and Disability. 36*(2), 175–183. https://doi.org/10.1007/s11195-017-9499-3

Grieveo, A., McLaren, S., & Lindsay, W. R. (2007). An evaluation of research and training resources for the sex education of people with moderate to severe learning disabilities. *British Journal of Learning Disabilities, 35*(1), 30–37. https://doi.org/10.1111/j.1468-3156.2006.00401.x

Gurza, A. (2019). Disability after dark. Retrieved from: http://www.andrewgurza.com/

Harader, D., Fullwood, H., & Hawthorne, M. (2009). Sexuality among adolescents with moderate disabilities: Promoting positive sexual development. *The Prevention Researcher, 16*(4), 17–20. https://doi.org/10.1037/e630642009-006

Harrison, L. D., & Inciardi, J. A. (2000). *Harm reduction: National and international perspectives*. Sage Publications.

Hassouneh-Phillips, D., & Curry, M. A. (2002). Abuse of women with disabilities: State of the science. *Rehabilitation Counseling Bulletin, 45*(2), 96. https://doi.org/10.1177/003435520204500204

Hayashi, M., Arakida, M., & Ohashi, K. (2011). The effectiveness of a sex education program facilitating social skills for people with intellectual disability in Japan. *Journal of Intellectual and Developmental Disability, 36*(1), 11–19. https://doi.org/10.3109/13668250.2010.549463

Healy, E., McGuire, B. E., Evans, D. S., & Carley, S. N. (2009). Sexuality and personal relationships for people with an intellectual disability. Part I: Service-user perspectives. *Journal of Intellectual Disability Research, 53*(11), 905–912. https://doi.org/10.1111/j.1365-2788.2009.01203.x

Holstrom, A. M. (2015). Sexuality education goes viral: What we know about online sexual health education. *American Journal of Sexuality Education, 10*, 277–294. https://doi.org/10.1080/15546128.2015.1040569

Houdek, V., & Gibson, J. (2017). *Treating sexual abuse and trauma with children, adolescents, and young adults with developmental disabilities: A workbook for clinicians.* Springfield, Illinois: Charles C Thomas.

Jahoda, A., & Pownall, J. (2014). Sexual understanding, sources of information and social networks: The reports of young people with intellectual disabilities and their non-disabled peers. *Journal of Intellectual Disability Research*, 430. https://doi.org/10.1111/jir.12040

Karellou, J. (2003). Laypeople's attitudes toward the sexuality of people with learning disabilities in Greece. *Sexuality and Disability*, *21*, 65–84. https://doi.org/10.1023/a:1023562909800

Katz, J., Mirenda, P., & Auerbach, S. (2002). Instructional strategies and educational outcomes for students with developmental disabilities in inclusive "multiple intelligences" and typical inclusive classrooms. *Research and Practice for Persons with Severe Disabilities*, *27*(4), 227–238. https://doi.org/10.2511/rpsd.27.4.227

Kellerman, T. (2002). *FAS and inappropriate sexual behavior.* Accessed 26 February 2010 from http://www.come-over.to/FAS/InappropriateSexualBehavior.htm

Kijak, R. (2011). A desire for love: Considerations on sexuality and sexual education of people with intellectual disability in Poland. *Sexuality and Disability*, *29*(1), 65–74. https://doi.org/10.1007/s11195-010-9184-2

Knight, J. (2009). Songs for learning. *Nursing Standard*, *23*(43), 22–23. https://doi.org/10.7748/ns.23.43.22.s27

Landman, A. (2014). "A counterfeit friendship": Mate crime and people with learning disabilities. *The Journal of Adult Protection*, *16*(6), 355–366. https://doi.org/10.1108/jap-10-2013-0043

Lindsay W. R., Bellshaw E., Culross G., Staines C., & Michie A. M. (1992) Increases in sexual knowledge following a course of sex education for people with intellectual disabilities. *Journal of Intellectual Disability Research*, *36*, 531–539. https://doi.org/10.1111/j.1365-2788.1992.tb00571.x

Löfgren-Mårtenson, L. (2004). "May I?" About sexuality and love in the new generation with intellectual disabilities. *Sexuality and Disability*, *23*(3), 197–207. https://doi.org/10.1023/B:SEDI.0000039062.73691.cb

Löfgren-Mårtenson, L. (2009). The invisibility of young homosexual women and men with intellectual disabilities. *Sexuality and Disability*, *27*(1), 21–26. https://doi.org/10.1007/s11195-008-9101-0

Malacrida, C. (2015). *A special hell: Institutional life in Alberta's eugenic years.* University of Toronto Press.

Maurer, J. (2007). Modelling socioeconomic and health determinants of health-care use: A semiparametric approach. *Health Economics*, *16*(9), 967–979. https://doi.org/10.1002/hec.1253

McCabe, M., & Schreck, A. (1992). Before sex education: An evaluation of the sexual knowledge, experience, and feelings and needs of people with mild intellectual disabilities. *Australia and New Zealand Journal of Developmental Disabilities, 16*, 75–82. https://doi.org/10.1080/07263869200034831

McCarthy, M. (1996). The sexual support needs of people with learning disabilities: A profile of those referred for sex education. *Sexuality & Disability, 14*(4), 265–279. https://doi.org/10.1007/bf02590099

McCarthy, M. (2014). Women with intellectual disability: Their sexual lives in the 21st century. *Journal of Intellectual & Developmental Disability, 39*(2), 124–131. https://doi.org/10.3109/13668250.2014.894963

McCarthy, M. (2017). "What kind of abuse is him spitting in my food?": Reflections on the similarities between disability hate crime, so-called "mate" crime and domestic violence against women with intellectual disabilities. *Disability & Society, 32*(4), 595–600. https://doi.org/10.1080/09687599.2017.1301854

McRuer, R., & Mollow, A. (2012). *Sex and disability*. Durham: Duke University Press.

McRuer, R., & Wilkerson, A. (2003). Introduction. Symposium: Desiring disability: Queer theory meets disability studies. *Journal of Lesbian and Gay Studies, 9*(1–2), 1–24.

Munro, B. E., Selman, J., Esmail, S., & Ponzetti, J., James. (2007). Are we there yet?: Using theatre in sexual education: A combination of academic and theatre groups. *The International Journal of Diversity in Organizations, Communities, and Nations: Annual Review, 7*(3), 131–138. https://doi.org/10.18848/1447-9532/cgp/v07i03/39376

Niederbuhl, J. M., & Morris, C. D. (1993). Sexual knowledge and the capability of persons with dual diagnoses to consent to sexual contact. *Sexuality and Disability, 11*(4), 295–307. https://doi.org/10.1007/bf01102174

Noonan, A., & Taylor Gomez, M. (2011). Who's missing? Awareness of lesbian, gay, bisexual and transgender people with intellectual disability. *Sexuality and Disability, 29*(2), 175–180. https://doi.org/10.1007/s11195-010-9175-3

O'Callaghan, A.C., & Murphy, G.H. (2007). Sexual relationships in adults with intellectual disabilities: Understanding the law. *Journal of Intellectual Disability Research, 51*(3), 197–206. https://doi.org/10.1111/j.1365-2788.2006.00857.x

Parchomiuk, M. (2013). Model of intellectual disability and the relationship of attitudes towards the sexuality of persons with an intellectual disability. *Sexuality & Disability, 31*(2), 125–139. https://doi.org/10.1007/s11195-012-9285-1

Parsons, A., Reichl, A., & Pedersen, C. (2016). Gendered ableism: Media representations and gender role beliefs' effect on perceptions of disability and sexuality. *Sex and Disability*. doi:10.1007/s11195-016-9464-6

Plummer, S.-B., & Findley, P. A. (2012) Women with disabilities' experience with physical and sexual abuse: A review of the literature and implications for the field. *Trauma, Violence, and Abuse, 13*(1), 15–29. https://doi.org/10.1177/1524838011426014

Pownall, J. D. (2010). Health knowledge and expected outcomes of risky behaviour: A comparative study of non-disabled adolescents and young people with intellectual and physical disabilities. Unpublished doctoral dissertation, University of Glasgow. Glasgow, UK.

Ramage, S. (2015). Sexual health education for adolescents with intellectual disabilities: A literature review. Prepared for the Saskatchewan Prevention Institute. https://skprevention.ca/wp-content/uploads/2017/01/7-527 -Sexual-Health-Education-for-Adolescents-with-Intellectual-Disabilities.pdf

Ryan, G., & Lane, S. (1997). *Juvenile sexual offending: Causes, consequences, and correction.* New and revised edition. San Francisco, California: Jossey-Bass Publishers.

Saxton, M., Curry, M. A., Powers, L. E., Maley, S., Eckels, K., & Gross, J. (2001). "Bring my scooter so I can leave you": A study of disabled women handling abuse by personal assistance providers. *Violence Against Women, 7*(4), 393–417. https://doi.org/10.1177/10778010122182523

Silberman, S. (2015). *Neurotribes: The legacy of autism and the future of neurodiversity.* New York: Avery, an imprint of Penguin Random House.

Smith, K., Wheeler, B., Pilecki, P., & Parker, T. (1995). The role of the pediatric nurse practitioner in educating teens with mental retardation about sex. *Journal of Pediatric Health Care, 9*(2), 59–66. https://doi.org/10.1016 /s0891-5245(05)80003-3

Stoffelen, J. M. T., Herps, M. A., Buntinx, W. H. E., Schaafsma, D., Kok, G., & Curfs, L. M. G. (2017). Sexuality and individual support plans for people with intellectual disabilities. *Journal of Intellectual Disability Research, 61*(12), 1117–1129. https://doi.org/10.1111/jir.12428

Swango-Wilson, A. (2008). Caregiver perceptions and implications for sex education for individuals with intellectual and developmental disabilities. *Sexuality and Disability, 26*(3), 167–174. https://doi.org/10.1007/s11195-008-9081-0

Swango-Wilson, A. (2011). Meaningful sex education programs for individuals with intellectual/developmental disabilities. *Sexuality and Disability, 29*(2), 113–118. https://doi.org/10.1007/s11195-010-9168-2

Sweeney, L. (2007). The importance of human sexuality education for students with disabilities. *Exceptional Parent, 37*(9), 38–39.

Trace, K. (2014). *Hot, wet & shaking: How I learned to talk about sex.* Halifax & Toronto: Invisible Publishing.

Travers, J., & Tincani, M. (2010). Sexuality education for individuals with autism spectrum disorders: Critical issues and decision making guidelines. *Education and Training in Autism and Developmental Disabilities, 45*(2), 284–293. Retrieved from https://www.jstor.org/stable/23879812

Turner, G. W., & Crane, B. (2016). Sexually silenced no more, adults with learning disabilities speak up: A call to action for social work to frame sexual voice as a social justice issue. *British Journal of Social Work, 46*(8), 2300–2317. https://doi.org/10.1093/bjsw/bcw133

Walter-Brice, A., Cox, R., Priest, H., & Thompson, F. (2012). What do women with learning disabilities say about their experiences of domestic abuse within the context of their intimate partner relationships? *Disability & Society*, 27(4), 503–517. https://doi.org/10.1080/09687599.2012.659460

Watson, N., Shakespeare, T., Cunningham-Burley, S., & Barnes, C. (1999). *Life as a disabled child: A qualitative study of young people's experiences and perspectives. Final report.* University of Edinburgh and University of Leeds, ESRC Research Programme.

Wells, J., Clark, K. D., & Sarno, K. (2012). A computer-based interactive multimedia program to reduce HIV transmission for people with intellectual disability. *Journal of Intellectual Disability Research*, 56(4), p. 371–381. https://doi.org/10.1111/j.1365-2788.2011.01482.x

Whitehouse, M. A., & McCabe, M. P. (1997). Sex education programs for people with intellectual disability: How effective are they? *Education and Training in Mental Retardation and Developmental Disabilities*, 32(3), 229–240. https://www.jstor.org/stable/23879152

Williams D (1999) *Like colour to the blind.* London: Jessica Kingsley Publishers.

Wolfe, P. (1997). The influence of personal values on issues of sexuality and disability. *Sexuality & Disability*, 2, 69. https://doi.org/10.1023/a:1024731917753

World Health Organization (WHO). (2006). Defining sexual health: Report of a technical consultation on sexual health, 28–31 January 2002, Geneva. Retrieved July 01, 2019, fromhttps://www.who.int/reproductivehealth/publications/sexual_health/defining_sexual_health.pdf?ua=1

16 Teachable Moments: The Intersections of Disabilities and Sexualities

MICHELLE OWEN AND BADEN GAEKE-FRANZ

For some time, I, Michelle, had been thinking about teaching a course on the topics of sexuality and disability. On their own both disability and sexuality exist on the margins of academe (if they exist at all), but together they become almost unimaginable. Combining these two subjects represents an exciting new field of study in higher education, and there are few courses available in this area. I decided to develop a course to fill this significant knowledge gap. Additionally, I suspected that this would be an important addition to the disability studies program that I coordinate at the University of Winnipeg. However, I had no idea how popular the course would be until I taught the first class in 2016.

The course, Disabilities, Sexualities, and Rights, is a second-year undergraduate course cross-listed between disability studies (DS) and women's and gender studies (WGS). There are no prerequisites, and it can be used as a humanities credit that some students need to fulfil their degree requirements. For these reasons, it attracts a diverse range of students, including those who want to pursue careers in social work and medicine. Plus, it has the word "sex" in the title, which has ended up being a big draw. Many of the people who took Disabilities, Sexualities, and Rights had never thought before about disabled people as sexual, let alone queer or into kink. In this chapter, Baden, a student from the inaugural class, and I will share and critically reflect on our experiences. Baden troubles my account by adding their perspective. We will also present some key theories and ideas about disability, sexuality, gender, and sex.

Course Development

In terms of course design, the description of Disabilities, Sexualities, and Rights in the course calendar reads as follows:

> Links between living with disabilities and risk of disadvantage or discrimina-
> tion are clear, yet focus on equity, employment access, services, and physi-
> cal health needs may render invisible issues of sexual health, identity, and
> expression of people with disabilities. This course embraces social models
> and explores human rights implications of challenging bio-medical views
> of sexualities and disabilities, focusing on how people with disabilities
> embrace their sexualities and/or are prevented from doing so. Students
> explore these topics from critical disability, feminist, and queer perspec-
> tives. Recognizing and balancing complex and sometimes apparently
> competing self-identities and needs are integral from a human rights per-
> spective. (University of Winnipeg, 2019, p. 70)

Guided by these words, I set out to find course materials, but this proved to be more difficult than I anticipated. To begin with, there are not a lot of books available about sexuality and disability, and even fewer that are appropriate for a course at this level. Some of what I reviewed was too theoretically advanced, such as *Sex and Disability* (McRuer & Mollow [Eds.], 2012) and *The Right to Maim: Debility, Capacity, Disability* (Puar, 2017). Other sources I came across were either too clinical or rehabilita-tion focused for my purposes. In the end, I decided on two very different texts for the course: *The Ultimate Guide to Sex and Disability: For All of Us Who Live with Disabilities, Chronic Pain & Illness* (Kaufman, Silverberg, & Odette, 2007); and *Loneliness and Its Opposite: Sex, Disability, and the Ethics of Engagement* (Kulick & Rydström, 2015). I also assigned selections from the journals *Disability Horizons* (n.d.) and *Sexuality and Disability* (n.d.).

My objective in this course, as in all the classes I teach, was to stimulate critical thinking. I did not want to just give my students facts and fig-ures to memorize and regurgitate back to me. Hence, our meetings were structured to allow space for group and class discussion, as opposed to lectures only. Students were advised to come to class prepared to discuss the assigned readings in a critical fashion. I emphasized that their par-ticipation mark was based not just on attendance but also on the ability to thoughtfully discuss assigned material. In addition to participation, students were assessed based on the following assignments.

First, everyone had to create a profile on Nexus, the UW online learn-ing platform. Even though we met in person, I used Nexus for assign-ment submission and grading. I also posted Power Point presentations and videos that were shown in class. Students were asked to upload a picture of themselves or something that represented or expressed who they were. I also asked them to fill in as many of the question boxes as possible. These included queries about favourite music, books, and so forth. This helped me to identify the students online.

The next assignment was a short paper (maximum 750 words), where students were asked to write about their experience with and/or knowledge of the subject matter. They were also encouraged to write about their lack of experience or knowledge in particular areas. Finally, I asked them to describe their interest in the course topics. This helped me to get to know the students a bit better. I was also able to get a sense of what they already knew about the subject matter and what their expectations were for the course. We revisited the question of what they learned at the end of the term so that the students could evaluate their own progression. I also wanted to know if they thought their knowledge of sex and disability had increased and if they had learned what they had hoped to at the beginning of the course. This assignment allowed me to evaluate how well students could write and if they needed to get some assistance from our writing centre.

Most weeks, students were asked to submit reading reports before class. The focus of these 250-word accounts was critical analysis of the assigned material. I emphasized that I was not interested in basic summaries; rather, I wanted to know what they thought about the readings. Writing in the first person was strongly encouraged. I also suggested that students include questions about concepts and issues they did not understand. The purpose of this assignment was twofold. Students needed to both read the assigned materials before class and formulate some thoughts about what they had read. This facilitated and enriched our discussions.

Reflection papers (five to seven pages) were designed to give students a chance to contemplate their learning experience in the class. These were not meant to be research papers but, instead, a critical consideration based on class materials, including readings, suggested websites, films, and discussions. I wanted students to have the opportunity to write a longer paper, but I have found research-based assignments with large first- and second-year classes somewhat unfruitful. Moreover, the interdisciplinary composition of this class meant that students had various understandings of what constituted a research-based essay. This assignment afforded students the opportunity to review our time together and write about what they had learned. Or what they did not learn – I also encouraged critique and suggestions for what could be done differently. I received lots of interesting information, including what Baden will expand on in this chapter.

The final examination was a cumulative assignment comprised of five questions. Students were instructed to choose three questions and answer them in essay style, including proper references. They had one week to complete the exam, and because it was not being written in the classroom, any number of materials could be consulted. I tend to have finals like this, especially in my second-year DS courses. It reduces stress and anxiety, and results in few, if any, requests for accommodation. Moreover, students can compose more thoughtful, critical answers instead of what they have been able to commit to memory. This latter skill is of course not the same for everyone and can be impacted by time pressure.

All in all, these assignments created a strong foundation, built on each other, and allowed me to get to know the students and assess their learning process. I have, however, continued to refine the class work in Disabilities, Sexualities, and Rights since it was first offered. In fall 2020, when universities were closed due to COVID-19, the course was adapted to online delivery.

Disability Studies, Women's and Gender Studies, and Sex 101

The Ultimate Guide has proven to be a good way to introduce the topics of disability and sexuality, because it is clearly written and does not assume people know about sexuality or disability before reading. Interestingly, some students reported feeling awkward reading the book in front of their families or in public because of the bright cover with the word "sex" on it. From the onset, I knew that I could not assume that students in the class would know anything about disability or DS, so I would have to do an overview. While some DS majors and minors signed up, as well as WGS students, there were also students from a variety of departments and faculties (e.g., business, science, kinesiology, conflict resolution, education, and human rights). While UW is primarily an undergraduate university, students may go on to obtain graduate degrees in fields such as social work. Having people from so many academic backgrounds presented a great opportunity to educate students about, and get them interested in, DS and WGS. In turn, their diverse experiences enriched the course. However, it also presented some challenges in that the students did not have a shared disciplinary knowledge or language. I attempted to counter this by lecturing about the biomedical and social models of disability (Withers, 2012) and providing information pertaining to disability history, terminology, and disability activism where appropriate.

I began by encouraging students to think about this common example. People who use wheelchairs (they are not "wheelchair bound") attempt to enter the university but are confronted by stairs and cannot find another entrance. According to the older biomedical model, they cannot walk and are thus prohibited from entering. The solution to this problem is to cure them so they can walk again. From the perspective of the charity model (Withers, 2012), which is connected to the medical model, people who cannot use their legs should be pitied. Developed in the 1960s by disability activists and scholars, the social model deconstructs this thinking so that structures become the problem rather than bodies using them. The inaccessible building is deemed as the source of the disability. Therefore, people with nonconformist bodies are disabled by society, rather than disability being inherent to their bodies. In this way, the social model is inherently political and advocates for social change. Bodies do not need to be fixed or cured; instead, environments need to be altered. From a social model perspective, the term "disabled person" is more appropriate than "person with a disability" because people are disabled by things that are external to them (Barnes & Mercer, 2003).

When I first taught this course, I was also unaware of two other important pedagogical issues. First, apart from the WGS and DS students, many of the students had not been exposed to gender theory or feminisms. Therefore, I needed to provide another primer on these topics. Second, I had not realized how little undergraduates know about sexuality and their own bodies. I was dismayed that my students seemed to know only as much as, or even less, than I did at their ages. According to their accounts, most of the sex education they had received prior to this course had been focused on avoidance of pregnancy and disease, with little discussion of pleasure, desire, or technique. In class, and in an online forum, they discussed what they learned from their parents about sex, which, for most of them, was very little. Some parents spoke to their children about menstruation and reproduction or provided informational literature. Very few offered any more information than this. I can remember only one or two students who reported that their parents broached the topic of sexual fulfillment. The majority of parents who spoke to their children about sex at all were mothers rather than fathers, so students often only had a one-sided perspective.

Alas, their schools did not seem to do a lot better. From my students, I learned the acronym "HAM" for the issues that their high school teachers were not supposed to talk about: homosexuality, abortion, and masturbation. When asked to think about how they learned about sex (if they had), students of various genders mainly said friends and pornography. Some added that they wished they had received accurate information from parents and teachers. Fortunately, *The Ultimate Guide* goes over the basics of anatomy, and even provides pictures. I learned from the first time this course was taught that I needed to provide basic information pertaining to disabilities and DS, feminisms and WGS, bodies, and sexualities, before I could even start teaching the rest of the course.

Themes

Based on my recollections and reflections of papers, discussions, and online posts, I will now examine a number of themes that emerged from the first four times I taught this course. To begin with, each year, many students confessed that they did not realize that they would be learning about sex – "real sex" and "sex-sex" (predominantly defined as heteronormative penis-in-vagina penetrative activity). This kept happening, despite the fact that after the first time teaching the course, I attempted to make the topics very clear. Not only is the word "sexualities" in the course title, but the syllabus also contains the aforementioned university course description. In addition, the objectives include "learning about the intersection of disability and sexuality studies, and gaining tools to reflect critically on this knowledge." Finally, both required texts contain the word "sex" in their titles, and the names of the assigned journals include the terms "sex" and "sexual."

Due to the confusion over these terms, I made sure to include a lecture about the differences between the terms "sex," "gender," and "sexuality." I explained that as a place to start, "sex" is about biology (female or male), "gender" is a social construction (girl/boy, woman/man), and "sexuality" is an identity or choice about attraction (heterosexual/ LGBTQ+). Simone de Beauvoir wrote in 1949 that "one is not born, but rather becomes a woman" (1949/1973, p. 301). This early distinction, a rupture, really, between sex and gender, the biological and the social, was of immense importance to the women's movement. However, as Judith Butler (1990) contends, this significant theoretical moment is ultimately meaningless. Sex and gender, biology and social construction, ultimately collapse into one another. Sex is gendered, and gender is sexed. They are inextricably intertwined.

And, as I explained to the class, it just gets more complicated from there: some people are born intersex; and gender can be de- and re-constructed (by transgender people for instance). In fact, as was discussed in class, biological sex is difficult to ascertain. We are usually labelled according to our primary external genitalia (i.e., what is between our legs), but there are many other components to "sex" determination, such as chromosomes, gonads, hormones, and internal reproductive anatomy (World Health Organization [WHO], n.d.). Many people do not know how many of these categories align unless they have been tested for (in)fertility or have competed in high-level sports. For example, South

African runner Caster Semenya has higher-than-average testosterone levels for a woman, but did not know about this condition until she was given sex-testing at the 2009 Olympics (North, 2019). In addition, the unstable category of "sex" is what gender is built on and what informs our expected sexuality (e.g., girl – woman – heterosexual wife and mother).

Moreover, "sexuality" can be an identity, a choice, or something unlabelled and fluid (as with bisexual, two-spirit, and gender non-binary people). The word "sex" is also used to describe the things (predominantly heteronormative things) that bodies do: they "have sex." With so many definitions for these related words, no wonder students were unsure what the term "sexualities" meant in the course title! Some thought it referred to gender, others to biological sex, and some guessed it was about being lesbian or gay. And, in a way, they were all correct. The course covered all aspects of sexuality for disabled people, including gender identity, biology, orientation, and activities. Every year, some students drop the course early, and I wonder if confusion over what "sexuality" encompasses in the context of this course or discomfort with disabled people being sexual beings are factors in their decision to leave.

What I do know is that the sex part of the course becomes a reality for students early on in a section about sex toys, and again a little further on, when BDSM (bondage, discipline, dominance, submission, and sadomasochism), devotees (people who desire people with disabilities and fetishize disability), and sexual relations with attendants are studied. Some students reported feeling shocked and uncomfortable with these topics, while others were captivated. One person who was studying to become an occupational therapist became excited by the possibilities she had not thought about, such as adapting sex toys, such as dildos and vibrators.

Many students, with and without disabilities, reported that they learned a lot about their own bodies. For example, some revealed that they had never masturbated and that this course had inspired them to try. The term "solo sex" was discussed, and the notion that masturbating constituted cheating on your partner was dismissed. Others visited sex toy stores or sex toy websites for the first time. Needless to say, these activities were not part of my official learning objectives, but I was happy that students gained practical knowledge and reported feeling empowered. This is not always the case in academe.

Overall students, even those with disabilities, had some myths dispelled. The authors of *The Ultimate Guide* begin by outlining 14 common misconceptions about disability and sex. Some examples include that disabled people are not sexual or desirable; they cannot have "real sex"; they do not make good partners; they have to pay for sex; or that sex should be spontaneous and private. Most importantly, nondisabled students were made aware that disabled people are, or can be, sexual beings.

I was initially struck by these words from the introduction of *The Ultimate Guide*: "sexual independence is an extremely potent form of empowerment" (Kaufman et al., 2007, p. xii). However, the first time I offered this course, some of the students who identified as asexual rejected the notion that all people are, or should be, sexual. This was a learning experience for me, as well as for the rest of the class. Obviously, this is another important myth with which to contend. Some students also brought up the concern that the class materials lacked information on mental health, autism, and developmental disabilities. Now when I teach the course, one of these students, Baden, the co-author of this chapter, does a presentation about autism and sexuality. This is always a popular presentation, and students ask a lot of questions.

A Student Perspective

When Baden signed up to take Disabilities, Sexualities and Rights the first time it was offered, they were excited. They looked forward to engaging in discussion about interesting topics related to sexuality, and also to learning things in class that they could apply to their own life and relationships. As the course progressed, however, Baden found that while there was no shortage of interesting discussion, the parts of the course that applied to their life as an autistic person on the asexual spectrum were few and far between.

The subtitle of *The Ultimate Guide* claims that the book is "for all of us who live with disabilities, chronic pain & illness" (Kaufman et al., 2007, cover). Yet the contents of the book do not apply to "all of us" as promised in the title. The authors go into detail about many aspects of disability and how they can affect sexuality, including dealing with chronic pain, lack of sensation, difficulty holding positions, and other concerns with mobility and pain disabilities. However, they only touch briefly on mental health, intellectual disability, and developmental disabilities. For example, they note that sexual excitement is a similar sensation to a panic attack or asthma attack, and give suggestions to avoid asthma attacks during sex, but fail to address how to avoid panic attacks (Kaufman et al., 2007). While *Loneliness and Its Opposite* (Kulick & Rydström, 2015) did more fully bring intellectual disability into the conversation, its focus was largely on people who lived in group homes and institutions, and thus also failed to address large portions of disabled people.

The dearth of information relating to their life as an autistic person was disappointing to Baden. This lack is not because there is nothing to say about autistic sexuality. There are many aspects of autism that transform people's experience of sexuality and relationships. For example, autistic people may experience overstimulation from sexual touch (After Hours Autism, 2015), find meeting places such as bars too loud to be accessible (Shire, 2013), have trouble expressing emotion in ways neurotypical partners can understand (Shire, 2013), have difficulty understanding what a partner is feeling (Hannah and Stagg, 2016), or develop what the Center for Autism Research terms "love fixations" (2017, p. 4): feelings so intense that they frighten off neurotypical or nonautistic partners. Furthermore, people who are both autistic and queer find that "ableism gets in the way of [their] access to the queer community […] while […] in autistic spaces, [they] do not always feel visible and affirmed as a queer […] person" (Tan, 2017, para. 6). These differences and barriers could and should be addressed in a course about disabilities and sexualities, as well as in the published works from which the course drew, but in the first iteration of this course, they were not.

Including autism and other developmental disabilities in discussions about sexuality is important because, as Bargiela et al. (2016) point out, autistic people are often socially isolated due to lack of acceptance of their differences. Thus, while neurotypical people may supplement poor sex education curriculum through conversations with their peers, autistic people rarely have this opportunity. Thus, it is even more important to give relevant sex education to autistic people.

Baden raised these concerns with me, and in subsequent times that I have taught the course, I have invited them to help fill these gaps by doing a presentation to the class about autism and sexuality. In these presentations, Baden covers a wide range of autistic traits that may affect sexuality, giving both information for people who may not have considered autistic sexuality before, as well as advice for people who may be autistic themselves or have an autistic partner. They also emphasize the aspects of autistic embodiment and neurology that can be a benefit in relationships, rather than focusing only on deficits. This is important because what little research there is on autistic sexuality tends to focus only on problems and not on strength or exploration (Lawson, 2005). For example, they may discuss tensions in marriages with an autistic spouse (Myhill & Jekel, 2008) or difficulties autistic people face in finding a partner (Center for Autism Research, 2017). Very rarely does writing on autistic sexuality consider that autism may be a positive aspect of a relationship or discuss the pleasure of autistic sexuality. Baden's presentation disrupts this normative view of autism as tragedy, challenging people to think of autism and pleasure together.

The other gap Baden saw in this course was a lack of acknowledgment of people on the asexual spectrum. The texts we examined in this course, as well as videos and class discussions, worked from the assumption that all people desire sex and romance. The insistence that disabled people are sexual beings is understandable, given a social context in which disabled people are often denied autonomy over their sexuality. However, frustration with the desexualization of disabled people too often comes in the form of people insisting that disabled people are not asexual, with no acknowledgment that asexuality is an identity that some people, disabled and not, choose to claim.

In *The Ultimate Guide*, this insistence on disabled sexuality went so far as to say, "We think *asexual* is a terrible term because we feel everyone has the potential to have sexual feelings. Even when we aren't being sexual or feeling sexual [...] we are still sexual beings" (Kaufman et al., 2007, p. 333, emphasis in original). Not allowing people with disabilities to explore their sexual identity is, of course, unacceptable, and needs to be addressed. However, challenging that oppression by referring to asexuality as "a terrible term" erases a large portion of the population who openly choose to identify as asexual and disallows those people's exploration of their own sexual identity.

This belief that all people are inherently sexual is an example of what Elizabeth Brake dubs amatonormativity: "assumptions that a central, exclusive, amorous relationship is normal for humans, in that it is a universally shared goal, and that such a relationship is normative, in that it should be aimed at in preference to other relationship types" (n.d., para. 4). This assumption excludes asexual people, but may also marginalize polyamorous people, people from cultures with different ideas about family and sexuality, and people who choose to remain single for many other reasons. Overvaluing sexual and romantic relationships can devalue other types of relationships, such as familial and friendship relationships.

The relationship between asexuality and disability is further complicated by the fact that asexuality is often pathologized under the name "Hypoactive Sexual Desire Disorder" (American Psychiatric Association, 2013, p. 440). Many asexual people have advocated against the medicalization of asexuality, saying that asexuality is not a disability (Elizabeth, 2008). However, this can leave many people who are both asexual and disabled having to choose between allying themselves with either the disabled or the asexual community, since both groups are invested in distancing themselves from the other (Liebowitz, 2015). Any discussion of disabled sexuality should include all disabilities and sexualities. Having Baden present to the class about autistic sexuality and asexuality has filled gaps in the initial course plan and opened important conversations about the diversity of disabled sexuality.

Reflections

First printed in 2003, and then again 2007, *The Ultimate Guide* is unfortunately outdated. I am pleased that many of the students noticed this and levelled legitimate critiques. In addition to its focus on so-called "physical" disabilities rather than mental health, intellectual disabilities, or autism, the book also lacks intersectional analysis as well as coverage on current topics like trans and nonbinary genders, and so forth. Reproduction is also left out, although this seems to be on purpose, challenging literature about sexuality that is often heteronormative and centres on reproductive issues. However, this trend is not necessarily the case for disabled people, who are sometimes denied reproductive care due to lack of accessible medical facilities (Tarasoff, 2017), as well as societal attitudes that disabled people will not make good parents or ought not to risk passing on congenital disabilities to future generations (Kuttai, 2010). Fortunately, one of my colleagues, Dr. Nadine LeGier, gives guest lectures in this course on disabled women's reproductive health to help fill that gap.

I have spoken to one of the authors of *The Ultimate Guide* (all three are Canadian) about updating and revising this textbook. Unfortunately, according to the author, the press (Cleis) is not interested in a revised edition. Despite these issues, I will continue to use the book until something better is written. Many students have told me that *The Ultimate Guide* is unlike anything else they have read in university, which delights me (especially when it is accompanied by comments that this course is unlike any other class they have taken). Overall, *The Ultimate Guide* is an excellent introduction to sex and disability/chronic illness and lays a foundation for the next text.

Loneliness and Its Opposite (2015) is a more academic book that weaves together history, politics, philosophy, and interviews. However, the topics are far from traditional: namely, the sex lives of people with intellectual disabilities. The authors compare two Scandinavian countries, Denmark and Sweden, both liberal welfare states portrayed as progressive in terms of both sexuality and disability. In many ways, they are not so different from Canada. However, what readers learn is that despite the similarities between these countries located in such close geographical proximity, the sex lives of disabled people are treated very differently. In Denmark, the sexuality of people with disabilities is "acknowledged, discussed, and facilitated" (p. 4), whereas in Sweden, it is "denied, repressed, and discouraged" (p. 4). Moreover, in Sweden only mobility and other "physical" disabilities are recognized, whereas in Denmark the focus is on intellectual disability and group living situations.

This is significant for at least two reasons. One, sex – with ourselves or others – is often considered a private affair in the more privileged parts of the Western world and global north. And two, the topic of sexuality and intellectual disability in particular is taboo. Reading *Loneliness and Its Opposite* with this class presented me with more learning opportunities. While the authors, Kulick and Rydström, make the assumption that disabled people are all potentially sexual, their focus on intellectual disability is courageous and vital. Many disability workers, as well as academics, shy away from this topic because of legal and ethical implications or communications difficulties, but this leaves a large group of disabled people out of the discussion about sexuality and reinforces the myth that sex requires independence and privacy. I had to ask myself why I had not thought much before about intellectual disability and sexuality, or about the implications of well-meaning parents (such as myself) telling children that playing with their genitals is fine, as long as they do it in private. What would I do, I wondered, if my child needed help masturbating? In *Loneliness and Its Opposite*, the class read about parents, mainly mothers, who thought about offering assistance and who hired sex-trade workers. The students also learned about people with intellectual disabilities in Denmark who were able to get help from government sexual advisors, had workers facilitate by positioning them and/or their partners and/or sex toys, and were able to hire sex-trade workers themselves. According to Kulick and Rydström, "Providing disabled adults with access to sexual lives is not just crucial for a life with dignity. It is an issue of fundamental social justice with far reaching consequences for everyone" (2015, p. 292).

Conclusion

Ultimately, I could not have imagined how complex and rewarding this academic endeavour would become. As a feminist, sex-positive professor, I encourage open dialogue and debate. For example, are devotees perverts or do they have just another type of fetish? Should care workers and/or the government assist disabled people with solo and partner sex? Most students appreciated this type of critical pedagogy, even or especially those who come from cultures that forbid such openness, especially for women. Students, like Baden, who challenge what is being studied serve to enrich the classroom experience for everyone. It is my hope that my comfort with sexuality will spread and stay with my students in their future roles as lovers, partners, parents, and perhaps even educators or service providers.

In terms of recommendations for teaching about sexuality in higher education, not just in social work but across many disciplines, this chapter contains examples pertaining to content, curriculum, and methods. Needless to say, disability should always be included. And above all, being at ease with the topic is crucial. If instructors want students to learn about sexuality, we must show that we are comfortable with the topic, especially when confronted with something new that pushes our boundaries. Furthermore, we must be open to students who challenge us. This interaction makes for a dynamic pedagogical experience that goes far beyond learning the facts.

REFERENCES

After hours autism (Adults Only). (2015). Retrieved from http://afterhoursautism.tumblr.com/post/169596033485/every-time-i-get-anywhere-close-to-climaxing-i

American Psychiatric Association. (2013). *Diagnostic and statistical manual of mental disorders* (5th ed.). Arlington, VA: Author.

Bargiela, S., Steward, R., & Mandy, W. (2016). The experiences of late-diagnosed women with autism spectrum conditions: An investigation of the female autism phenotype. *Journal of Autism and Developmental Disorders, 46*(10), 3281–3294. https://doi.org/10.1007/s10803-016-2872-8

Barnes, C., & Mercer, G. (2003). *Disability*. Cambridge: Polity Press.

Brake, E. (n.d.). Amatonormativity. Retrieved from https://elizabethbrake.com.

Butler, J. (1990). *Gender trouble: Feminism and the subversion of identity*. New York: Routledge.

Center for Autism Research. (2017). Romance 101: Dating for adults with ASD. Retrieved from https://www.carautismroadmap.org/romance-101-dating-for-adults-with-asd/

De Beauvoir, S. (1949/1973). *The second sex* (H. M. Parshley, Trans.). New York: Vintage Books.

Elizabeth. (2008, June 4). Asexuality as a disability? Prismatic entanglements. Retrieved from https://prismaticentanglements.com

Hannah, L. A., & Stagg, S. D. (2016). Experiences of sex education and sexual awareness in young adults with autism spectrum disorder. *Journal of Autism and Developmental Disorders, 46*(12), 3678–3687. https://doi.org/10.1007/s10803-016-2906-2

Kaufman, M., Silverberg, C., & Odette, F. (2007). *The ultimate guide to sex and disability: For all of us who live with disabilities, chronic pain & illness*. San Francisco: Cleis Press.

Kulick, D., & Rydström, J. (2015). *Loneliness and its opposite: Sex, disability, and the ethics of engagement.* Durham, NC: Duke University Press.

Kuttai, H. (2010). *Maternity rolls: Pregnancy, childbirth and disability.* Nova Scotia and Winnipeg: Fernwood Publishing.

Lawson, W. (2005). *Sex, sexuality and autism spectrum.* London: Jessica Kingsley Publishers.

Liebowitz, C. (2015, November 12). 3 ways you might be marginalizing disabled asexual people (and what to do about it). Everyday Feminism. Retrieved from https://everydayfeminism.com

McRuer, R., & Mollow, A. (Eds.). (2012). *Sex and disability.* Durham, NC: Duke University Press.

Myhill, G., & Jekel, D. (2008). Asperger marriage: Viewing partnerships thru a different lens. Retrieved from https://www.pathfindersforautism.org /wp-content/uploads/2017/01/Asperger-Marriage.pdf

North, A. (2019, May 3). "I am a woman and I am fast": what Caster Semenya's story says about gender and race in sports. *Vox.* Retrieved from https:// www.vox.com

Puar, J. K. (2017). *The right to maim.* Durham, NC: Duke University Press.

Relationships & Sex. (n.d.). *Disability horizons.* Retrieved from http:// disabilityhorizons.com/category/relationships-and-sex/

Sexuality and Disability. (n.d.). Retrieved from http://sexualityanddisability .org/

Shire, E. (2013, August 5). Dating on the autism spectrum. *The Atlantic.* Retrieved from https://www.theatlantic.com/

Tan, C. (2017, October 30). I'm autistic and sick of feeling excluded from queer spaces: "I do not exist as a fraction, and I cannot extricate my queerness from my autism." *Them.* Retrieved from https://www.them.us

Tarasoff, L. A. "We don't know. We've never had anybody like you before": Barriers to perinatal care for women with physical disabilities. (2017). *Disability and Health Journal, 10*(3), 3426–433. https://doi.org/10.1016 /j.dhjo.2017.03.017

University of Winnipeg. (2019). Course descriptions [PDF file]. Retrieved from https://www.uwinnipeg.ca/academics/calendar/docs/all-course -descriptions.pdf

Withers, A. J. (2012). *Disability politics & theory.* Black Point, NS: Fernwood Publishing.

World Health Organization (WHO). (n.d.). Gender and Genetics. https:// www.who.int/genomics/gender/en/

17 Developing a Sexual Education Workshop: Addressing a Gap in Social Work Education

CHRISTOPHER STERLING-MURPHY AND RICK CSIERNIK

Introduction

Sex research has been derived from various fields including medicine, biology, psychology, sociology, epidemiology, and criminology. As a result, much of the existing literature has been described as medical and pathologizing (Myers & Milner, 2007). This has historically led social workers and other counselling professionals to approach sexuality in terms of "problems to be solved," which can further stigmatize service users, many of whom are already marginalized. Helping professionals have the potential to influence sex research, education, and training in a manner that is less pathologizing and more service-user focused. Examining sexuality from a person-in-environment lens is advantageous compared to traditional approaches that have been based primarily on medical or, contrarily, religious teachings. It can provide more accurate descriptions of sexual behaviours, as well as their implications and origins, that can not only ease service users' anxiety regarding sex and their sexuality(ies) but also enrich their lives, given the importance that sex plays in the human condition, while exploring topics that remain taboo and stigmatized such as polyamoury. Hawkes and Scott (2005) exemplify some critical social influences in their definition of human sexuality:

> Human sexuality is distinct from non-human sexuality in that it is neither immutable nor static but is highly responsive to social forces. Human sexuality is imbued with symbolic meaning and social significance ... given that humans are social beings, human sexuality is inevitably influenced by a person's social location ... forms of social stratification, relating to class, status, gender, ethnicity, age and so on, will influence modes of individual self-expression. (p. 7)

While this chapter focuses on a social work specific study, the findings should be considered in context of what is offered and what is needed in higher education for other helping professions. Sex research in social work remains limited; an increase in such scholarship has been noted (Dunk, 2007; Myers & Milner, 2007).

In the Canadian Association of Social Workers' ([CASW], 2017) description of social work practice, sex therapy is explicitly indicated as a critical service offered by social workers, and yet sex research, education, and training have been widely neglected by the field. CASW's (2005) Code of Ethics states that social workers "uphold the right of clients to be offered the highest quality service possible," and further that they "[limit] professional practice to areas of demonstrated competence" (p. 8). This begs an important question: What do social workers rely on to support service users' sexuality, if not their formal education and training?

To demonstrate this gap in social work education, Glass (2016) examined 67 individual social workers' attitudes regarding sexuality, what informed their response to sexually orientated content and disclosures, as well as the different ways sexuality was addressed in their practice. She found that "88% [of] participants were not required to take any courses that specifically addressed sex and sexuality during their social work program" (p. 20). With regard to elective courses, "66% [of] respondents likewise reported taking no courses that specifically addressed sex and sexuality" (p. 20). As such, "57% [of] participants felt their program had not adequately prepared them to address topics of sex and sexuality with clients" (Glass, 2016, p. 20). Participants overwhelmingly endorsed the inclusion of several topics in social work education, which included sexual pleasure; sexual health; sexual orientation; BDSM (bondage and discipline [B&D]; dominance and submission [D&S]; sadism and masochism [S&M]); and sexual transference and countertransference (Glass, 2016, p. 22). Glass also reported that "94% [of] respondents said that sexuality-related topics are relevant to their clients" (p. 23).

In examining courses offered at accredited Canadian social work programs during the 2019 winter term, the authors likewise found a distinct gap in the availability of sexual education content. Of 41 Canadian BSW programs, 49% (n = 20) offered at least one course that specifically examines sex or sexuality. Twenty-two BSW courses that address sexuality were identified; 18 (82%) examined gender and sexual diversity, three (14%) examined the prevention of or response to sexual violence, while one (5%), explored human sexuality more generally.

A total of eight Canadian MSW courses were identified in the review and only six of 32 (19%) MSW level programs offered at least one course in human sexuality. Five (63%) of these focused on sexual and gender diversity, two (25%) explored sexual health, while one (13%) examined sexual abuse. An analysis of Canadian social work doctoral programs revealed that only two of the 15 programs currently offer courses relating to human sexuality. A total of four courses were identified in our review; three (75%) of which examine sex and gender diversity, while one (25%) examined sexual abuse. Note that no social work course, at either the graduate or undergraduate level, specifically examines sex therapy or sexual desire, pleasure, or wellness.

Needs Assessment

Background

The Professional Development Series at King's University College was designed to provide applied MSW education to graduate students on topics not covered adequately in the curriculum. Students are required to attend a minimum of three out of five annual workshops, each of which is three hours long. As human sexuality was not part of the current curriculum, a workshop, Social Work's Role in Human Sexuality, was proposed for presentation during the winter 2019 academic term to fill gaps in student knowledge. The committee responsible for workshop development approved the proposal that led to the development of a Needs Assessment as the first step in creating the sexuality workshop.

Instrument

The needs assessment instrument (Appendix B) developed by the authors asked students what education, pertaining to human sexuality they had received thus far in their postsecondary studies, which topics relating to sexuality they wished to learn about, and the means through which they wished to be taught. Ethics approval was obtained from the King's University College Research Ethics and Review Committee. The instrument was administered during class time in required courses during the fall 2018 term. This led to a response rate of 100% among MSW candidates (n = 46) and 95% among BSW students (n = 82).

Results

The majority of MSW (72%) and BSW (60%) students described their knowledge of topics related to sexuality as adequate, 13% of MSWs and 22% of BSWs reported extensive knowledge, while 11% of MSWs and

16% of BSWs indicated limited knowledge. Respondents were also asked how comfortable they felt in discussing sexually orientated materials. The majority indicated they were somewhat comfortable (58%), with 25% reporting feeling very comfortable, 16% indicating they felt uncomfortable, and only 1% feeling very uncomfortable.

When asked what topics graduate and undergraduate social work students have learned about thus far as part of their training at King's University College, the most common responses were the social construction of human sexuality (69%), sexual health (30%), and social workers' role in service users' sexuality (20%). Nonetheless, results indicated that less than 5% of respondents identified having learned about sexual dysfunction, sex therapy, sex scripts, or the sexual response cycle as part of their social work education (Figure 17.1).

Students were next asked to identify which topics they would find most beneficial to be included in a professional development workshop regarding their current or future practice. In order of most to least frequent, responses were best practices for common sexual concerns (92%); social workers' role in clients' sexuality (91%); best practices for supporting sexual health (89%); working with specific populations (87%); sex positivity (79%); future issues in human sexuality (78%); best practices for supporting sexual dysfunctions (72%); critical analyses of modern sex scripts (52%); and the history of sex research (38%). Seven per cent of respondents reported other topics in an open-text field. These included sex work, childhood sexual behaviours, sexuality on campus, and how to properly discuss sexual identity. Interestingly, two respondents indicated that they did not see any benefit in continuing training in the area of human sexuality (Figure 17.2).

When asked which specific service-user populations on which they needed to receive additional education or training with regard to supporting sex and sexuality, respondents indicated LGBT2Q+ communities (87%), youth (81%), sex workers (74%), people with (dis)abilities (68%), aging populations (56%), and people with paraphilias (i.e., intense sexual arousal to atypical objects, situations, fantasies, behaviours, or individuals [APA, 2013]) 47%. Conservative religious individuals, sex offenders, sex "addicts," and polyamorous and palliative populations were also identified as groups for which students desired more education.

Students were additionally asked to identify how they would most prefer to learn about sexually orientated material in a workshop setting. This question raised the greatest amount of variability from respondents. The most preferred approach was case studies (82%), followed by lecture style (69%), panel discussion (66%), videos (54%), small group discussions (52%), large group discussions (46%), roleplay/practice exercises

Figure 17.1. Topics social work students have learned during their education at King's

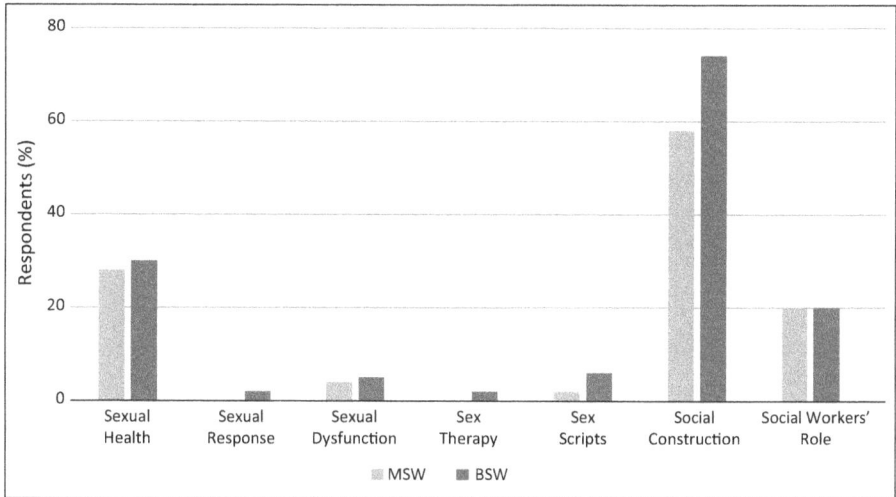

(19%), independent reflection exercises (18%), and taking sexuality questionnaires (15%) (Figure 17.3).

The final needs assessment question was qualitative in nature and asked participants what questions they would want addressed at the professional development workshop. A total of 41 (32%) students responded. Fourteen responses were general comments, primarily pertaining to the importance of sex education or comments acknowledging current lack of knowledge, exemplified by one participant's response: "I don't know what I don't know." The main themes that arose were ethical considerations when working in this field of practice, the desire for more knowledge regarding specific groups (e.g., LGBT2Q+, youth, aging and palliative populations, and those with ability issues), best practices, appropriate resources, and questions relating to sex, consent, and safety (n = 3). Examples of responses to this question included "how to confront your own bias" and "how far can you go ... and still be ethical?" Of those questions concerning LGBT2Q+ individuals, four were concerned with supporting service users who make disclosures about their sexual orientation and two referred to the use of appropriate or nonstigmatizing language. An example of a question asked in this theme was "How do I support someone questioning her/his/their sexuality?"

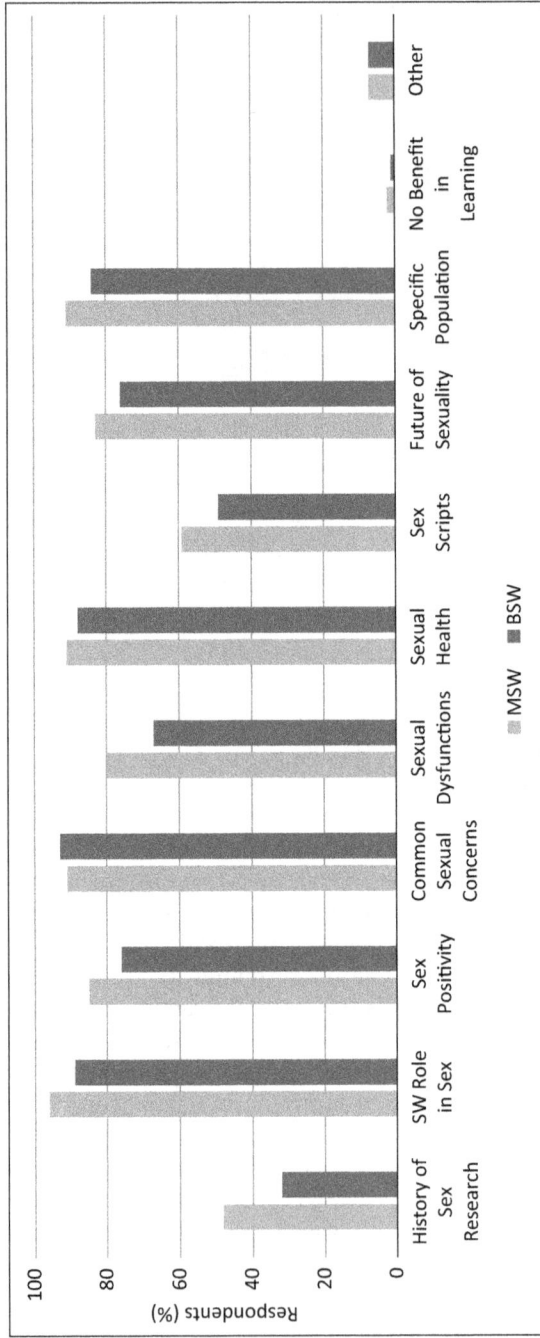

Figure 17.2. Topics to include in a workshop on sexuality

Figure 17.3. Preferred method of instruction

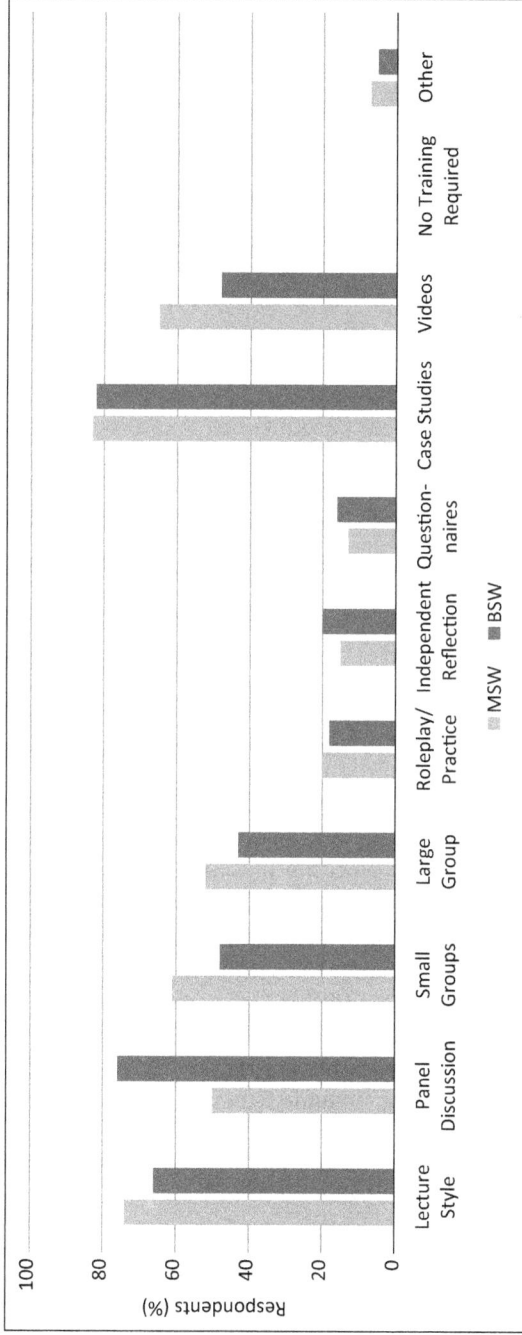

Theoretical Orientation

The insights obtained through the needs assessment informed the selection of which topics would be included in the workshop and the medium through which they would be presented. As presenter, the first author was tasked with selecting a theoretical framework from which the material could be presented. As mentioned previously, traditional sexuality scholarship and education have been described as medicalizing and pathologizing, with little input from the social work profession (Myers & Milner, 2007). People have unique relationships to their own sexuality, and these are informed by culture, gender, sexual orientation, ethnicity, race, residential status, and past experiences of trauma. It was important to the researchers to discuss sexuality in a manner that recognized that people differ widely in their responses to sexual content (Myers & Milner, 2007). The presenter, who is also first author, therefore chose three principles to guide how the material would be presented and discussed. They included being 1) anti-oppressive; 2) trauma informed; and 3) sex positive. The following section discusses application of these principles.

Anti-oppressive Instruction

An anti-oppressive perspective also informed the workshop's construction. Bhuyan, Bejan, and Jeyapal (2017) state, "[Anti-oppressive practice] in social work aims to educate against multiple forms of oppression, usually defined by identity characteristics (race, gender, class) in order to address structural inequalities that impact service users and the social worker" (p. 376). This position aligns with the CASW's Code of Ethics (2005), which identifies the pursuit of social justice as a guiding principal for social work practice. Evoking an anti-oppressive lens is particularly important when educating about sex and is appropriate for all helping professionals as it calls for a more accepting lens that celebrates diversity and inclusion. In addition, it makes students more aware that unexamined heteronormative attitudes, beliefs, and discourses reinforce discrimination, harassment, and stigma directed toward various groups based solely on their sex, sexuality(ies), and identity. Anti-oppressive instruction increases the likelihood that participants understand how a variety of social influences and intersecting oppressions work to maintain these problems in marginalized communities.

Anti-oppressive education was demonstrated from the onset of the presentation to encourage a climate of safety and critical thinking. Initially, the presenter chose to read an Indigenous land acknowledgment to recognize the traditional and rightful owners of the land where the presentation was hosted. This acknowledgment was regionally specific and named the local First Nations communities. An anti-oppressive framework was further actualized by requesting participants to share their pronouns. This recognized and validated individuals' identities by respecting the gender pronouns they chose to use and attempted to mitigate the harmful effects people experience when they are misgendered. In addition, inviting a discussion about preferred pronouns raises consciousness for participants who are cisgender or use the pronouns that correspond with the gender they were assigned at birth and who may not understand the importance of inquiring about pronouns.

As anti-oppressive practice emphasizes the importance of social location and cultural identity, the presenter chose to disclose his identities to provide participants with more context. As a young, cisgender, Caucasian gay male, the speaker shared that despite having many identities and personality traits, being gay is often identified by others as the central piece of his identity. The audience was encouraged to think about the ways they discuss queer people and people with "othered" sexuality, and to consider the language they use and the ways it may strip others of their identity.

Trauma-Informed Instruction

A trauma-informed lens was central to the workshop's construction (Levinson, 2017) and, as with an anti-oppressive approach, is applicable to all academic disciplines. Within service delivery, trauma-informed care includes providing a safe and collaborative environment that is free from physical threats and potential re-traumatization for both service providers and service users (Wilson & Nochajski, 2016). The intent of using a trauma-informed instruction approach in education is to provide students with an understanding of how trauma impacts their own lives and the lives of service users. Further, trauma-informed education encourages the use of trauma-informed interventions with service users, while also prioritizing self-care for the worker, regardless of profession. Fallot and Harris (2009) outline five components to facilitating a trauma-informed environment: safety; trustworthiness; choice; collaboration; and empowerment. Adopting a trauma-informed stance is particularly important when discussing personal and intimate themes related to sexuality, as it recognizes that trauma is pervasive.

Central to trauma-informed instruction is the idea that classroom behaviours, characteristics, discussions, and content can be triggering to learners. Bentley (2017) argues that "triggering is a complex phenomenon and adverse reactions can be caused by factors as random and unexpected as a particular smell" (p. 472). As triggers are so individualized and are based on the experience of individual trauma, there is no way to know exactly what will be triggering for participants. Common triggering themes related to sexuality include homo-, bi- and trans-phobia, racism and sexism, fertility issues, and discussion related to incest, sexual abuse, intimate-partner violence, and pornography (Banyard, Williams, & Siegel, 2003; Kammerer & Mazelis, 2006; Kearns & Calhoun, 2010). To foster an educational climate of safety for participants, the presenter read a trigger warning at the onset of the presentation:

> The following presentation will contain themes related to sexuality, which some people may find triggering. If you feel you have been triggered, you are welcome to take a break, or leave the presentation at any time. Common triggering topics include sexual assault; child abuse; pornography; pregnancy/childbirth; homo-/bi-/trans-phobia; sexism; and racism. While no topic is explicitly "off-limits," please be mindful that these topics could be triggering throughout your discussions.

During a discussion regarding body image, the presenter was reporting that women's most common body image concern is "degree of fat" (Wiederman & Sarin, 2014). The presenter chose to disclose his own personal discomfort with the word "fat," based on previous life experience of being overweight. Participants were cautioned that there will be times that we are triggered by service users and that one way we can counter this negative experience is to better understand our own triggers.

Sex-Positive Instruction

Sex positivity was a third foundation of the workshop. This should be part of any sex education training, regardless of academic discipline. It refers to a nonpathologizing attitude toward sexuality. Burnes, Singh, and Witherspoon (2017) explain, "Sex positive approaches begin with the assumption that a wide variety of sex practices and desires are an inherently healthy and important component of human development and connection" (p. 472). Sex-positive education emphasizes sexual pleasure as an integral piece of sex and sexuality. As presenter, the first author supported a sex-positive approach using intentional language, a focus on wellness and pleasure, as well as a nonjudgmental approach and professional presentation of the material. Accordingly, the ways in which sexuality is conceptualized and spoken about have substantive consequences on social work practice (Myers & Milner, 2007). The use of a sex-positive lens aligns with the World Health Organization's (2006) call for all health professionals to adopt sex-positive models and shift toward nonpathologizing sexuality frameworks. Williams, Christensen, and Capous-Desyllas (2016) further demonstrated that social workers and other counselling professionals who adopted a sex-positive framework expanded their awareness of sexual diversity and therefore were better equipped to empower service users who were sexually marginalized.

As many of the desired topics identified in the needs assessment deal primarily with sexual risk, the presenter was tasked with presenting this information in a way that was congruent with a sex-positive approach. As an example, participants identified assessing participants' sexual health as a desired topic of instruction. Traditional approaches to sexual health education have been identified as being sex negative, risk focused, and in many ways oppressive. These claims are the result of too heavy a focus on sexually transmitted infections and targeted populations identified as being at increased risk, and an omission of discussion related to pleasure, desire, and wellness. One provincial sexual-health campaign designed for men who have sex with men (MSM), The Sex You Want (Gay Men's Sexual Health Alliance, 2019), challenged the traditional approach to sexual health education by working from an anti-oppressive and sex-positive approach. A central tenet of the campaign is that people can still have pleasurable and desirable sex while making decisions regarding their own sexual health. Central to this campaign is affording agency to individuals to make their own informed choices regarding sexual health.

Assessing Sexual Health: Three-Stage Model

In the workshop, a three-stage model for assessing sexual health was presented, which was similarly sex positive and respected the self-determination of service users. More specifically, the first stage encourages participants to first assess for risk by asking service users what they know about their own sexual health and offering supplementary information. The second involves listening to service users' sexual-health decisions and supporting them, and the third requires developing an action plan that addresses potential barriers outlined by the service user. Workshop participants were additionally made aware about the ways in which some service users can be made to feel marginalized when too many sexual risk-assessment questions are asked. For example, MSM carry an increased burden of HIV transmission. Consequently, when interacting with healthcare professionals, many MSM feel that their sexuality is viewed as inherently and stereotypically "risky." When evoking sex-negative and risk-oriented assessments of sexual health, well-intentioned clinicians therefore run the risk of further marginalizing already oppressed service users.

Workshop on Sexuality[1]

As stated earlier, students' feedback from the needs assessment informed the development of a three-hour workshop. The goals of the presentation became five-fold: to

1. establish a climate of comfort and safety;
2. have participants begin to confront their own values and biases related to sex and sexuality;
3. help participants better understand their role as social workers in service users' sexuality;
4. enter a conversation about what "normal" and "abnormal" sexuality is, if such distinctions exist; and
5. provide specific and practical information to participants on the topics identified in the needs assessment.

Workshop attendees were welcomed, then read the trigger warning mentioned earlier, followed by the Indigenous land acknowledgment. Next, participants were asked to introduce themselves to those around them and to share their names, preferred pronouns, comfort level in discussing sexuality, and one thing they find attractive in a prospective partner. As a large group, in order to demonstrate the diversity of motivations people have for engaging in sexual activity, participants were invited to share why people have sex. In small groups, participants were given the CASW Code of Ethics (2005) and were invited to pick one principle and determine how it could be interpreted with regard to their role in service users' sex and sexuality. Participants were then introduced to the nine sexual dysfunctions outlined in the *Diagnostic and Statistical Manual-5* ([*DSM-5*] American Psychiatric Association, 2013). Descriptions, prevalence, and critiques for each of the disorders were derived from Binik and Hall's (2014) *Principles and Practice of Sex Therapy*. Throughout this discussion, the presenter encouraged participants to consider the ways that the diagnostic criteria are oppressive, heteronormative, and medically biased. As an example, the presenter discussed how Sexual Sadism Disorder and other sexual dysfunctions outlined in the *DSM-5* are often misinterpreted to include any and all individuals who enjoy sadism as part of a healthy and consensual sex life.

---

1 For more specifics regarding actual content of the workshop, please send an e-mail to rcsierni@uwo.ca.

The second half of the presentation began with a discussion about how to assess sexual health, in which participants were introduced to the assessment model outlined above, then asked to explore the concepts through the use of a case study. Next, the presenter focused on two populations that emerged as the most desired topics in the needs assessment: namely, youth and LGBT2Q+ communities. The presenter discussed porn literacy for youth and discussed the ways social workers can be sex positive while remaining ethical and professional. In discussing LGBT2Q+ communities, participants were encouraged to take a stance of curiosity, to not make assumptions, and to not view queer sexuality as inherently risky. Respecting the findings from the needs assessment, the final component of the presentation addressed two common problems social workers are likely to face: negative body image and infidelity.

Critique

While participants' feedback for the workshop was overwhelmingly positive, the authors acknowledge that, as a work in progress, there were areas necessary for improvement. Key omissions were the lack of inclusion of feminist, disability, and queer theories. O'Quinn and Fields (2019) discuss how these theories add another layer of understanding of sex and sexuality: "Queer health science scholars, like Black feminist and other critical scholars, delineate the social construction of normative understandings of healthy bodies: hegemonic discourse on race, gender, and able-bodiedness informs scientific understandings of health and pathologizes certain racialized, sexualized, and gendered bodies" (p. 5). By including feminist, disability, and queer theories of sexuality in future presentations, participants could gain a broader understanding of the various ways social location interacts with sexual experience, increase their ability to take a not-knowing stance, and potentially be better able to provide better service to service users. Reflecting the above-noted critique, core features of the presentation have since been added to an elective offering in the program, with the goal of making this presentation an ongoing part of graduate student professional development moving forward.

Conclusion

This chapter explored the need for the social work profession to better educate new social workers about sexuality(ies); however, the findings are certainly applicable to other helping professions. Research suggests that social work students are currently inadequately trained in the area of practice and do not know how to discuss sex and issues of sexuality with service users, despite most expressing an interest in obtaining more knowledge and training in this area (Dunk, 2007; Glass, 2016; Grady & Abramson, 2011). Our needs assessment identified students' previous exposure to postsecondary sex education; areas in which they needed more knowledge; preferred method of instruction when learning about sexually orientated material; and comfort levels in discussing this content with service users. The results of the needs assessment were used in the construction of a three-hour professional development workshop that was taught from a sex-positive, anti-oppressive, and trauma-informed approach. The workshop's evaluation indicated that the material was well received by participants, as was the manner of presentation. Their major critique was that more time was needed to cover the material in greater depth, particularly the specific populations, given the dearth of education in this area due to a lack in the core curriculum of their school of social work. This process could be easily repeated with other helping professions to likewise ascertain their specific educational needs pertaining to sexual education, as well as to ascertain how students would like to be better informed on these important issues and topics, which range from abortion to contraception to normalizing sexual pleasure.

REFERENCES

American Psychiatric Association. (2013). *Diagnostic and statistical manual of mental disorders* (5th ed.). Arlington: Author.

Banyard, V., Williams, L., & Siegel, J. (2003). Retraumatization among adult women sexually abused in childhood: Exploratory analyses in a prospective study. *Journal of Child Sexual Abuse, 11*(3), 19–48. https://doi.org/10.1300/j070v11n03_02

Bentley, M. (2017). Trigger warnings and the student experience. *Politics, 37*(4), 470–485. https://doi.org/10.1177/0263395716684526

Bhuyan, R., Bejan, R., & Jeyapal, D. (2017). Social workers' perspectives on social justice in social work education: When mainstreaming social justice masks structural inequalities. *Social Work Education, 36*(4), 373–390. https://doi.org/10.1080/02615479.2017.1298741

Binik, Y. M., & Hall, K. S. K. (Eds). (2014). *Principles and practices of sex therapy.* New York: Guilford Press.

Burnes, T. R., Singh, A. A., & Witherspoon, R. G. (2017). Sex positivity and counseling psychology: An introduction to the major contribution. *The Counseling Psychologist, 45*(4), 470–486. https://doi.org/10.1177/0011000017710216

Canadian Association of Social Workers. (2005). *Code of ethics.* Retrieved from
https://www.casw-acts.ca/files/documents/casw_code_of_ethics.pdf

Canadian Association of Social Workers. (2017). *What is social work?* Retrieved
from https://www.casw-acts.ca/en/what-social-work

Dunk, P. (2007). Everyday sexuality and social work: Locating sexuality in
professional practice and education. *Social Work & Society, 5*(2).

Fallot, R. D., & Harris, M. (2009). *Creating cultures of trauma-informed
care (CCTIC): A self-assessment and planning protocol.* Washington, DC:
Community Connections. Retrieved from https://www.theannainstitute
.org/CCTICSELFASSPP.pdf.

Gay Men's Sexual Health Alliance. (2019). The sex you want. Retrieved from
https://thesexyouwant.ca/

Glass, S. R. (2016). It's time to talk about sex and social work: Why human
sexuality education matters for social work practice. *Theses, Dissertations,
and Projects.*1695. Retrieved from https://scholarworks.smith.edu/cgi
/viewcontent.cgi?article=2788&context=theses.

Grady, M. D., & Abramson, J. M. (2011). Has social work heeded the call?
Sex offender content in social work. *Social Work Education, 30*(4), 440–453.
https://doi.org/10.1080/02615479.2010.500659

Hawkes, G., & Scott, J. G. (Eds.). (2005). *Perspectives in human sexuality.* South
Melbourne: Oxford University Press.

Kammerer, N., & Mazelis, R. (2006). After the crisis: Trauma and retraumatization.
Paper presented at *After the crisis: Healing from trauma after disasters expert panel,*
24–25, April 2006, Bethesda MD. Retrieved from: https://www.homelesshub
.ca/resource/after-crisis-trauma-and-retraumatization-issue-brief

Kearns, M., & Calhoun, K. (2010). Sexual revictimization and interpersonal
effectiveness. *Violence and Victims, 25*(4), 504–517. https://doi.org/10.1891
/0886-6708.25.4.504

Levinson, J. (2017). Trauma informed social work practice, *Social work, 62*(2),
105–113.

Myers, S., & Milner, J. (2007). *Sexual issues in social work.* Bristol: Policy Press.

O'Quinn, J., & Fields, J. (2019). The future of evidence: Queerness in
progressive visions of sexuality education. *Sexuality Research and Social Policy.*
doi:10.1007/s13178–019–00395-z

Wiederman, M. W., & Sarin, S. (2014). Body image and sexuality In Y. M. Binik
& K. S. Hall (Eds.), *Principles and practice of sex therapy,* 5th ed. New York:
Guildford Press.

Wilson, B., & Nochajski, T. H. (2016). Evaluating the impact of trauma-informed
care (TIC) perspective in social work curriculum. *Social Work Education, 35*(5),
589–602. https://doi.org/10.1080/02615479.2016.1164840

Williams, D., Christensen, M. C., & Capous-Desyllas, M. (2016). Social
work practice and sexuality: Applying a positive sexuality model to

enhance diversity and resolve problems. *Families in Society: The Journal of Contemporary Social Services, 97*(4), 287–294. https://doi.org/10.1606 /1044-3894.2016.97.35

World Health Organization. (2006). *Defining sexual health: Report of a technical consultation on sexual health.* Retrieved from https://www.who .int/reproductivehealth/topics/gender_rights/defining_sexual_health .pdf?ua=1

18 Can We Just Stop Faking It? Real Talk about Sex and Sexualities in the Classroom

SUSAN HILLOCK

As demonstrated across this book, the topic of human sexuality is important and an integral part of our emotional, physical, social, and psychological well-being. Despite progress in terms of developing sex theory/research and sex-positive approaches, as well as the growth of sexuality programs, specializations, and courses, many of the book's contributors have argued that colleagues remain reticent about discussing the topic or teaching about it and may not necessarily have the skills or training to do so. As well, particularly in professional programs and the helping professions, there remains a significant lack of discipline-specific theoretical and/or applied literature, research, exemplars, and scholarship available on what to teach and how to best teach sexuality(ies). Additionally, although it is evolving, what has been historically available has tended toward sex negativity, cisgenderism, and heteronormativity. Accordingly, this book has made a comprehensive effort to fill gaps in higher education, demonstrate the need for multidisciplinary approaches to this area of study, and encourage real talk (and teaching) about sex and sexuality(ies) in the classroom.

This concluding chapter continues these efforts by highlighting key themes. Based on the preceding chapters, as well as my own experience and research, I present recommendations regarding what sex education content should be taught in higher education, suggest helpful sources and models that readers can replicate in their teaching and practice, and explore how best to teach sexuality(ies) in higher education.

Key Themes

In this book, several key themes have been highlighted. In my view, the contributors have successfully demonstrated that many disciplines in higher education, particularly in professional programs and the helping professions, would benefit from the inclusion (and/or increase) of sex education; outlined the merits of multidisciplinary approaches to teaching sex; and emphasized the need to utilize inclusive approaches that interrogate heteronormativity, monogamy, and cisgenderism, while also celebrating diversity. Going forward, I would like to expand further on three significant themes: sex-positive versus sex-negative approaches, common barriers to teaching sex education, and comfort with sexuality(ies).

Sex-Positive versus Sex-Negative Approaches

This book has highlighted the problems associated with using a risk-averse/sex-negative approach and has instead promulgated sex-positive/sex-forward approaches as a better fit for this work. Before the twentieth century, most sex- and sexuality-related discourse focused on sex negativity and abstinence, the dominant perspective of the time (Mosher, 2017). Discussions that focused on sex negativity presented sex, its activities, and sexualities that differed from the societal norm of heterosexism as "risky, problematic … [and] adversarial" (Williams, Prior, & Wegner, 2013, p. 1). In fact, these views, some of which are still encouraged in discussions today, have emphasized "sexism, racism, homophobia, and ageism" (p. 1).

Historically, in terms of sex education, especially in the helping professions, as well as in some disciplines within higher education, there was scant content and information available, and what was available tended to be from sex-negative/risk approaches, focusing on problems, differences, and dysfunction, stopping violence, and treating heterosexuality and monogamy as the "norm." Accordingly, this sex-negative or risk-based approach, emphasizing vulnerability, violence, and abuse, dominated the helping professions, many professional programs, and healthcare for years. And although currently there has been significant progress and research within specific disciplines such as sexuality, psychology, disability, gender, porn, and queer studies, many academic and professional programs, as well as the helping professions, still have minimal content about pleasure, desire, bodies, masturbation, or other diverse sexual identities and behaviours such as the BDSM community, polyamoury, nonmonogamous relationships, and folks who identify as asexual, intersex, trans, pansexual, and queer (Hillock & Mulé, 2016). Specifically, in terms of social work education, one could even argue that coverage of sex topics – if there is any at all – tends to be based on a Western white heteronormative monogamous dominant paradigm that excludes, through invisibility, judgement, and shaming, as well as active repression and oppression, many other modes of sexuality (Dunk, 2007;

Hicks, 2008; Hillock & Mulé, 2016; Jeyasingham, 2008). In addition, common (and somewhat controversial and stigmatized) areas of counselling, medicine, and social work and human-service practice (such as referral to abortion, contraception, trans/surgery, STI and HIV testing, family planning, and fertility services) are still not widely discussed in classrooms.

In contrast, sex positivity emphasizes sexual pleasure and desire as integral parts of sex and sexuality. Incorporating positive sexuality into higher education provides students with accurate basic information about sex, breaks the silence, interrogates heteronormativity, and smashes taboos (Johnson, 2009; Williams, Prior, & Wegner, 2013). As Burnes, Singh, and Witherspoon (2017) explain, "sex positive approaches begin with the assumption that a wide variety of sex practices and desires are an inherently healthy and important component of human development and connection" (p. 472). Comparatively, societies that encompass healthier, more positive discourses of sex and sexuality(ies) have broader and more inclusive perspectives. As Agocha, Asencio, and Decena (2014) argue, historically, sex education tended to be West- and andro-centric, compared to differing sexual constructs and histories from around the world. Schwartz and Rubel-Lifschitz (2009) found that people in countries that are more sex positive and have greater sexual equality – and that teach forms of sex education that shame less and are more representative of all genders and sexuality(ies) – tend to have healthier sexual relationships.

From an inclusive perspective, Shuttleworth (2007) also notes that when "sexuality studies and the sexual rights movement [embrace] disability," this further promotes ethical inclusion and education of the entire community (p. 3). Another example of diversity is from the LGBTQI+ community. Rather than engaging in heteronormative views about what is "normal," we celebrate all kinds of diverse sexual desires, behaviours, and identities (e.g., sex before and outside of marriage/relationships, multiple or zero sexual partners, kink, and so on) (Hillock & Mulé, 2016; Williams et al., 2013). According to Williams et al. (2013),

A sex-positive approach means being open, communicative, and accepting of individuals' differences related to sexuality and sexual behaviour. Sex positivity is not about having frequent sex or condoning sexual activity per se ... A sex-positive approach is about allowing for a wide rage of sexual expression that takes into account sexual identities, orientations, and behaviours; gender presentation; accessible health care and education and multiple dimensions of human diversity ... It is important that the topic of sex can be discussed in an open, respectful, and non-judgemental manner ... When sex is a taboo topic or when it is talked about in whispers or hushed tones (signs of sex negativity), it severely restricts the range of human diversity generally and contributes to marginalization and other-ing. (p. 1)

However, although the sexual liberation era of the 1960s is long gone, this does not mean that today all students (or, for that matter, instruc-tors) are comfortable with sex-positive discourse and content. Indeed, teachers can run into difficult classroom situations when some students, for a variety of reasons, are resistant to this curriculum content.

Common Barriers to Teaching Sex Education

There is a variety of reasons why instructors might avoid the topic of sex in their courses, including instructor discomfort; embarrassment/ shame; trauma histories; a lack of training and education/preparation; limited knowledge; no sense of competency or confidence in the sub-ject matter; repression related to family background or diverse religious and cultural contexts; as well as differing and shifting religious, moral, and spiritual views (Schaub, Willis, & Dunk-West, 2017; Stayton, 1998). It can also depend on where instructors reside and where they teach, as well as the support (or lack thereof) of colleagues and administration (Sloane, 2014). In terms of healthcare professionals, Monteiro-Cesnik and Zerbini (2017) found that they "may feel insecure addressing issues of sexuality" and identified a "need for professional development" (p. 2). In addition, depending on the academic discipline, educators and practitioners may think that sexual teaching is out of their discipline-specific domain or scope of practice (Sloane, 2014). Academics also note that there can be a stigma attached to sex research, scholarship, and teaching that may result in less departmental, collegial, and institutional support, and negatively effect tenure, promotion, and publication out-comes (Fletcher, Dowsett, Duncan, Slavin, & Corboz, 2013; Hammond & Kingston, 2014). As well, sex education is "highly contentious ... political and politicized" (Fletcher, Dowsett, Duncan, Slavin, & Corboz, p. 319), thus making teaching sex a risky proposition, as mentioned earlier in Chapter 1.

Moreover, students can be resistant to sex education for many of the same reasons outlined above. The same analysis can also be applied to understanding why some patients/service users feel uncomfortable dis-cussing sex with a care provider. As Athol, Rosen, Perelman, and Rubio-Aurioles (2013) point out, they may think that they are bothering the care provider or that sex is not an appropriate subject to bring up in cer-tain settings. They may feel a sense of embarrassment and shame because of social and cultural taboos, think they are imposing, or believe that there is no opportunity to openly discuss sex. On the other hand, clinicians report a variety of reasons for not bringing sex up, including a lack of time, fear of offending, and lack of proficiency related to interviewing and communication skills (ibid.).

Comfort with Sexuality(ies)

As I explained in Chapter 1, it is critical that social workers and other care providers feel comfortable with sexually explicit content, intimate topics, and words and phrases that the general public may use (e.g., pussy instead of vagina or cock instead of penis). It is also essential that we demonstrate comfort in terms of our own sexuality(ies), identity(ies), and bodies, so that in therapeutic encounters, we are not startled, shocked, or judgmental when service users talk about sexuality. If we are uncomfortable, they are likely to sense our anxiety. We might react nonverbally in ways that give people the message that we are not open to hearing their story, are negatively judging them, or are trying to blame and shame them. As a result, not only will service users choose not to share their intimate and private thoughts, beliefs, and experiences with us, but also they might emotionally shut down or minimize/deny their experiences and pain. Therefore, even if we do not to intend to cause harm, people may leave our offices feeling ashamed and judged.

Although we are not in therapeutic relationships, the same principles can apply to teaching and how we handle student disclosures, especially in terms of diverse sexual practices, sexual violence, and trauma experiences. As instructors, we need to feel comfortable with our own sexuality(ies) in order to handle these situations and effectively teach this content. One interesting suggestion from the literature that aims to increase people's comfort with talking and teaching about sex is outlined by Glickman (2000). He advises that we need to find new ways of speaking and teaching about sex. To do this, he utilizes variations of a metaphor that compares sex to food. According to Glickman, this "takes much of the reaction out of the discussion" (para. 1). For instance, it is culturally and socially acceptable to ask people what food they like or dislike, how often they prefer to eat, and where they like to eat. One can also ask people if they prefer to eat alone or with others. Another variation in terms of diversity in food is that personal choice is supported, so some people are vegan, some prefer breakfast rather than dinner, and so on. He argues that this food–sex metaphor uses humour to encourage creativity and ease conversations about a controversial subject.

Sex Education Content in Higher Education: Knowledge, Attitude, and Skills

As recommended in this book's introduction, in my view, the book's contributors have successfully demonstrated that the helping professions and some disciplines in higher education would benefit from including and/or increasing education about sex and sexuality(ies) in their programs and courses. If we accept that premise, then what follows next are practical questions about the content we should be teaching and how we should teaching it. In terms of planning what sex education content may be required, it is also important to consider differences across disciplinarian lines, as well as differences across bachelor, master, and doctoral programs.

According to Sloane (2014), without the inclusion of formal direct sex training, education, and discussion in higher education, the default position then is to "rely on knowledge, skill, and attitudes that are the result of limited personal experience, sex education as adolescents, and representations of sex in popular culture" (p. 45). In addition, Monteiro-Cesnik and Zerbini (2017) found that even "higher education courses in health care do not provide adequate training, and therefore the students are insufficiently prepared to deal with sexuality issues" (p. 7). Obviously, these educational gaps can have detrimental effects on students, service users, and society at large. To remedy this, the literature recommends that instructors incorporate the following sexual content areas: knowledge gains (i.e., cognition); attitude shifts (i.e., affect); and skill development (i.e., behaviour), sometimes referred to as KAS (Monteiro-Cesnik & Zerbini, 2017; Stayton, 1998; Werley, 2016).

Knowledge Gains

More broadly, although the following reference is from the 1970s, geared to medical students, couched in a traditional gender binary, and problem based, the basic goals of good sex education have not changed much over the last five decades. In fact, educators can adapt the following basics to fit more current language choices, timelines, content, and academic disciplines, so that after participating in sexuality education programming, the student is

> able to listen to and talk with patients about sex without experiencing embarrassment and anxiety; has an appreciation and acceptance of a wide variety of sexual behaviors outside his or her own range of experience; is sufficiently self aware about his or her own prejudices and biases, and to appreciate the ways in which these can interfere with professional objectivity; is aware of the subtleties of non-verbal communication that might indicate the presence of a sexual problem underlying other presenting symptoms; has sufficient

---

Box 18.1: Basic Sex Education Components

Historical, cultural, and social theories and perspectives
Anatomy and physiology
Reproduction, fertility, contraception, and abortion
Psychosexual development and functioning over the life cycle
Physical, psychological, emotional, and behavioural aspects
Sexual response cycle: Discourses of desire and pleasure
Heteronormativity, cisgenderism, and sex/gender identity(ies)
Sexual diversity
Intersectional analysis: Gender, race, disability, age, and class
Sexual violence and trauma
Common sexual concerns and symptoms (organic, psychological, and
    socio-cultural causes)
Effects of medication
Sexual wellness, citizenship, and global human rights
Policy, politics, and social justice
Permission asking/consent seeking/confidentiality
Communication, interviewing, and therapy skills
Education and research methodologies
Media and technology

Source: Adapted from Dunk, 2007; Fletcher, Dowsett, Duncan, Slavin, &
Corboz, 2013; Monteiro-Cesnik & Zerbini, 2017; Rowntree, 2014; Sangra,
2016; Stanley, 1979; Stayton, 1998.

---

knowledge and interviewing skills to be able to take an accurate and sensitive
history in which the sexual problem is clearly defined. (Stanley, 1979, p. 184)

Of course, not all academic disciplines, programs, and courses require this
depth of knowledge, have the time to dedicate to comprehensive coverage, nor is the content above always appropriate or a good fit for everyone.
Each discipline needs to decide what basic sex education knowledge its
students need to competently practise in their respective fields. Indeed,
the following content suggestions are not meant to provide a cookie-cutter
one-size-fits-all formula but to provide a starting point for instructors to cre-
atively think about how to integrate relevant pieces into their teaching and
curriculum planning. Although not an exhaustive list, Box 18.1 identifies
basic sex education components that are recommended in the literature.

In professional programs, along with these components, we also tend to teach more advanced and discipline-specific skills. Examples include more in-depth assessment, interviewing, communication, and therapeutic skills; detailed reviews of our legal, moral, ethical, and professional boundaries and standards, obligations, and duties; teaching students how to ask for permission, seek consent, and maintain confidentiality, as well as how to ask services users about sex, take a sex history, and determine what service users need. It is also critical that we know the limits of our skills and abilities, knowledge, professional domains, and scopes of practice. Knowing how, when, and to whom to refer is also very important (Stayton, 1998). To some extent (dependent on discipline), beginner and/or front-line practitioners may also need to know "available treatment models and the appropriateness and effectiveness of each" (Stayton, 1998, p. 29). However, this depth may beyond the scope of many bachelor and college programs. For some, such as specialists in the medical field or sex therapists, basic sex education will not be adequate: they require more intensive training and supervision at master and doctoral levels, and may need to fulfil continuing education and professional development requirements over the spans of their careers.

Attitude Shifts

In terms of sex education for caregiving professions, students' attitudes should be explored, reflected on, and perhaps shifted before students are deemed competent to work with vulnerable individuals and groups. Specifically, Stayton (1998) argues that "the health care professional needs to be keenly aware of his or her own attitudes, feelings, and judgments about all areas of sexuality, and should have a basic knowledge and the skills to address the sexual concerns of the patient, client, or student" (p. 26). Indeed, this self-awareness can assist students to "more effectively assist clients with their sexuality" (p. 29).

If this is accurate, what attitudes, then, do we want to target for change and how can we support this transformational learning? Stayton (1998) proposes that the best way to change/shift people's attitudes about sex is "desensitization and resensitization" (p. 28). The aim of these processes is "desensitization to hasty or emotional overreaction" and a move "toward gentle, humanistic, and professional understanding of the sexuality of both self and others" (Chilgren, Rosenberg, & Cole, 1971, as cited in Stayton, 1998, p. 28). There are various methods to achieve this "implosion," including being exposed to explicit films, open and direct sex talk, and "the use of fantasy, experiential exercises, and guided imagery followed by discussion" (p. 28). In fact, Stayton's (1998) research determined that "medical students who participated in the implosion model were significantly more comfortable in confronting sexual issues in patients than those who saw no films" (p. 28). Of course, not everyone responds well to explicit materials (nor are quality materials always available), so instructors need to be respectful and sensitive, flexible in their approaches, and prepared to handle a diverse range of student reactions.

Ideally, sexuality(ies) content and frank sex talk in the classroom set up conditions to encourage students to better understand their own attitudes and beliefs; desensitize them to sexual talk, diverse content, and terms; encourage reflection on their own sexualities, identities, fears, desires, and behaviours; deepen their understandings of the dynamic, intersectional, and diverse nature of sexuality; for some, help them feel more comfortable and less alone; and teach them how to speak about private and sometimes uncomfortable things (e.g., masturbation, fellatio, cunnilingus, and anal sex) (Fahs, Plante, McClelland, 2018; Hicks, 2008; Oswalt, Wagner, Eastmann-Mueller, & Nevers, 2014; Satterly & Dyson, 1998). These attitudinal challenges have particular application in the helping professions. These shifts may not only be helpful for potential future service users but can also have positive impacts on students' own lives. For instance, research has repeatedly demonstrated that openness about sexuality is connected to improved outcomes in sexual health, wellness, and self-esteem (Fahs, Plante, & McClelland, 2018; Jeyasingham, 2008; Steinauer et al., 2009; Williams, Prior, & Wegner, 2013). For information about scales that measure sex education outcomes, please see Appendix C.

Skills Development

Once students are comfortable with "sexual development, behavior, and expression, they [sic] must then learn how to apply this new attitude and knowledge to help another person" (Stayton, 1998, p. 29). This often requires learning new skills. As mentioned previously, each discipline must determine what specific skills, related to sex, are necessary to prepare their students in their particular field. In terms of most care providers, basic sexuality(ies) skills include learning how to establish trust and safety; bring the subject up; ask relevant questions; interview, assess, and take a sex history, as well as knowing what our professional boundaries are, and when and whom to refer. Learning to work with others, particularly in a multidisciplinary format, can also be useful. Indeed, Sloane (2014) has found that "team approaches to incorporating sexuality ... tend to be more successful" (p. 458).

Sexuality(ies) Assessment: Taking a Good Sex History

Although many social workers, healthcare professionals, and care providers are required to complete a structured bio-psycho-social assessment that should include a sexual history of service users, many practitioners (and educators in higher education settings) often ignore sexuality as a required assessment domain (Ribeiro, Alarcao, Simoes, Leao Miranda, Carrieira, & Galvao-Teles, 2014). Even in medicine, where one might expect general practitioners (GPs) to have a sense of comfort as well as a certain level of skill and expertise in handling sexuality(ies) concerns, Ribeiro et al. (2014) report that most GPs preferred "open conversation rather than a structured one" (p. 388), and that "only 9% of men and women report having been asked by their GP about sexual difficulties" (p. 390). Moreover, Athol, Rosen, Perelman, and Rubio-Aurioles (2013) conclude that most "healthcare professionals (HCPs) are typically reluctant, disinterested, or unskilled in sexual problem management and regrettably disinclined to inquire about sexual issues" (p. 26). They blame this apathy on the fact that HCPs, "receive variable, non-standardized, or inadequate training in sexual history taking and its treatment" (p. 26). This highlights the critical need for professional and educational standards, guidelines, training, and research in this area. In terms of integrating sexuality(ies) into bio-psycho-social assessments, please see Appendix C for more information on how to take a sex history (Risen, 1995) and related useful sex education resources.

Teaching Sexuality(ies)

Although this book is a good start, we need further research into what are the most effective ways of teaching sexuality(ies) as well as discipline-specific and professional standards, resources, and guidelines. Informed by multiple disciplines, suggestions and recommendations have been made across the book to aid readers in improving their sex education teaching, decide what sex content to include/increase, and help prepare students for their respective fields of practice. For other helpful resources, please see the Appendices.

Of course, there are many creative methods to introduce and teach sexuality(ies) content. The research clearly demonstrates that once students feel like they have a sense of confidence and efficacy in the subject, and have opportunities to practice and ask appropriate questions, they are more likely to bring up sex, be open to diverse sexuality(ies) and identity(ies), do a proper assessment and take a good sex history, as well as be more accepting and less judgmental (Clegg, Pye, & Wylie, 2016;

Dwyer & Thornhill, 2010; Stayton, 1998). In a broad study of health-care professionals, Monteiro-Cesnik and Zerbini (2017) showed "significant and lasting improvement in practitioner knowledge, attitude, and comfort in dealing with patients sexuality concerns after completing the training provided" (p. 8).

Therefore, in terms of higher education, interested instructors can start by advocating for the inclusion of sex education and also examine where and how sexuality is already being taught and where it should be introduced across the curriculum. Of course, there is lots of variation in the format and structure of sexuality courses. Faculty can assess whether sex education content should be taught: in specific required courses; situated solely as part of elective offerings; infused across all courses; or held in stand-alone sexuality, sexual health, and sexual wellness courses. In addition, we need to explore which methods and topics are best suited for undergraduate versus graduate education. Moreover, in terms of time constraints, courses do not have to be lengthy, as Dixon-Woods, Regan, Robertson, Yong, Cordie, and Tobin (2002) demonstrate that "sex education courses, in a relatively short space of time, can be extremely successful in helping students feel more comfortable and skilled in handling issues around sexuality in their practice" (p. 12).

Although not an exhaustive list, Box 18.2 highlights several interactive and experiential sex education teaching methods that emphasize cognitive, affective, and behavioural learning approaches.

On a final note, another suggestion, borrowed from medicine, is that we adopt the PLISSIT model to teach sex education and help us better determine when – and if – students or service users are ready to learn sexual content (Annon, 1976; Gil & Hough, 2007; Montgomery, Marshall, Sanders, Phillips, Cline, & Snowden, 2018). First developed by Annon in 1976, Smyth (2018) posits that "the PLISSIT model offers a framework to assess sexuality of adults." It involves four stages: "obtaining permission; providing the limited information needed to function sexually; giving specific suggestions for the individual to proceed with sexual relations; and providing intensive therapy" (para. 3). These stages can be adapted to teach sex education in higher education as well as to prepare students for the field. To be clear, this model is not meant to be used as a simplistic, linear, step-by-step process but rather requires active engagement in the classroom that constantly renegotiates "understandings, acceptance of contradiction, and ongoing assessment of perceptions of power relationships by all involved" (Fletcher, Dowsett, Duncan, Slavin, & Corboz, 2013, p. 331). Other models that can be adapted are BETTER, which stands for "bring up, explain, tell, time, educate, and record" (Mick, Hughes, & Cohen, 2004, as cited in Monteiro-Cesnik & Zerbini, 2017, p. 9), ALARM: "activity;

Box 18.2: Sex Education Teaching Methods

Tools, checklists, and scales to assess knowledge and attitudes

Videos, YouTube, and explicit films

Service user case histories/vignettes for assignments, analysis, and class discussion

Large and small group exercises and discussion

Listening and reflecting exercises and worksheets

Instructor role modelling

Co-teaching, guest lectures, local experts, and community panels

Roleplays, mock scenarios, and reciprocal pair interviews (where students take turns interviewing/assessing each other and playing the professional)

Power Point presentations and handouts with guidelines

Lecture materials, discussion, and tests on basic sex education components (see Box 18.1)

Practice and field opportunities (communication and interviewing skills, and how to take a sex history)

Individual and group presentations

Required readings and research

Technology, social media, and online learning

Interdisciplinary and teamwork projects

Source: Adapted from Clegg, Pye, and Wylie, 2016; Dixon-Woods, Regan, Robertson, Yong, Cordie, & Tobin, 2002; Dwyer & Thornhill, 2010; Hillock, 2021; Monteiro-Cesnik & Zerbini, 2017; Nicholson, Carter, Savage, & Collinson, 2000; Rowntree, 2014; Stayton, 1998; Westberg & Jason, 1985; Wineberg, 2015; Wylie & Weerakoon, 2010.

---

libido; arousal; resolution; and medical information" (Quinn, Happell, & Welsh, 2013, p. 18), and PLEASURE: "Partner; Lovemaking; Emotions; Attitude; Symptoms; Understanding; Reproduction; and Energy" (p. 18).

Finally, as mentioned in this book's preface, one area of sex education that has not been covered in great detail in this book – and is definitely less developed than most other academic and professional areas – is supervision and training in the field. From social work, one example that could be adapted is the "Field Model: Field Instructors Extending EBP Learning in Dyads" (Tennille, Solomon, & Bohrman, 2014, p. 469). Using "motivational interviewing techniques," this model "imparts sexuality and intimacy practice competencies for collaboration with persons living with psychiatric disabilities" (p. 469). Moreover, as evidenced in this book, the adoption of a multidisciplinary approach to teach about sex is useful, as various disciplines can learn from each other; guest lecture in each others' classrooms; work together to create sex research and publications, effective teaching methods, and effective curriculum; and adapt and improve others' resources to use in their own fields.

Conclusion

This concluding chapter has briefly highlighted key themes. Based on the preceding chapters, as well as my own experience and research, I have presented recommendations regarding sex education content that should be taught in the helping professions, professional programs, and higher education; suggested helpful sources and models that readers can replicate in their teaching and practice; and explored how best to teach sexuality(ies) in higher education. Overall, I think that the book has made the case for the value of teaching about sex in higher education and, hopefully, provided readers with the opportunity to learn helpful new theories, skills, tools, and techniques.

In the end, though, it is not enough to assume that others are going to do this necessary work or are covering this material. Yes, I know that it can be challenging to be viewed as "the sex person." Students and colleagues may get upset. Sometimes our research is not valued or taken seriously. As a consequence, we need to become sex education leaders and champions in our faculties, departments, institutions, and communities. As champions, we can recruit our colleagues and administrators to ensure sexuality(ies)' "core content and placement in the curriculum, inter-professional education and training for integrated care, evaluation mechanisms, faculty development, and cooperative strategies" (Coleman, Elders, Satcher, Shindel, Parish, Kenagy, Bayer, Knudson, Kingsberg, Clayton, Lunn, Goldsmith, Tsai, & Light, 2013, pp. 1–2).

In order for our individual efforts not to falter, we must also work toward "providing a forum for expanding and developing sexuality as a legitimate area of scholarship" (Fletcher, Dowsett, Duncan, Slavin, & Corboz, 2013, p. 321). Additionally, we need to "increase quality and diversity of research and training, develop and enhance existing skill levels, connect with multidisciplinary investigations, create wider network[s] of researchers and practitioners, contribute to increased global dialogue on human sexuality" (p. 326). These recommendations align with what I argued in Chapter 1 that to protect ourselves, feel less isolated, and mitigate risk, it is essential that we build collegial support, develop provincial and national teaching and research networks, and continue to grow the sex education literature, research, and scholarship.

REFERENCES

Agocha, V. B., Asencio, M., & Decena, C. U. (2014). Sexuality and culture. In D. L. Tolman, L. M. Diamond, A. Bauermeister, W. H. George, J. P. Pfaus, & I. M. Wards (Eds.), *APA handbook of sexuality and psychology, Vol. 2, Contextual approaches* (pp. 183–228). Washington, D.C.: American Psychological Association.

Annon, J. (1976). The PLISSIT model: A proposed conceptual theme for the behavioral treatment of sexual problems. *Journal of Sex Education and Therapy, 2*(2), 1–15. https://doi.org/10.1080/01614576.1976.11074483

Athol, S. E., Rosen, R. C., Perelman, M. A., & Rubio-Aurioles, E. (2013). Standard operating procedures for taking a sexual history. *Journal of Sexual Medicine, 10*, 26–35. https://doi.org/10.1111/j.1743-6109.2012.02823.x

Burnes, T. R., Singh, A. A., & Witherspoon, R. J. (2017). Sex positivity and counseling psychology: An introduction to the major contribution. *The Counseling Psychologist, 45*(4), 470–486. https://doi.org/10.1177/0011000017710216

Clegg, M., Pye, J., & Wylie, K. R. (2016). Undergraduate training in human sexuality: Evaluation of the impact on medical doctors' practice ten years after graduation. *Sexual Medicine, 4*, 198–208. https://doi.org/10.1016/j.esxm.2016.04.004

Coleman, E., Elders, J., Satcher, D., Shindel, A., Parish, S., Kenagy, G., Bayer, C. R., Knudson, G., Kingsberg, S., Clayton, A., Lunn, M. R., Goldsmith, E., Tsai P., & Light, A. (2013) Summit on medical school education in sexual health: Report of an expert consultation. *Journal of Sexual Medicine, 10*(4) 924–938. https://doi.org/10.1111/jsm.12142

Dixon-Woods, M. Regan, J., Robertson, N., Yong, B., Cordie, C., & Tobin, M (2002). Teaching and learning about human sexuality in undergraduate medical education. *Medical Education.* Doi.org/10.1046/j.1365–2923.2002.01198.x

Dunk, P. (2007). Everyday sexuality and social work: Locating sexuality in professional practice and education, *Social Work and the Society: International Online Journal, 5*(2), https://www.researchgate.net/publication/26585076_Everyday_Sexuality_and_Social_Work_Locating_Sexuality_in_Professional_Practice_and_Education

Dwyer, R. G., & Thornhill, J. T. (2010). Recommendations for teaching sexual health: How to ask and what to do with the answers. *Academic Psychiatry, 34*(5), 339–341. https://doi.org/10.1176/appi.ap.34.5.339

Fahs, B., Plante, R. F., & McClelland, S. I. (2018). Working at the crossroads of pleasure and danger: Feminist perspectives on doing critical sexuality studies. *Sexualities, 21*(4), 503–519. https://doi.org/10.1177/1363460717713743

Fletcher, G., Dowsett, G., Duncan, D., Slavin, S., & Corboz, J. (2013). Advancing sexuality studies: A short course on sexuality theory and research methodologies. *Sex Education, 13*(3), 319–335. https://doi.org/10.1080/14681811.2012.742847

Gil, K. M., & Hough, S. (2007). Sexuality training, education and therapy in the healthcare environment: Taboo, avoidance, discomfort or ignorance? *Sex and Disability, 25*, 73–76. https://doi.org/10.1007/s11195-007-9033-0

Glickman, C. (2000). The language of sex positivity. *Electronic Journal of Human Sexuality.* http://www.ejhs.org/

Hammond, N., & Kingston, S. (2014). Experiencing stigma as sex work researchers in professional and personal lives. *Sexualities, 17*(3), 329–347. https://doi.org/10.1177/1363460713516333

Hicks, S. (2008). What does social work desire? *Social Work Education, 27*(2), 131–137. https://doi.org/10.1080/02615470701709451

Hillock, S. (2021). Femagogy: Centring feminist knowledge and methods in social work teaching. In R. Csiernik & S. Hillock (Eds.), *Teaching social work in Canada: Reflections on pedagogy and practice.* Toronto: University of Toronto Press.

Hillock, S., & Mulé, N. J. (Eds.) (2016). *Queering social work education.* Vancouver: UBC Press.

Jeyasingham, D. (2008). Knowledge/ignorance and the construction of sexuality in social work education. *Social Work Education, 27*(2), 138–151. https://doi.org/10.1080/02615470701709469

Johnson, S. (2009). II. Between a rock and a hard place. *Feminism & Psychology, 19*(2), 186–189. https://doi.org/10.1177/0959353509102195

Monteiro-Cesnik, V., & Zerbini, T. (2017). Sexuality education for health professional: A literature review. *Estudos de Psicologia (Campinas), 34*(1). https://doi.org/10.1590/1982-02752017000100016

Montgomery, B.E.E., Marshall, S. A., Sanders, S. E., Phillips, M.M., Cline, M., & Snowden, M. (2018). Stakeholder identification of barriers and facilitators to sexual health education for female survivors of violence: A mixed methods study. *American Journal of Sexuality Education, 13*(10), 18–39. https://doi.org/10.1080/15546128.2017.1410870

Mosher, C. M. (2017). Historical perspectives of sex positivity: Contributing to a new paradigm within counseling psychology. *The Counseling Psychologist, 45*(4), 487–503. https://doi.org/10.1177/0011000017713755

Nicholson, S., Carter, Y. H., Savage, W., & Collinson, S. (2000). Let's talk about sex: A description of an interactive sexual history taking session. *Medical Teacher, 22*(4), 412–414. https://doi.org/10.1080/014215900409537

Oswalt, S. B., Wagner, L. M., Eastmann-Mueller, H.P., & Nevers, M. (2014). Pedagogy and content in sexuality education course in US colleges and universities. *Sex Education, 15*(2), 172–187. https://doi.org/10.1080/14681811.2014.991958

Quinn, C., Happell, B., & Welsh, A. (2013). The 5-As framework for including sexual concerns in mental health nursing practice. *Issues in Mental Health Nursing, 34*, 17–24. https://doi.org/10.3109/01612840.2012.711433

Ribeiro, S., Alarcao, V., Simoes, R., Leao Miranda, F., Carrieira, M., & Galvao-Teles, A. (2014). General practitioners' procedures for sexual history taking and treating sexual dysfunction in primary care. *Journal Of Sexual Medicine, 11*, 386–393. https://doi.org/10.1111/jsm.12395

Risen, C. B. (1995). A guide to taking a sexual history. *The Psychiatric Clinics of North America, 18*(1), 39–53. https://doi.org/10.1016/s0193-953x(18)30069-8

Rowntree, M. R. (2014) Making sexuality visible in Australian social work education. *Social Work Education: The International Journal, 33*. https://doi.org/10.1080/02615479.2013.834885.

Sangra, N. (2016). Let's talk about sex: Counsellors' experiences of actively integrating sexuality into counselling practice, Masters Thesis, Athabasca University, Alberta, 1–154.

Satterly, B. A., & Dyson, D. A. (1998). The use of self-disclosure as an educational intervention in the graduate social work human sexuality classroom. *Journal of Sex Education and Therapy, 23*(1), 55–61) https://doi.org/10.1080/01614576.1998.11074207

Schaub, J., Willis, P. B., & Dunk-West, P. (2017). Accounting for self, sex and sexuality in UK social workers' knowledge base: Findings from an exploratory study. *British Journal of Social Work, 47*(2), 427–446. https://doi.org/10.1093/bjsw/bcw015

Schwartz, S. H., & Rubel-Lifschitz, T. (2009). Cross-national variation in the size of sex differences in values: Effects of gender equality. *Journal of personality and social psychology, 97*(1), 171–185. https://doi.org/10.1037/a0015546

Shuttleworth (2007). Disability and sexuality: Toward a constructionist focus on access and the inclusion of disabled people in the sexuality rights movement. In N. Tuenis & G. Herdt (Eds.), *Sexual inequalities and social justice* (pp. 174–207). Los Angeles: University Of California Press.

Sloane, H. M. (2014). Tales of a reluctant sex radical: Barriers to teaching the importance of pleasure for well-being. *Sex and Disability, 32*, 453–467. https://doi.org/10.1007/s11195-014-9381-5

Smyth, C. (2018). Sexuality assessment for older adults. *Try This: Best Practices in Nursing Care to Older Adults*, 10. https://consultgeri.org/try-this/general-assessment/issue-10.pdf

Stanley, E. (1979). The way we teach human sexuality. *Medical Teacher, 1*(4), 184–189. https://doi.org/10.3109/01421597909012598

Stayton, W. (1998). A curriculum for training professional in human sexuality using the sexual attitude restructuring (SAR) model. *Journal of Sex Education and Therapy, 23*(1), 26–32. https://doi.org/10.1080/01614576.1998.11074203

Steinauer, J., La Rochelle, F., Rowh, M., Backus, L. Sandahl, Y., & Foster, A. (2009). First impression: What are preclinical medical students in the US and Canada learning about sexual and reproductive health. *Contraception, 80*, pp. 74–80.

Tennille, J., Solomon, P., & Bohrman, C. (2014). Using the FIELD model to prepare social work students and field instructors on sexuality and intimacy for persons with psychiatric disabilities. *Sexuality and Disability, 32*. https://doi.org/10.1007/s11195-014-9380-6

Werley, J. (2016). Sex ed all grown up: The benefits of teaching human sexuality at the collegiate level, department of liberal studies. *IUSB Graduate Journal, 3*, 99–102.

Westberg, J., & Jason, H. (1985). Teaching human sexuality. *Medical Teacher, 7*(1), 53–61. https://doi.org/10.3109/01421598509036791

Williams, D. J., Prior, E., & Wegner, J. (2013). Resolving social problems associated with sexuality: Can a "sex-positive" approach help. *Social Work, 58*(3). https://doi.org/10.1093/sw/swt024

Wineberg, H. R. (2015). Social work and human sexuality: An examination of the country's top 25-CWSE ranked MSW curricula. *Theses, Dissertations, and Projects.* 663, 1–41.

Wylie, K., & Weerakoon, P. (2010). International perspectives on teaching human sexuality. *Academic Psychiatry, 34*(5), 397–402. https://doi.org/10.1176/appi.ap.34.5.397

Appendix A: Course Outline for Social Work Elective

HEATHER PETERS

SOCW 449: GENDER & SEXUALITY

Course Description

This course critically examines constructions of gender and sexuality that include cross-cultural and class analyses. It also focuses on the historical character of sexual relations and gender and begins to challenge what is taken for granted in contemporary society, specifically as these notions affect social work policy and practice.

Learning Outcomes

- Develop a critical awareness of the social construction of gender, sexuality, sexual relations, and oppression
- Base this understanding in an examination of the historical character and social construction of gender and sexuality
- Understand how this "common sense" and socially constructed knowledge of gender and sexuality influences professional practice and policy
- Examine the interaction of personal perspectives, values, and beliefs with our behaviour and actions on personal, professional, and societal levels
- Develop an ability to talk openly and appropriately with service users and others about these topics

Required Texts

1. Ferber, A. L., Holcomb, K., & Wentling, T. (Eds.). (2013). *Sex, Gender, and Sexuality: The New Basics* (second edition). Oxford: Oxford University Press.
2. Hickling, M. (2002). *Boys, Girls & Body Science: A First Book about Facts of Life.* Madeira Park, BC: Harbour Publishing Co. Ltd.
3. Hickling, M. (2005). *The New Speaking of Sex: What Your Children Need to Know and When They Need to Know It.* Kelowna, BC: Northstone.
4. Rutter, V., & Schwartz, P. (2012). *The Gender of Sexuality: Exploring Sexual Possibilities* (second edition). Plymouth, United Kingdom: Rowman & Littlefield Publishers Inc.

Additional Readings

- Optional text: Fitzgerald, K. J., & Grossman, K. L. (2018). *Sociology of Sexualities.* Thousand Oaks, CA: SAGE Publications, Inc.

Note: The topic of sexuality is often seen as controversial and is linked to concepts of personal morality and values. We will be exploring ideas that may be uncomfortable for some. It is important to maintain a supportive classroom environment that allows room for discussion and differences of opinion, while not perpetuating discrimination and oppression. We do not have to agree with each other, but we do have to disagree in a way that treats people with respect. During our first class together, we will jointly set some boundaries for this process.

Each of the following classes is 3 hours in length.

Part I: Introduction, Anatomy, Norms, and Social Constructions

Class #1

- Introductions
- Review course outline and assignments
- Setting classroom boundaries
- Language, terms, and terminology
- Introduction to gender, sex, and sexuality
- Norms and societal values
- Learning how to talk about sex and sexuality

Required readings
1. Ferber text: Introduction: Rethinking foundations: Theorizing sex, gender, and sexuality (p. xv–xx)
2. Ferber text: Chapter 1: Dueling Dualisms
3. Payne, M. (2005). Chapter 8: Social psychology and social construction. In text titled: *Modern Social Work Theory* (third edition). Chicago: Lyceum Books, Inc.
4. Canada's laws on the age of consent for sexual activity: http://www .justice.gc.ca/eng/rp-pr/other-autre/clp/faq.html

Class #2

- Guest speaker: Reproductive anatomy and physiology
- Social construction theory
- Social construction of gender, sex, and sexuality
- Biology and gender as affected by social construction

Required Readings
1. Ferber text: Chapter 27: The egg and the sperm: How science has constructed a romance based on stereotypical male-female roles
2. Hyde, J. S., DeLamater, J. D., & Byers, E. S. (2012). Chapter 4: Sexual anatomy. In text titled: *Human Sexuality* (Fifth Canadian Edition). McGraw-Hill Ryerson.
3. Rutter & Schwartz text: Chapter 1: Sexual desire and gender

Class #3

- Media and the portrayal of gender
- Constructions of masculinity and femininity. Optional videos/ DVDs:
  - *The Mask You Live In* (2016, DVD, approx. 90 minutes)
  - Or in-class DVD: *The Strength to Resist: Media's Impact on Women and Girls* (2006, 30 minutes, in UNBC library)
  - Or in-class video: *Tough Guise: Violence, Media and the Crisis in Masculinity*, Part Two (1999, 57 minutes – Part One is the first 30 minutes; Part Two is the last 30 minutes; in UNBC library)

Required Readings
1. Ferber text: Chapter 23: How do you fuck a fat woman?
2. Ferber text: Chapter 4: Heterosexuality: It's just not natural!

3. Ray, R., & Rosow, J. A. (2011). Chapter 15: Getting off and getting intimate: How normative institutional arrangements structure Black and white fraternity men's approaches toward women. In text: *Gender Through the Prism of Difference* (Fourth Edition). Oxford: Oxford University Press.

Part II: Sexual Orientation, Sexual and Gender Identities, and Sexuality

Class #4

- Guest speaker on concepts and issues related to sexual orientation and identity
- Historical views of sexual orientation
- LGBTQ perspectives (lesbian, gay, bisexual, transgender, and questioning/queer)
- LGBTQ and the school system
- Sexual identity as a continuum

Required Readings
1. O'Neill, B. (2003). Chapter 7: Heterosexism: Shaping social policy in relation to gay men and lesbians. In *Canadian Social Policy: Issues and Perspectives* (Third Edition). Anne Westhues (Editor). Waterloo: Wilfrid Laurier University Press. (pp. 128–144)
2. Ferber text: Chapter 9: Heterosexism in research: The heterosexual questionnaire
3. Ferber text: Chapter 11: O au no keia: Voices from Hawai'I's Mahu and transgender communities
4. Ferber text: Chapter 12: What is bisexuality?

Class #5

- Discussion of yesterday's presentation
- Gender spectrum
- Being an ally with clients and others: Connections to practice
- Sexual behaviour and gender
- Intersections of race, gender, class, and sexuality

Required Readings
1. Ferber text: Chapter 52: We are all works in progress
2. Ferber text: Chapter 40: "Personal preference" as the new racism: Gay desire and racial cleansing in cyberspace

3. Ferber text, second edition: Chapter 7: Keeping sex in bounds: Sexuality and the deconstruction of race and gender

Class #6

- Sexual relationships and expectations
- Gender identity, gender expression, sexual identity, and sexual orientation
- In-class DVD: *Assume Nothing* (2009, 80 minutes, in UNBC library)

Required Readings
1. Ferber text: Chapter 29: Intersex narratives: Gender, medicine and identity
2. Ferber text: Chapter 18: Loving outside simple lines
3. Ferber text: Chapter 19: Whose body is this anyway?
4. Rutter & Schwartz text: Chapter 3: Uncommitted sexual relationships

Class #7

- Historical perspectives of women, orgasm, men and sexuality
- In-class DVD: *Hysteria* (2012, 1.5 hours, in UNBC library)
- From past to present: Expectations of gender and sexuality and effects on individuals and relationships
- The role and function of marriage in sexuality and gender roles

Required Readings
1. Ferber text, second edition: Chapter 24: The function of the orgasm
2. Ferber text: Chapter 32: Arab American femininities: Beyond Arab virgin/American(ized) whore
3. Ferber text: Chapter 43: State of our unions: Marriage promotion and the contested power of heterosexuality
4. Rutter & Schwartz text: Chapter 4: Sex and marriage

Class #8

- Guest speaker: Sexually transmitted infections and safer sex (1.5 to 2 hours)
- How to talk with others about safer sex
- Negotiating sexual boundaries between partners

Required Readings
1. Rutter & Schwartz text: Chapter 2: Sexual behaviour and gender

Part III: Challenging the Policing, Politicizing, and Pathologizing of Sexuality

Class #9

- Policing and politicizing sexuality
- Sex work
- Effects of "moral" and "legal" discourses of sexuality on individuals
- Legalization of sex work
- Discussion of presentation assignment
- In-class DVD: *Hysteria: Special features documentary* (1 hour)

Required Readings
1. Ferber text: Chapter 24: Women of color and the global sex trade: Transnational feminist perspectives
2. Pivot Legal Society. (2017). Evaluating Canada's Sex Work Laws: The case for repeal. (Read first 4 pages; review the rest) Retrieved from Pivot web site: https://www.pivotlegal.org /evaluating_canada_s_sex_work_laws_the_case_for_repealb
3. Ralston, M. (2013). Selling sex: A tale of two films. First chapter in section IV of textbook: *Talk About Sex: A Multidisciplinary Discussion*, pp. 156–181. Edited by R. S. Stewart. Nova Scotia: Cape Breton University Press.

Class #10

- Sexuality and politics
- Pathologizing and depathologizing gender identity over time
- Safety and identity

Required Readings
1. Rutter & Schwartz text: Chapter 5: The politics of sexuality
2. Ferber text: Chapter 30: Am I obsessed? Gender identity disorder, stress and obsession

Class #11

- Student presentations
- Sex education with children and youth

- Sex education, awareness-raising, and challenging gender and sexual oppression at individual and community levels
- Possible DVD: Meg Hickling (one of the four programs in the series) (UNBC Quesnel Social Work office)

Required Readings
1. Hickling, M. (2005). *The New Speaking of Sex: What Your Children Need to Know and When They Need to Know It.* Read the whole book.
2. Hickling, M. (2002). *Boys, Girls & Body Science: A First Book about Facts of Life.*
3. Ferber text: Chapter 50: A world without gender: Making the revolution (8 pages)

Class #12

- Sexual variations and talking with clients
- Social work and other practice with adults around sexuality and gender
  - Talking with clients; what questions to ask and how; answering questions clients may have; reading between the lines when clients are nervous about asking questions
- The future of sexuality and gender
- Any leftovers from previous classes and discussion of any questions/topics from students
- Discuss the take-home exam

Required Readings
1. Ferber text: Chapter 31: The privilege of perversities: Race, class and education among polyamorists and kinksters
2. Lorde, Audre. (1984). The uses of the erotic: The erotic as power. In text: *Sister Outsider.* Berkeley: The Crossing Press.
3. Westerfelhaus, R. G. (2007). Chapter 19: The spirituality of sex and the sexuality of the spirit: BDSM erotic play as soulwork and social critique. In text: *Sexualities and Communication in Everyday Life: A Reader.* Editors: K. E. Lovaas & M. M. Jenkins. Thousand Oaks: SAGE Publications.

Details of Assignments

1. Presentation and development of a teaching workshop. (25%)
   - As social workers we are often asked to present information on a variety of topics to clients, colleagues, the public, parents or

family members of clients, or other professionals. Working either individually or in pairs, select a topic within the area of sexuality and gender, then identify your target audience; identify these on your written assignment and at the start of your presentation.

- You are to develop a one-hour teaching workshop on your topic, appropriate to your audience, although you will present only a small portion of the workshop in class. You are to hand in a two-page outline and description of the workshop, including topics, resources, and estimated time for each section. A separate list of resources you will draw on for your topic must be added (e.g., a references list) in addition to the two-page outline.
- The presentation should be age appropriate (pretend the class is the age of your intended audience) and engaging, as well as demonstrate your knowledge of the content.
- Both the presentation and the document you hand in will be marked. Visuals used during the presentation should also be handed in and will form a part of the presentation marks (e.g., handouts, PowerPoint slides, etc.).
- Do not simply repeat topics and information already covered in class. You may choose a similar topic, but should present new information and develop material for a different target audience.

2. Midterm assignment: Review and analysis of a book, movie, documentary, or TV show. (35%).
- Much of what we learn and know about gender and sexuality comes from popular culture and the media, including (but not limited to) TV shows, movies, documentaries, music lyrics and videos, magazines, the news, advertising, etc.
- You are to choose a book, movie, documentary or TV show to review in the context of the literature on the topic. You may choose to review a work of fiction in the popular media (i.e., a movie or novel), or a work of nonfiction (i.e., a documentary or educational book, or an autobiography, etc.).
- Provide a brief review of the item (one page) describing what it is and the content. The rest of the paper should be an analysis that may address the following points. What is the purpose of the item? What point is it trying to make? What points may it be unintentionally making? What are the potential positive and negative repercussions? Could this item be used in an educational way? If so, with what population, for what purpose and how? If not, why not? What social constructions are embedded in it? Cover other aspects that you see as relevant and link your analysis to the literature. References are required.

- Your written analysis is to be four to five (max.) pages long (1,000 to 1,250 words), not including the cover page and references list.
3. Journals (Pass/Fail – but lose one mark per journal if not completed)
    - Write approximately one-and-a-half to two pages (double-spaced, typed, as per assignment guidelines) about your thoughts on the classes and readings for each weekend of classes.
    - Journals are pass/fail. You are to do one for each weekend of classes (for a total of four). You will lose one mark for each journal entry that is missed or not submitted (to a maximum of four marks off your final grade).
    - Do not just repeat or list the topics covered in class. Highlight something that stood out for you and why. Did you learn something new? Will you practice in your field of work differently because of something from class? Were you challenged or offended by something in class and why?
4. Take-home exam (40%).
    - The take-home exam will be given to you at the end of the last day of classes.
    - Connect your answers to the critical investigations we have done through course readings and in-class material (including lectures, presentations, videos, and discussions). Citations, references, and connections to the literature are required. Give only one reference list at the end of the exam.

Appendix B: An Evaluation of Social Work Students' Competency Working with Sexuality

CHRISTOPHER STERLING-MURPHY AND RICK CSIERNIK

1. How would you describe your current knowledge of human sexuality?
   a) Extremely limited
   b) Limited
   c) Adequate
   d) Extensive
   e) Unsure
2. Do you have experience working with clients' sexuality?
   a) No
   b) Yes – some
   c) Yes – extensive
3. Which of the following have you learned about throughout your social work education at King's University College? (Please check all that apply.)
   ☐ Sexual health information
   ☐ Sexual response cycle
   ☐ Sexual dysfunctions
   ☐ Current sex therapy orientations
   ☐ Sex scripts/sex narratives
   ☐ Social construction of sexuality
   ☐ Social workers' role in sexuality
4. What topics would you find most beneficial in learning about sexuality? (Please check all that apply.)
   ☐ History of the study of human sexuality
   ☐ Social work's role in sexuality
   ☐ Sex positivity and introducing sex-positive policies (macro-level applications)
   ☐ Best practices: sex therapy with common sexual concerns (body image, desire, sexual scripts)

- ☐ Best practices: sex therapy with sexual dysfunctions (erectile dysfunction, vaginismus, etc.)
- ☐ Best practices: supporting clients' sexual health
- ☐ Critical analyses of modern sexual scripts
- ☐ The future of human sexuality (emerging issues related to digisexuality, online dating, fourth-wave feminism, porn accessibility, pharmacological interventions)
- ☐ Working with specific populations (youth, LGBT2Q+, aging populations)
- ☐ I do not see the benefit in learning about human sexuality as part of the ongoing professional development component of social work education at King's
- ☐ Other (please describe)

5. Some specific client populations have different needs than the general population with regard to human sexuality. If specific populations were to be discussed, which topics would be most pertinent to you? (Please check all that apply.)
- ☐ Youth
- ☐ Aging populations
- ☐ LGBT2Q+
- ☐ Cultural humility when working with sex
- ☐ People with disabilities
- ☐ Men & women (as a comparison)
- ☐ Sex workers
- ☐ People with paraphilias
- ☐ I do not see the benefit in learning about specific populations as part of the ongoing professional development component of social work education at King's
- ☐ Other (please describe)

6. What training style would be best suited to teach you about human sexuality? (Select all that apply.)
- ☐ Lecture style
- ☐ Panel discussion Q & A
- ☐ Small group discussion
- ☐ Broader group discussion
- ☐ Practice exercises (roleplays)
- ☐ Guided independent reflection
- ☐ Taking sexuality questionnaires
- ☐ Case studies
- ☐ Videos
- ☐ I do not require additional training regarding human sexuality
- ☐ Other (please describe)

7. Given the sensitive nature of the (potential) topics to be explored, how comfortable are you sharing your own feelings, values, biases and experiences related to sexuality?
   a) Very comfortable (Open book!)
   b) Somewhat comfortable (I might exercise my right to pass for some topics.)
   c) Uncomfortable (Learning about sexual themes is alright, but I prefer to keep my own values and experiences private.)
   d) Very uncomfortable (I'm not comfortable discussing sexually-laden content.)
   e) Prefer not to answer

What question(s) do you have about social work and human sexuality that you would like addressed in the workshop on [date]?

Thank you for your time in completing this questionnaire.

Appendix C: Taking a Sex History and Related Sex Education Resources

SUSAN HILLOCK

Taking a Sex History

Before taking a sex history, it is recommended that practitioners develop a caring relationship with service users; establish safety, trust, respect, and confidentiality; consider cultural sensitivity, sexual diversity, and gender differences; and demonstrate openness and nonjudgement (Athol, Rosen, Perelman, & Rubio-Aurioles, 2013). Interestingly, taking a sexual history can not only improve health outcomes and interpersonal satisfaction, but also serve to "strengthen the therapeutic alliance" (p. 27). Once this relationship and atmosphere have been established, the practitioners can begin by asking simple but direct questions about sex. At this point, it is important to seek consent. For instance, we can say something like "At this point in the exam, I usually ask some questions regarding your sex life. Is that okay" (p. 29)? Then we can use prompts to further explore sexuality(ies). Examples include "Are you sexually active?" "Do you have any sexual concerns or problems you would like to discuss?" "Are you satisfied with your sex life?" and "How much does this issue bother you" (ibid., pp. 26–32)?

Other tips include avoiding medical jargon, mirroring service users' language, using a sex-positive approach, and asking service users what they want (Glickman, 2000; Hillock, 2021; Risen, 1995). As well, practitioners would be wise to expand their focus from a singular interest in biological-, disease-, and risk-based discourse to think broadly about social, cultural, philosophical, and psychological contexts, implications, and issues. Thus, a more global assessment is essential, one that includes sexuality(ies) and body image, as well as sexual identity, orientation, relationships, desire, and well-being.

Recommended Guides for Taking a Sex History

Readers can refer to the following excellent guides for taking a comprehensive sex history:

1. Risen. (1995). *A guide to taking a sexual history.*
2. Nicholson, Carter, Savage, and Collinson. (2000). *Let's talk about sex: A description of an interactive sexual history taking session.*
3. Athol, Rosen, Perelman, and Rubio-Aurioles. (2013). *Standard operating procedures for taking a sexual history.*
4. Ribeiro et al. (2014). *General practitioners' procedures for sexual history taking and treating sexual dysfunction in primary care.*

Scales as Useful Sex Education Tools

In the literature, there are several scales for creating baseline data and measuring knowledge and attitude outcomes that are useful in sex education courses. Here are some popular ones:

1. The Knowledge, Comfort, Approach, and Attitudes Sexuality Scale (KCASS) (Monteiro-Cesnik & Zerbini, 2017, p. 6)
2. The Sex Attitude Scale (Hudson, Murphy, & Nurius, 1983, as cited in Monteiro-Cesnik & Zerbini, 2017, p. 6)
3. The Learning Needs for Addressing Patients' Sexual Health Concerns Scale (LNAPSHC) (Tsai, Huang, Liao, Tseng, & Lai, 2013, as cited in Monteiro-Cesnik & Zerbini, 2017, p. 6)
4. Sexual Attitude Restructuring (Developed by McIlvenna, first reported by Roseberg & Chilgren, 1975, as cited in Stanley, 1979, p. 186)
5. Sexual Knowledge and Attitude Test (SKAT) (Originally developed by Lief and Reed in 1967, as cited Dwyer & Thornhill, 2010, p. 339)

Curriculum Exemplar

Please refer to the University of Minnesota's *Curriculum in Human Sexuality Manual* as it is "regarded by many as a model in the field" (Stayton, 1998, p. 28).

Online Sex Education Sites

1. For other useful sex education resources, *Mashable* provide links to 20 free online sex education sites (https://mashable.com/article/online-sex-ed-resources/).

2. In 2019, SIECCAN (Sex Information and Education Council of Canada) published "The Canadian Guidelines for Sexual Health Education": http://sieccan.org/sexual-health-education/.

3. Another excellent resource is called Action Canada for Sexual Health Rights: https://www.actioncanadashr.org/topics/comprehensive -sexuality-education?gclid=EAIaIQobChMIhuHjmfT05wIVC47ICh2NkA -gEAAYAiAAEgI65fD_BwE.

4. The Society of Obstetricians and Gynaecologists of Canada also have a comprehensive Q&A site called "Sex and U": https://www.sexandu.ca.

5. Although primarily aimed at K-12 teachers, The Alberta Health Network has a website called "Teaching Sexual Health" that provides useful resources: https://teachingsexualhealth.ca.

6. Manitoba also has an online Sexuality Education Resource Centre: https://serc.mb.ca/about/.

Sexuality Conferences

1. The Canadian Sex Research Forum (CSRF) is held annually in different Canadian cities. It "aims to be Canada's leading organization dedicated to interdisciplinary theoretical and applied research in the field of sexuality, fostering sexual science, and improving the sexual health and well-being of Canadians" (p. 1, para. 1) (http://www .canadiansexresearchforum.com).

2. The Guelph Sexuality Conference "is recognized as Canada's leading, annual training and education forum for sexual health professionals" (p. 1, para. 1) and "provides opportunities to share information, research, skills, experiences, programming, and strategies that includes an anti-oppression framework that fosters health and wellness and resists shame" (p. 2, para. 1) (https://www .guelphsexualityconference.ca).

3. The Annual International Social Work and Sexualities Conference strives to raise awareness of the relevance of sexuality issues, increase the social work knowledge base, and enrich people's lives. The planning group has also produced two special journal issues: *Social Work Education* (2008) and *Practice: Social Work in Action* (2009). For more information, please see https://www.sexualityandsocialwork.com/.

4. An international online social work forum, called the *Sexuality & Social Work: Special Interest Group* has recently been developed for practitioners, educators, and students to research and discuss sexuality(ies). They offer annual international conferences on various topics related to sexuality(ies): https://www.sexualityandsocialwork .com.

REFERENCES

Annual International Social Work and Sexualities Conference: https://www
.sexualityandsocialwork.com/

Athol, S. E., Rosen, R. C., Perelman, M.A., & Rubio-Aurioles, E. (2013).
Standard operating procedures for taking a sexual history. *Journal of Sexual Medicine, 10,* 26–35. https://doi.org/10.1111/j.1743-6109.2012.02823.x

Canadian Sex Research Forum: http://www.canadiansexresearchforum.com

Dwyer, R. G., & Thornhill, J. T. (2010). Recommendations for teaching sexual health: How to ask and what to do with the answers. *Academic Psychiatry, 34*(5), 339–341. https://doi.org/10.1176/appi.ap.34.5.339

Glickman, C. (2000). The language of sex positivity. *Electronic Journal Of Human Sexuality*.http:/www.ejhs.org/

Guelph Sexuality Conference Website: https://www.guelphsexualityconference.ca

Hillock, S. (2021). Femagogy: Centring feminist knowledge and methods in social work teaching. In R. Csiernik & S. Hillock (Eds.), *Teaching social work: Reflections on pedagogy and practice.* Toronto: University of Toronto Press.

Monteiro-Cesnik, V., & Zerbini, T. (2017). Sexuality education for health professional: A literature review. *Estudos de Psicologia (Campinas), 34*(1). https://doi.org/10.1590/1982-02752017000100016

Ribeiro, S., Alarcao, V., Simoes, R., Leao Miranda, F., Carrieira, M., & Galvao-Teles, A. (2014). General practitioners' procedures for sexual history taking and treating sexual dysfunction in primary care. *Journal of Sexual Medicine, 11,* 386–393. https://doi.org/10.1111/jsm.12395

Risen, C. B. (1995). A guide to taking a sexual history. *The Psychiatric Clinics of North America, 18*(1), 39–53. https://doi.org/10.1016/s0193-953x(18)30069-8

Sexuality & Social Work: Special Interest Group. https://www.sexualityandsocialwork
.com.

Stanley, E. (1979). The way we teach human sexuality. *Medical Teacher, 1*(4), 184–189. https://doi.org/10.3109/01421597909012598

Stayton, W. (1998). A curriculum for training professional in human sexuality using the sexual attitude restructuring (SAR) model. *Journal of Sex Education and Therapy, 23*(1), 26–32. https://doi.org/10.1080/01614576.1998.11074203

Contributors

Editor

Susan Hillock (BA, BSW, MEd, PhD) is a professor of social work at Trent University, Durham, Ontario, and a faculty member of Trent's Graduate Studies and Master of Education Program. Her education, research, and direct service methods stem from and build upon experiential, liberation, and anti-oppressive theories, including feminist, antiracist, and critical theory, structural social work, queer theory, and Marxism. She was recently awarded the Ontario Confederation of University Faculty Association (OCUFA)'s Status of Women and Equity Award of Distinction for outstanding contributions of members whose work has contributed meaningfully to the advancement of professors, academic librarians, and/or academic staff who are Indigenous, women, racialized, LGBTQ2S+, living with disabilities, and/or belong to other historically marginalized groups. Her solo-edited book *Teaching about Sex and Sexuality(ies) in Higher Education* (University of Toronto Press, In Press) and her two co-edited books – *Teaching Social Work: Reflections on Pedagogy and Practice* (University of Toronto Press, 2021) and *Queering Social Work Education* (UBC Press, 2016) – are the first of their kind in North America.

Other Contributors

Oreoluwa Adara (BA) is an emerging academic and scholar. They are interested in queer-of-colour critiques and Black feminisms. Oreoluwa received their bachelor's degree from the University of Toronto, in equity studies and sexual diversity studies. They have worked at the Sexual and Gender Diversity Office and have published an academic paper in the sexual diversity studies undergraduate journal, *Hardwire*.

Sadie Anderson (BA) is the lab manager for Morning Star Lodge. She is a proud member of the Peepeekisis First Nation in Saskatchewan. Her education and background are in anthropology. Her research focus areas include ethical engagement with and for Indigenous communities.

Carrie Bourassa (BA, MA, PhD) is a professor of community health and epidemiology, at the College of Medicine, University of Saskatchewan. She also is scientific director of the Institute of Indigenous Peoples' Health – Canadian Institutes of Health Research (CIHR-IIPH), an adjunct in the Faculties of Education and Kinesiology and Health Studies at the University of Regina, and the nominated principal investigator for the Canada Foundation for Innovation (CFI) funded Morning Star Lodge established in 2010, and also recently for the CFI-funded Cultural Safety, Evaluation, Training and Research Lab built in 2020, hosted at the University of Saskatchewan. She is a member of the College of New Scholars, Artists, and Scientists of the Royal Society of Canada; Royal College Council of the Royal College of Physicians and Surgeons of Canada; International Research Advisory Board (IRAB) for the Health Research Council (New Zealand); and Health Quality Council Board of Saskatchewan. She was appointed to the National Research Council of Canada Advisory Board (NRC) – Human Health Therapeutics Research Centre Advisory Board in May 2018. She is Métis and belongs to the Riel Métis Council of Regina Inc. (RMCR, Local #34).

El Chenier (BA, MA, PhD) is a historian of sexuality with expertise in queer history, oral history, and digital archives. They are the author of *Strangers in Our Midst: Sexual Deviancy in Postwar Ontario* (University of Toronto Press, 2008) and have published articles in journals such as *Radical History*, the *Journal of the History of Sexuality*, *Sexuality and Culture*, and *Left History*. In 2010, they created the Archives of Lesbian Oral Testimony, a radical experiment in open-access digital archives (alotarchives.org), and in 2020, they founded Gender Mentors (www.elechenier.com/), a community of support for non-binary people and those who support them.

Sheena Churla (BA, MScOT) graduated with a bachelor of arts with distinction in psychology from the University of Alberta in 2012. She went on to work with adults with intellectual disabilities for the next seven years before deciding to pursue her master's in occupational therapy, which she is currently completing. In her free time, Sheena enjoys art, reading, a hot cup of coffee, and travel.

Rick Csiernik (BSc, MSW, PhD, CCAC, RSW) is a professor, in the School of Social Work, King's University College and is a white settler currently living on Dish With One Spoon Treaty Territory. He has contributed to more than 200 peer-reviewed publications along with 15 books and has made more than 250 public presentations during his career.

Adam W. J. Davies (BMus, MA, PhD) is an assistant professor in family relations and human development (FRHD) at the University of Guelph in Guelph, Canada. Adam holds a PhD in curriculum studies and teacher development with collaborative specializations in women and gender studies and sexual diversity studies from the University of Toronto. Adam's research interests include queer masculinities, queer and trans schooling, sexuality education, early childhood education, and critical disability studies. Adam's PhD dissertation examined productions of queer masculinities and emotional intimacies within gay online networking applications. Adam has conducted research within the areas of gay men's sexual health, sexual health in early childhood education, critical disability studies, and queer and trans schooling. Adam is an Ontario Certified Teacher and Ontario Registered Early Childhood Educator.

Renee Dumaresque (BSW, MSW, PHD candidate) is a mad white settler who lives in Toronto/Tkaronto, where they work at the intersection of creative, critical, and chaotic thought as a community organizer, writer, and PhD student of social work at York University. Renee's research examines how sites of madness and disability figure into projects of race, colonialism, heteropatriarchy, and neoliberalism.

Shaniff Esmail (BA, BSc OT, MSc OT, PhD) is an associate chair and professor in the Department of Occupational Therapy, University of Alberta. Dr. Esmail is an occupational therapist with clinical and research interest focusing primarily on sexuality and disability. Specific areas of interest and research include couples impacted by disability and sexuality education for individuals with disabilities. He teaches a variety of human sexuality courses at the University of Alberta, in the faculties of Rehabilitation Medicine, Medicine, and Human Ecology and in an online sexuality course with Athabasca University. Dr. Esmail designed and established the first Canadian post-graduate certificate in sexual health at the University of Alberta. He is also the VP for both the Alberta Society for the Promotion of Sexual Health and Alberta Council of Professionals for Sexual Health.

Baden Gaeke-Franz (BA) is an autistic self-advocate and served from 2014 to 2020 as Manitoba chapter president of Autistics United Canada: a grassroots organization dedicated to raising the voices of autistic people in social and political conversations about autism. Their advocacy work has led to exciting opportunities, including giving presentations to clinical staff of the Manitoba government, travelling to Ottawa to consult on accessibility legislation, and writing documents for the United Nations. They are a graduate of the University of Winnipeg with a BA (Honours) in women's and gender studies, minoring in disability studies and human rights.

Lorna Guse (RN, BN, MA, PhD) is an adjunct professor in the College of Nursing, Rady Faculty of Health Sciences, at the University of Manitoba. She is a registered nurse and her interdisciplinary PhD is in gerontology. Her research has been conducted primarily in nursing homes examining quality of life issues for residents who are living with dementia. She is interested in the relationship among sexuality, aging, and ageism, and the expression of sexual being in nursing homes. Currently, she is part of an interdisciplinary team of researchers who are evaluating the transformation of nursing home units into more homelike and socially supportive environments for residents living with dementia.

Mikayla Hagel (BHS) is a research assistant for the Morning Star Lodge, Saskatchewan. Her educational background includes Indigenous health research and the natural sciences. Her research interests are to meaningfully contribute to the Indigenization of the Canadian healthcare system with leadership and guidance from community. As an Indigenous ally, she is dedicated to and passionate about ethical engagement with community.

Terry Humphreys (BA, MA, PhD) is a full professor in the Department of Psychology at Trent University, Peterborough, Ontario. He is the editor of the *Canadian Journal of Human Sexuality* (CJHS), a consulting editor for the *Journal of Sex Research*, and sits on the advisory board of the World Association for Sexual Health. He is also a past president of the Society for the Scientific Study of Sexuality (SSSS), the Canadian Sex Research Forum, and a long-standing planning-committee member of the Guelph Sexuality Conference (Canada's largest and longest running sexuality conference). His academic and research interests focus broadly on sexual communication in intimate relationships. Specifically, his expertise is in the negotiation of sexual consent in multiple contexts; sexting behaviour in young adults; first sexual experiences; and unwanted/coercive sexual encounters.

Jennifer L. Johnson (BA, MSt, PhD) is an associate professor of women's, gender, and sexuality studies, Thorneloe University, federated with Laurentian University in Sudbury, Ontario. She holds a PhD in women's studies from York University and degrees from the University of Oxford (United Kingdom) and Queen's University. Her research and teaching include feminist geographical approaches to the study of social reproduction and global economies, including food economies, gender, race, and racism, and feminist pedagogies. She is co-editor of *Feminist Issues: Gender, Race, and Class*, 6th edition (Pearson Education, 2016), *Feminist Praxis Revisited: Critical Reflections on University-Community Engagement* (WLUP, 2019), and *Maternal Geographies: Mothering in and out of Place* (Demeter Press, 2019). She is an editorial board member of *Atlantis: Critical Studies in Gender, Culture, & Social Justice.*

Miranda Keewatin (BSW) holds a bachelor's of Indigenous social work from the University of Regina and focused her studies on Indigenous spirituality, philosophies, ideology, knowledges, and methodologies. Miranda is a research assistant at the Morning Star Lodge, working with Treaty Four communities in Saskatchewan, and a Cree woman from Peepeekisis Cree Nation. She has a strong interest in health equity for Indigenous people and the social and structural determinants of health.

Maryam Khan (SSW, BSW, MSW, and PhD) is an assistant professor at Wilfrid Laurier University's Faculty of Social Work. Maryam identifies as a queer Muslim and is passionate about producing critical knowledges and working with racialized LGBTQ individuals and communities and religious and spiritual sexual minorities on the following topics: LGBTQ policy and education; Islam, sexuality, and gender diversity; gender variance and (dis)ability; social construction and representation of race and otherness; sex workers; HIV/AIDS; and intersectional identities of ethnic minorities. Theoretically, Maryam draws on critical pedagogies including intersectionality and standpoint feminisms, transnational and critical race feminisms, holistic knowledges and decolonization perspectives, liberatory Islamic perspectives, anticolonial, postcolonial and critical approaches to social work practice, education, and research.

Amie Kroes (BA, MSW/RSW) has been working in the field as a helping professional for more than 10 years. In the course of earning her degrees, Amie dedicated much of her time and energy to the issue of sexual violence prevention. As a strong advocate for the topic, Amie has worked in a variety of contexts within community not-for-profit organizations and in higher education. Her roles have included counselling, education facilitation, consultation, clinical supervision, investigations of complaints, and policy writing. Amie uses her trauma-informed, anti-oppressive, feminist lens to provide education, prevention, and response in her current roles as an independent consultant and as the manager of the Youth Justice Programs at Peterborough Youth Services.

Jennifer Langan (BA, MSc) is a research assistant at Morning Star Lodge, Saskatchewan. Jen's master of science degree explored the experiences and health of Indigenous grandmothers who are caring for their grandchildren. She also holds a bachelor of arts degree with a focus in women's and gender studies and Indigenous studies. She has spent the majority of her life volunteering with various community-based projects. As an ally, Jen is dedicated to working with Indigenous communities on projects that benefit the health outcomes of Indigenous communities.

Mike Lee-Poy (MD, CCFP, FCFP) is an associate clinical professor in the Department of Medicine, DeGroote School of Medicine, McMaster University, and a family physician at the Centre for Family Medicine, Kitchener, Ontario. He actively seeks leadership opportunities that combine patient care, teaching, and advocacy. A leader in transgender health in his community, he worked alongside his University of Waterloo School of Pharmacy colleagues in 2016 to develop TransEd – an online education program to help students provide high-quality care to transgender patients. He has received awards for his teaching and mentorship of family practice residents.

Marlin Legare (BSc) works as a research assistant who aids in the development and production of research projects at the Morning Star Lodge, Saskatchewan. He is also a citizen of the Métis Nation of Saskatchewan and was raised in the Northeast area of Saskatchewan in a rural community called Mistatim. He is excited to be working with the Morning Star Lodge studying health sciences, as he is someone who has seen first hand the positive and negative health outcomes for Indigenous individuals in rural communities.

Sarah Lima (BA) is currently a master's of global affairs candidate at the University of Toronto's Munk School of Global Affairs and Public Policy. Prior to her MA candidacy, she earned an honours BA with distinction at the University of Toronto focused on critical disability studies.

Hai Luo's (BA, MSW, PhD) work addresses social and health issues of older adults of diverse cultural backgrounds and the implications to social work theory and practice. Her research and publications include cross-cultural aging, end-of-life issues from cultural perspectives, barriers for older immigrants to access healthcare, gambling in older adults and all age groups, elder abuse in culturally minoritized groups and in the general aging population, and social capital and social support for older adults. Currently, she is involved in local and international projects to study cross-cultural active aging, cultural minority and Indigenous older adults in global aging, elder abuse, and transformation of nursing homes. Dr. Luo is active in gerontological social work education and facilitates a working group of gerontological social workers and graduate students.

Stuart MacLeod is a women's studies and sexual diversity studies undergraduate student at the University of Toronto. He is interested in HIV/AIDS advocacy, criminalization, and the role of stigma in the lives of people living with HIV. Stuart is currently working with Planned Parenthood Toronto's PEAK Project – a peer-led youth HIV education program.

Carys Massarella (MD, FRCPC, Emergency Medicine) is an assistant clinical professor, Department of Medicine, DeGroote School of Medicine, McMaster University, attending emergency physician, St Joseph's Healthcare, Hamilton, and lead physician, Transgender Health Program, Quest CHC, St Catharine's. She is an expert in transgender healthcare receiving the Women of Distinction Award in 2017. She has been recognized by the *Huffington Post* and *Maclean's* magazine as a national and international transgender icon. She was given the YWCA Women of Distinction Award for healthcare in 2012. She is a council member to the OMA and a member of the Hamilton Academy of Medicine Executive.

Cari McIlduff (BA, PHD) is a research fellow at Morning Star Lodge, Saskatchewan. Her PhD of psychology, at the University of Queensland, explored cultural sensitivity in working with Indigenous Peoples and communities, and developed and evaluated a model of culturally sympathetic methodology for community capacity building and social change. She also holds a bachelor of arts degree, with a focus on research in psychology, in families and education. As an ally, Cari is dedicated to working with Indigenous communities globally to support and promote their social change and research agendas for what is required in their unique communities.

Betty McKenna is from the Anishnaabae Nation, Shoal River Band in Manitoba, and is the Elder in Residence, First Nations and Métis Education at the Regina Public School Board, and a professor at the First Nations University of Canada as well as the Guiding Elder for RESOLVE (Research and Education to End Violence and Abuse) in Saskatchewan. She also provides leadership to many research projects concerned with culturally safe care for Indigenous people and families. Elder Betty is co-author of several peer-reviewed publications and sits on two graduate committees at the University of Regina.

Colleen McMillan (PhD, MSW, RSW) is an associate professor in the School of Social Work at the University of Waterloo and cross-appointed with the School of Pharmacy, and McMaster University Family Medicine. She combines teaching, research, and clinical practice, working interdisciplinarily with pharmacy, medicine, psychology, and applied health sciences. She is recognized for research, mentoring, and clinical contributions in advancing healthcare for vulnerable groups through provincial leadership and teaching awards.

Nick J. Mulé (SSW Dipl, BA, MSW, PhD) is an associate professor in the School of Social Work, cross appointed to the Faculty of Health and seconded to the School of Gender, Sexuality and Women's Studies, where he is currently serving as coordinator of the Sexuality Studies program at York University in Toronto, Ontario, Canada. His research interests include the social inclusion/exclusion of LGBTQ populations in social policy and service provision, critical analysis of the LGBTQ movement and the development of queer liberation theory. He has co-edited *LGBTQ People and Social Work: Intersectional Perspectives* (2015); *Queering Social Work Education* (2016); *The Shifting Terrain: Nonprofit Policy Advocacy in Canada* (2017); *Envisioning Global LGBT Human Rights: (Neo)colonialism, Neoliberalism, Resistance and Hope* (2018); and directed the feature documentary *Queer Edge: From Gay to Queer Liberation* (2019).

Michelle Owen (HBA, MA, PhD) is a professor in women's and gender studies and coordinator of the Disability Studies Program at the University of Winnipeg in Manitoba. Their research interests include gender, disability, chronic illness, violence, and sexuality. Their latest project is a collection entitled *Not a New Problem: Violence in the Lives of Women with Disabilities*, co-edited with Diane Hiebert-Murphy and Janice Ristock (Fernwood 2018). That year, they also co-authored "How Crip Is Too Crip?: Reimagining the Presence of Disabled Professors in the Academy" with Nadine LeGier (in *International Perspectives on Teaching with Disability*, edited by Michael Jeffress, New York: Routledge, 2018). In 2014, they co-edited *Working Bodies: Chronic Illness in the Canadian Workplace* with Sharon Dale Stone and Valorie Crooks (Kingston: McGill-Queens University Press).

Heather Peters (BA-Psyc, BSW, MSW, PhD) is an associate professor, School of Social Work, University of Northern British Columbia and has been there since 2001. Her research and teaching interests include working with marginalized populations, homelessness and affordable housing, social policy, and structural social work theory and practice. She seeks to understand the roles of gender and sexual identity, sexual orientation, and healthy sexuality in the context of all of these fields. Prior to academia, she worked extensively as a social worker with children, youth, and families in a variety of capacities, including child welfare work with an Indigenous organization and as executive director of a youth centre, where she worked to create a safe and informal drop-in centre with services and programs designed to support at-risk youth. During her work at the youth centre and volunteer work with HIV/AIDS prevention organizations, she became increasingly aware of the need for professionals to be trained to talk and work with service users about the topics of sexuality, sexual health, gender identity, and sexual orientation.

Danette Starblanket (MIS, PhD, ABD) is Lab Co-Lead for Morning Star Lodge, Saskatchewan. She is currently completing her PhD in Public Policy with the University of Saskatchewan. Her research background includes treaty history and Indigenous health issues. She holds a master's degree in Indigenous Studies with a focus on Treaty Four. She has worked extensively with treaty based Knowledge Keepers and is from the Star Blanket Cree Nation.

Christopher Sterling-Murphy (BA, MSW, RSW) is currently employed as a child and family therapist. To date, Christopher has worked as a child protection worker, sexual health educator, a group facilitator for an LGBT2Q+ support group, and has developed the curriculum for and implemented a peer support group for men at risk of perpetrating violence against women. Most recently, Christopher has examined the gap in social work education as it relates to educating prospective social workers on issues related to service-user sexuality.

Imogen Tam (BA) is currently working on her MSW at Factor-Inwentash Faculty of Social Work at the University of Toronto. Imogen's work focuses on holistic and intersectional approaches to health and mental health within LGBTQ+ populations. She has also worked with Asian Community AIDS Services, Mark S. Bonham Centre for Sexual Diversity Studies, and Egale Canada Human Rights Trust.

Meg Tronson (BSW) graduated with honours from the University of Victoria with a degree in social work and is currently completing her MscOT at the University of Alberta. She has worked as a support worker for people with intellectual and developmental disabilities since 2012 and in her spare time enjoys writing children's stories.

Laine Zisman Newman (PhD, MFA, MA, BA) is a post-doctoral research fellow in the Department of Geography and Tourism Studies at Brock University. She received her PhD from the University of Toronto in theatre and sexual diversity studies.

www.ingramcontent.com/pod-product-compliance
Lightning Source LLC
Chambersburg PA
CBHW030235030426
42336CB00009B/108